T0215268

PHOSPHATE METABOLISM

SECOND INTERNATIONAL WORKSHOP ON PHOSPHATE
HEIDELBERG, GERMANY, JUNE 28-30, 1976

ADVANCES IN EXPERIMENTAL MEDICINE AND BIOLOGY

Recent Volumes in this Series

PHOSPHATE METABOLISM

Edited by

Shaul G. Massry

University of Southern California
Los Angeles, California

and

Eberhard Ritz

Department of Internal Medicine
University of Heidelberg
Heidelberg, Germany

Springer Science+Business Media, LLC

Library of Congress Cataloging in Publication Data

Workshop on Phosphate, 2d, Heidelberg, 1976.
    Phosphate metabolism.

    (Advances in experimental medicine and biology; 81)
    Includes index.
    1. Renal osteodystrophy–Congresses. 2. Phosphates–Metabolism–Congresses. 3.
Vitamin D metabolism–Congresses. 4. Mineral metabolism–Congresses. I. Massry,
Shaul G. II. Ritz, Eberhard. III. Title. IV. Series
    RC931.R4W67 1976   616.7'1   77-1502

ISBN 978-1-4613-4219-9   ISBN 978-1-4613-4217-5 (eBook)
DOI 10.1007/978-1-4613-4217-5

Proceedings of the second international workshop on Phosphate held in Heidelberg,
Germany, June 28–30, 1976

© 1977 Springer Science+Business Media New York
Originally published by Plenum Press, New Y ork in 1977.
Softcover reprint of the hardcover 1st edition 1977

Preface

We present to our readers the proceedings of the Second International Workshop on Phosphate. A short account of the history of the effort led to the Phosphate Workshops is appropriate and can be of interest to the reader.

The idea for Phosphate Workshops was born in the early days of November, 1974. One of us (S.G.M.) suggested the thought to a group of scientists gathered for a luncheon in one of the attractive small restaurants in Weisbaden, Germany. The purpose of the workshop was to bring together interested scientists to discuss the newer developments and the recent advances in the field of phosphate metabolism and the other related minerals. An Organizing Committee made of Shaul G. Massry (USA), Louis V. Avioli (USA), Philippe Bordier (France), Herbert Fleisch (Switzerland), and Eduardo Slatopolsky (USA) was formed. The First Workshop was held in Paris during June 5-6, 1975 and was hosted by Dr. Philippe Bordier. Its proceeding was already published. The Second Workshop took place in Heidelberg during June 28-30, 1976 and was hosted by Dr. Eberhard Ritz.

Both of these workshops were extremely successful scientific endeavors, and the need for them was demonstrated by the great interest they generated among the scientific community. The Organizing Committee, therefore, decided to continue with the tradition to hold additional Workshops annually or every other year. The Third Workshop on Phosphate and other Minerals will be held in Madrid during July 13-15, 1977 and will be hosted by Dr. Aurelio Rapado.

The theme of the future Workshops will continue to focus on the pathophysiology of phosphate homeostasis and the metabolism of other minerals. As such, the Workshops are of interest to nephrologists, endocrinologists, metabolites, hormone researchers, bone scientists and all others who have interest in mineral metabolism.

The enthusiasm and interest noticed during the previous
Workshops generated the thought that the publication of a journal
dealing with mineral and electrolyte metabolism is timely and
needed. Plans have been made to publish such a journal with the
title "Mineral and Electrolyte Metabolism," by S. Karger, Basel,
Switzerland under the Editorship of Dr. Shaul G. Massry with
Drs. Louis V. Avioli and Eberhard Ritz as Associate Editors. An
Editorial Board of 40 distinguished scientists has been appointed
and the first issue of the Journal will appear in January 1978.

The list of individuals who assisted in all these endeavors
are too long to be detailed. We, therefore, would like to express
our deepest appreciation for all those who have stimulated, en-
couraged and helped us to bring the Phosphate Workshops into
reality. A special thank goes to Ms. Carla Schoenmakers,
Ms. Gracy Fick and Ms. Gwen Jones for their invaluable and tire-
less efforts in the organization of the Second International
Workshop on Phosphate.

Shaul G. Massry, M.D.
Eberhard Ritz, M.D.

Contents

CONTENTS

II. REGULATION OF VITAMIN D METABOLISM: ROLE OF PHOSPHATE

III. PHOSPHATE TRANSPORT
AND PHOSPHATE IN DISEASE STATES

IV.   PHOSPHATE AND RENAL OSTEODYSTROPHY

Renal Handling of

Phosphate and Other Minerals

RENAL HANDLING OF PHOSPHATE: UPDATE

Franklyn G. Knox, Rainer F. Greger, Florian C. Lang,
and Gary R. Marchand
Department of Physiology, Mayo Clinic, Rochester
Minnesota   U.S.A.

SITE OF REABSORPTION

Phosphate is predominantely reabsorbed in the proximal tubule (1,2) and this reabsorption is inhibited by parathyroid hormone (PTH) (3,4). However, in both normal and TPTX animals, phosphate delivery beyond the point of micropuncture in the late proximal tubule exceeds that excreted in the urine (3-11). Furthermore, most investigators report an increase in delivery of phosphate from the proximal tubule but only a moderate phosphaturia after saline expansion in TPTX animals (3,4,6,11). This blunting of the saline induced phosphaturia in TPTX animals has been interpreted as evidence for distal phosphate reabsorption. Similarly, the phosphaturia induced by acetazolamide is also blunted in TPTX animals. From these studies it was concluded that PTH, although it has effects similar to acetazolamide on the proximal tubule, also has a more distal site of action (10,12). Since these latter conclusions were derived from micropuncture studies where only proximal tubules were punctured, the site of altered phosphate reabsorption could be in any segment beyond the point of micropuncture.

In microinjection studies, Brunette et al found marked phosphate reabsorption in the loop of Henle in TPTX rats (16). In both TPTX and PTH loaded rats, there was no phosphate reabsorbed beyond the microinjection site in the distal tubule. Similarly, in free flow studies Kuntziger et al showed marked phosphate reabsorption between the late proximal tubule and the distal tubule in TPTX rats (7). On the other hand, they found a small discrepancy between distal delivery and urinary excretion in TPTX animals and a marked difference in TPTX animals given cAMP.

3

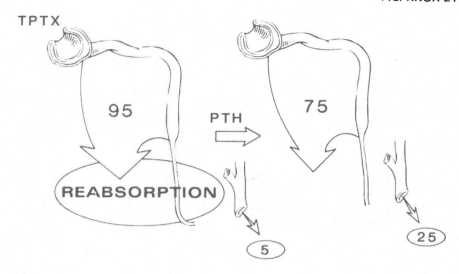

Fig. 1. Phosphate Regulation

Recently Chiu et al concluded that the main distal site of phosphate reabsorption is in the collecting duct system and that this
reabsorption is sensitive to PTH (8). Thus, there are major discrepancies with phosphate reabsorption alleged in the distal tubule and collecting system in free flow studies but not in microinjection studies. Such discrepancies are present in studies from
both intact and TPTX animals. As we have previously discussed,
these incompatible conclusions indicate the necessity for critical
evaluation of methodologies and reinvestigation of the nephron
sites for phosphate reabsorption (14). In studies in which we
used both free flow micropuncture and microinjection in the same
animal, we concluded that phosphate reabsorption is confined to
the proximal tubule including the pars recta (15). Further, this
phosphate reabsorption is inhibited by PTH as illustrated in figure 1.

UNIDIRECTIONAL PHOSPHATE REABSORPTION

Net reabsorption of phosphate can be predominantely characterized by a marked phosphate outflux with very little if any phosphate influx or "secretion". Again, this general statement can
serve as an introduction to the controversy which surrounds the
possibility that there may indeed be a necessity to postulate
phosphate secretion in some nephron segment. The fundamental
question is whether the net phosphate reabsorptive process is
predominantely unidirectional or whether there is a significant
secretory component. The relationship between plasma phosphate

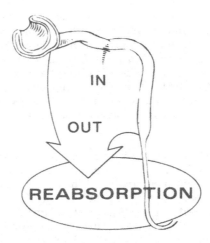

IN

OUT

REABSORPTION

Fig. 2.   Mechanism of Phosphate Reabsorption

concentration and phosphate reabsorption was first demonstrated
by Pitts in 1933 (16). At low plasma concentrations, phosphate
is reabsorbed from the filtrate, and as the plasma concentration
is raised, the phosphate clearance approached the xylose clearance
without exceeding it. Pitts concluded that phosphate was not
secreted since the phosphate clearance following phosphate infusions could be accounted for by filtered phosphate. Inspection of
his data indicates that several of the data points exceed the unity
clearance ratio for phosphate and xylose. Pitts did not interpret
these observations to indicate secretion, but rather the experimental error associated with two clearance determinations. However, others have interpreted similar data from experiments in
dog and man to indicate secretion of phosphate. For example,
Webster, Mann and Hill report that in seven out of thirty-one
human subjects phosphate clearance exceeded inulin clearance following phosphate loading (17). It is possible that these results
may have been due to an underestimation of the inulin clearance
since these patients had very low filtration fractions. Ginsburg
has also reported net secretion of phosphate with combinations of
phosphate and glucose loading (18). He emphasized, however, that
this demonstration of secretion was not consistently reproducible.
Further, Handler attempted to convincingly demonstrate phosphate
secretion in dogs by employing the phosphaturic procedures of
infusions of PAH, glucose, mannitol, parathyroid hormone, phosphate
and reductions in glomerular filtration rate (19). The filtered
load of phosphate exceeded the excreted phosphate despite vigorous

attempts to facilitate secretion. Thus, in contrast to other
species, in which net phosphate secretion has been clearly demonstrated, no such clear demonstration has been reported in intact
mammals. Nonetheless, it is important to note that each of these
studies report clearance ratios of phosphate over inulin which
approach unity. This indicates that the phosphate reabsorptive
process has been either virtually abolished by these procedures or
that there may be a secretory component to the net reabsorptive
process.

Although not net secretion per se, the possibility of a passive backflux of phosphate into the tubule lumen must be considered. Murayama, Morel and LeGrimellec have studied the bidirectional
flux of phosphate in the proximal tubule (20). The calculated
backflux, 17% of the net flux, was not significantly different
from zero. More recently, an influx of phosphate into the proximal tubules of the rat in microperfusion and micropuncture experiments has been reported (21). Since leakage of phosphate containing fluid into the perfused segment was not controlled for,
and could potentially account for the data interpreted to represent
secretion, we have repeated these microperfusion experiments using
systemic inulin as a marker for leakage (22). From our data, we
conclude that secretion is not a significant component of net
phosphate transport in the proximal tubule. Possible secretion of
phosphate in more distal nephron segments is difficult to evaluate,
however, it remains a possible explanation for phosphate clearance
ratios which approach unity.

KINETICS OF PHOSPHATE TRANSPORT

Phosphate reabsorption by the dog kidney has been described
as saturable, that is characterized by a maximal transport rate
or Tm, as established by the clearance studies of Pitts and
Alexander (23). This maximal transport rate has been reproduced
by a variety of investigators in clearance studies in man, dog
and rat and has yielded important information relating to the
regulation of phosphate excretion. However, the application of
clearance methods to further define the mechanism for regulation
of phosphate reabsorption has inherent limitations. First, the
filtered load of phosphate to the renal tubules is increased by
infusion of phosphate solutions in these clearance studies. This
phosphate infusion may stimulate PTH secretion through hypocalcemia
which in turn inhibits phosphate transport (24). Indeed, experiments in rats, dogs, and cats demonstrate a progressive decline
in maximal transport rate with continued phosphate infusion (25-28).
Even if the effect of PTH is ruled out, phosphate infusions may
alter the kinetics of phosphate reabsorption (29). In addition,
recent studies by Bonjour and colleagues indicate that dietary

phosphate activates an important mechanism for regulation of phosphate reabsorption other than parathyroid hormone and plasma phosphate concentration (30). These investigators showed that there were marked differences in phosphate excretion rates in thyroparathyroidectomized rats on low and high phosphate diets even though plasma phosphate was controlled by phosphate infusions. Similarly, phosphate infusions change other variables known to affect phosphate transport such as glomerular filtration rate (31). Thus it is impossible to determine whether the decline in maximal transport rate with continued phosphate infusions represents a "self-depression" of transport by phosphate itself or is a consequence of other uncontrolled factors identified above. Our recent microperfusion studies indicate that phosphate transport by superficial proximal tubules can be characterized by saturation kinetics.

ROLE OF CALCIUM IN PHOSPHATE REGULATION

Detailed review of the literature indicates a failure to reach consensus on a possible direct effect of calcium in regulation of phosphate reabsorption (14). Studies can be cited to support the position that hypercalcemia either stimulates, has no effect, or inhibits phosphate reabsorption. That calcium has an indirect role on renal phosphate regulation, through regulation of PTH release, is well established (35). Although increases in plasma calcium should decrease PTH and therefore increase phosphate reabsorption, data conflicting with this prediction have been reported in man and monkey (36-39). Levitt et al infused calcium gluconate in five normal men and observed a decrease in fractional phosphate reabsorption in each subject (37). This decrease could be due to an osmotic effect of calcium gluconate, to changes in plasma phosphate concentration, or to a direct effect of calcium (40). A direct effect of calcium to decrease phosphate reabsorption receives support from a study in hypoparathyroid patients in which a chronic calcium chloride infusion decreased phosphate reabsorption (41). On the other hand, infusions of calcium chloride in the renal artery of dogs increased phosphate reabsorption (42). Similarly, infusion of calcium increased phosphate reabsorption in patients with X-linked hypophosphatemia (43). Recently, Popovtzer reported that hypercalcemia stimulates phosphate reabsorption in saline loaded parathyroidectomized rats (44). Each of the above findings interpreted to indicate increased phosphate reabsorption following calcium infusions may have been due, at least in part, to the failure to recognize that calcium infusions decrease the ultrafilterability of phosphate (45). In our own laboratory, we accounted for this change in ultrafilterability and re-examined a possible intrarenal role of calcium on phosphate reabsorption both in the presence and absence of PTH (31). In the first series of experiments, TPTX dogs were given a constant infusion of bovine PTH. A 25% increase in plasma ionized calcium significantly decreased fractional reabsorption of phosphate when infused either intravenously or in the renal artery. In contrast a 75% increase in plasma ionized calcium did not significantly change fractional phosphate reabsorption perhaps due to changes in renal hemodynamics. In a second series of experiments in TPTX dogs, an injection of bovine PTH decreased fractional phosphate reabsorption to a greater extent in normocalcemic dogs than in either hyper or hypocalcemic dogs. Our results suggest that plasma calcium modulates the phosphaturic effect of PTH but has no effect on phosphate excretion in the absence of PTH.

In each of the above studies variables important in phosphate regulation were difficult to control. Thus, even though parathyroid hormone and calcitonin levels may be controlled it is exceedingly difficult to control and/or properly evaluate the consequences of calcium infusions on plasma phosphate, ultrafilterability of phosphate, and renal hemodynamics. Furthermore, the potentially important role of changes in intracellular calcium (46) has not been adequately approached in these experiments.

In vitro studies suggest that calcium is a prerequisite for the physiologic effect of PTH (47). In renal tubule preparations, PTH-induced gluconeogenesis is higher in the presence of calcium than in the presence of EDTA and low calcium. On the other hand, calcium inhibits this response when concentrations are increased in the medium (46). This is in agreement with the concept that calcium can inhibit cyclic AMP formation both in vitro and in vivo (48-50). Bikle, Murphy and Rasmussen have shown that increasing calcium concentration markedly increased 1α hydroxylase activity in kidney mitochondria from vitamin D deficient chicks (51). It is likely that these biochemicl components of phosphate regulation are not more fully expressed in the clearance studies because intracellular calcium concentrations are effectively buffered against acute changes in extracellular calcium concentrations.

ROLE OF pH IN PHOSPHATE REABSORPTION

The role of pH in the renal reabsorption of phosphate remains controversial. Although it is well recognized that the administration of sodium bicarbonate results in an increased excretion of phosphorus in the urine in dog and man, recent studies clearly show that this phosphaturia is due to expansion of the extracellular fluid volume and the release of parathyroid hormone and not to alkalinization of the urine (52). Similarly, Beck and Goldberg administered acetazolamide to dogs and found an inhibition of proximal phosphate reabsorption and a phosphaturia (53). In addition, we have shown that the effects of parathyroid hormone and acetazol-

amide to decrease phosphate reabsorption in the proximal tubule
are additive (12). Again, the phosphaturic effect of acetazolamide
is probably not due to alkalinization of the urine. Although
carbonic anhydrase inhibition decreases bicarbonate reabsorption
and alkalinizes the urine, proximal tubule fluid may be acidified
rather than alkalinized because of the resulting disequilibrium
pH (54). In turn, the effect of acidification of proximal tubule
fluid on phosphate reabsorption is difficult to predict. On the
one hand, in microperfusions, Bank, Aynedjian and Weinstein report
that acid phosphate is preferentially reabsorbed over the basic
form (55). The opposite conclusion was reached by Baumann and
coworkers from additional microperfusion studies in which they
report that basic phosphate is preferentially reabsorbed (56).
In our own experiments, acidification of proximal tubule fluid
which accompanies acidemia with either ammonium chloride on acetazolamide tended to increase phosphate reabsorption in the hamster.
These findings then are consistent with preferential reabsorption
of the acid form of phosphate in the proximal tubule. Thus, phosphate reabsorption is clearly not correlated with the pH of the
final urine but may be correlated either with the pH of proximal
tubule fluid or with hydrogen ion secretion per se.

References

1. Strickler JC, Thompson DD, Klose RM, and Giebisch G: Micropuncture study of inorganic phosphate excretion in the rat. J Clin Invest 43:1596-1607, 1964

2. Staum BB, Hamburger RJ, and Goldberg M: Tracer microinjection study of renal tubular phosphate reabsorption in the rat. J Clin Invest 51:2271-2276, 1972

3. Wen SF: Micropuncture studies of phosphate transport in the proximal tubule of the dog. J Clin Invest 53:143-153, 1974

4. Knox FG, and Lechene CP: Distal site of action of parathyroid hormone on phosphate reabsorption. Am J Physiol 229:1556-1560, 1975

5. Amiel C, Kuntziger HE, and Richet G: Micropuncture study of handling of phosphate by proximal and distal nephron in normal and parathyroidectomized rat. Evidence for distal reabsorption. Pflügers Arch 317:93-109, 1970

6. Maesaka JK, Levitt MF, and Abramson RG: Effect of saline infusion on phosphate transport in intact and thyroparathyroidectomized rats. Am J Physiol 225:1421-1429, 1973

7. Kuntziger HE, Amiel C, Roinel N, and Morel F: Effects of parathyroidectomy and cyclic AMP on renal transport of phosphate, calcium, and magnesium. Am J Physiol 227:905-911, 1974

8. Chiu PJS, Agus ZS, and Goldberg M: Effect of thyroparathyroidectomy (TPTX) on renal phosphate transport in the rat. Clin Res 32:520, 1974

9. Greger RF, Lang FC, Marchand GR, and Knox FG: Re-examination of renal phosphate handling in acutely thyroparathyroidectomized and normal rats with an ultramicromodification of a chemical phosphate method. Clin Res. 24:468, 1976.

10. Beck LH, and Goldberg M: Effects of acetazolamide and parathyroidectomy on renal transport of sodium, calcium and phosphate. Am J Physiol 224:1136-1142, 1973

11. Beck LH, and Goldberg M: Mechanism of the blunted phosphaturia in saline-loaded thyroparathyroidectomized dogs. Kidney Int 6:18-23, 1974

12. Knox FG, Haas JA, and Lechene CP: Effect of parathyroid hormone on phosphate reabsorption in the presence of acetazolamide. Kidney Int. 10:216-220, 1976.

13. Brunette MG, Taleb L, and Carriere S: Effect of parathyroid hormone on phosphate reabsorption along the nephron of the rat. Am J Physiol 225:1076-1081, 1973

14. Knox FG, Schneider EG, Willis LR, Strandhoy JW, and Ott CE: Site and control of phosphate reabsorption by the kidney. Kidney Int 3:347-353, 1973

15. Greger RF, Lang FC, Marchand GR, and Knox FG: Nephron sites of phosphate reabsorption in thyroparathyroidectomized rat. Fed Proc 35:466, 1976

16. Pitts RF: The excretion of urine in the dog. Am J Physiol 106:1-8, 1933

17. Webster GD, Mann JB, and Hills AG: The effect of phosphate infusions upon renal phosphate clearance in man: evidence for tubular phosphate secretion. Metabolism 16:797-814, 1967

18. Ginsburg JM: Effect of glucose and free fatty acid on phosphate transport in dog kidney. Am J Physiol 222:1153-1160, 1972

19. Handler JS: A study on renal phosphate excretion in the dog. Am J Physiol 202:787, 1962

20. Murayama Y, Morel F, and LeGrimellac C: Phosphate, calcium and magnesium transfers in proximal tubules and loops of Henle, as measured by single nephron microperfusion experiments in the rat. Pflügers Arch 338:1-16, 1972

21. Boudry J-F, Troehler U, Touabi M, Fleisch H, and Bonjour J-F: Secretion of inorganic phosphate in the rat nephron. Clin Sci Mol Med 48:475-489, 1975

22. Lang FC, Greger RF, Knox FG, and Lechene CP: Microperfusion studies of phosphate (PO4) and a calcium (Ca) influx in proximal tubules of rats and dogs. Fed Proc (in press), 1976

23. Pitts RF, and Alexander RS: The renal reabsorptive mechanism for inorganic phosphate in normal and acidotic dogs. Am J Physiol 142:648-662, 1944

24. Reiss E, Canterbury JM, Bercovita MA, and Kaplan EL: The role of phosphate in the secretion of parathyroid hormone in man. J Clin Invest 49:2146-2149, 1970

25. Frick A: Reabsorption of inorganic phosphate in the rat kidney. I. Saturation of transport mechanism. II. Suppression of fractional phosphate reabsorption due to expansion of extracellular fluid volume. Pflügers Arch 304:351-364, 1968

26. Hogben CA, and Bollman JL: Renal reabsorption of phosphate: normal and thyroparathyroidectomized dog. Am J Physiol 164:670-681, 1951

27. Foulks JG: Homeostatic adjustment in the renal tubular transport of inorganic phosphate in the dog. Can J Biochem Physiol 33:638-650, 1955

28. Eggleton MG, and Habib YA: Urinary excretion of phosphate in man and the cat. J Physiol (Lond) 111:423-436, 1950

29. Engle JE, and Steele TH: Renal phosphate reabsorption in the rat: effect of inhibitors. Kidney Int 8:98-104, 1975

30. Bonjour JP, Muhlbauer R, Troehler U, and Fleisch H: Regulation and site of the tubular transport of inorganic phosphate (P_i) in the rat kidney. Intern Symp Urolith Res March 29-April 1, 1976 Davos, Switzerland

31. Hellman D, Baird HR, and Bartter FC: Relationship of maximal tubular phosphate reabsorption to filtration rate in the dog. Am J Physiol 207:89-96, 1964

32. Cuche JL, Ott CE, Marchand GR, Diaz-Buxo JA, and Knox FG: Intrarenal role of calcium in phosphate handling. Am J Physiol 230:790-796, 1976

33. Massry SG, Coburn JW, and Kleeman CR: The influence of extracellular volume expansion on renal phosphate reabsorption in the dog. J Clin Invest 48:1237-1245, 1969

34. Lang FC, Greger RF, Marchand GR, and Knox FG: Saturation kinetics of phosphate reabsorption: Microperfusion studies on the renal proximal tubule of the thyroparathyroidectomized rat. Clin Res 24:405, 1976

35. Potts JT Jr, and Deftos LJ: Parathyroid hormone, thyrocalcitonins, vitamin D, bone, and bone mineral metabolism. In Duncan's Diseases of Metabolism. Sixth edition. Edited by PK Bondy. Philadelphia, W.B. Saunders, 1969, pp 904-1082

36. Bernstein D, Kleeman CR, Rockney R, Dowling JT, and Maxwell MH: Studies of the renal clearance of phosphate and the role of parathyroid glands in its regulation. J Clin Endocrinol Metabol 22:641-654, 1962

37. Levitt MF, Halpern MH, Pilimeros DP, Sweet AY, and Gribetz D: The effect of abrupt changes in plasma calcium concentrations on renal function and electrolyte excretion in man and monkey. J Clin Invest 37:294-305, 1958

38. Schussler GC, Verso MA, and Nemoto T: Phosphaturia in hyper-calcemicbreast cancer patients. J Clin Endocrinol Metab 35:497-504, 1972

39. DiBona GF: Effect of hypercalcemia on renal tubular sodium handling in the rat. Am J Physiol 220:49-53, 1971

40. Beck N, Singh H, Reed SW, and Davis BB: Direct inhibitory effect of hypercalcemia on renal actions of parathyroid hormone. J Clin Invest 53:717-725, 1974

41. Eisenberg E: Effects of serum calcium level and parathyroid extracts on phosphate and calcium excretion in hypoparathyroid patients. J Clin Invest 44:942-946, 1965

42. Lavender AR, and Pullman TN: Changes in inorganic phosphate excretion induced by renal arterial infusions of calcium. Am J Physiol 205:1025-1032, 1963

43. Glorieux F, and Scriver CR: Loss of a parathyroid hormone-sensitive component of phosphate transport in X-linked hypophos-phatemia. Science 175:997-1000,

44. Popovtzer MM, Robinette JB, McDonald KM, and Kuruvila CK: Effect of Ca++ on renal handling of PO_4 : evidence for two reabsorptive mechanisms. Am J Physiol 229:901-906, 1975

45. Hopkins T, Howard JE, and Eisenberg H: Ultrafiltration studies on calcium and phosphorus in human serum. Bull Johns Hopkins Hosp 91:1-21, 1952

46. Rasmussen H: Ionic and hormonal control of calcium homeo-stasis. Am J Med 50:567-588, 1972

47. Rasmussen H, and Tenenhouse A: Parathyroid hormone and calcitonin. In Biochemical Actions of Hormones. Vol. 1. Edited by F Litwick. New York, Academic Press, 1970, pp 365-413

48. Beck N, Singh H, Reed SW, and Davis BB: Direct inhibitory effect of hypercalcemia on renal actions of parathyroid hormone. J Clin Invest 53:717-725, 1974

49. Chase LR, Fedak SA, and Aurbach GD: Activation of skeletal adenyl cyclase by parathyroid hormone in vitro. Endocrinology 87:761-768, 1969

50. Streeto JM: Renal cortical adenyl cyclase: effect of para-thyroid hormone and calcium. Metabolism 11:968-973, 1969

51. Bikle DD, Murphy EW, and Rasmussen H: The ionic control of 1,25-Dihydroxyvitamin D_3 synthesis in isolated renal mitochondria. J Clin Invest 55:299-304, 1975

52. Mercado A, Slatopolsky E, and Klahr S: On the mechanisms responsible for the phosphaturia of bicarbonate administration. J Clin Invest 56:1386-1395, 1975

53. Beck LH, and Goldberg M: Effects of acetazolamide and parathyroidectomy on renal transport of sodium, calicum, and phosphate. Am J Physiol 224:1136-1142, 1973

54. Rector FC, Carter NW, and Seldin DW: The mechanism of bicarbonate reabsorption in the proximal and distal tubules of the kidney. J Clin Invest 44:278-290, 1965

55. Bank N, Aynedjian HS, Weinstein SW: A microperfusion study of phosphate reabsorption by the rat proximal renal tubule. Effect of parathyroid hormone. J Clin Invest 54:1040-1048, 1974

56. Baumann K, Rumrich G, Papavassiliou F, and Kloss S: pH dependence of phosphate reabsorption in the proximal tubule of rat kidney. Pflugers Arch 360:183-187, 1975

RENAL HANDLING OF CALCIUM : OVERVIEW

Roger A.L. Sutton and John H. Dirks

Department of Medicine, Royal Victoria Hospital &

McGill University, Montreal, Canada

There have been several comprehensive recent reviews of renal calcium handling, emphasising either clearance data, micropuncture data, or both (1-4). In this review we will be concerned particularly with the extent and possible mechanisms of calcium transport in successive segments of the nephron, from glomerulus to collecting system and with the sites of action of those factors - both physiological and pharmacological - which have specific effects upon tubular calcium transport.

The overall similarity between renal calcium and sodium handling is apparent from both clearance (5) and micropuncture (6) studies. Each ion is normally excreted in an amount equal to less than 2 percent of its glomerular filtered load. Since there is no evidence for tubular secretion of either calcium or sodium in the mammalian nephron, urinary excretion is presumably controlled by adjustment of tubular reabsorption of each ion.

Figure 1 indicates diagrammatically the extent of calcium, sodium and water reabsorption in successive nephron segments in the mammalian kidney. Since the figure is derived from several studies in different animal species, under different conditions of hydration, and since it ignores the possibility of important nephron heterogeneity in calcium and sodium reabsorption, the quantitation is only approximate.

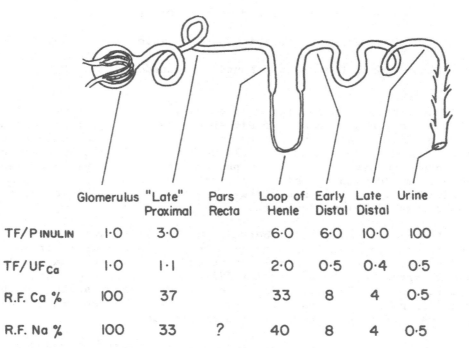

	Glomerulus	"Late" Proximal	Pars Recta	Loop of Henle	Early Distal	Late Distal	Urine
TF/P $_{INULIN}$	1·0	3·0		6·0	6·0	10·0	100
TF/UF$_{Ca}$	1·0	1·1		2·0	0·5	0·4	0·5
R.F. Ca %	100	37		33	8	4	0·5
R.F. Na %	100	33	?	40	8	4	0·5

Fig. 1. Segmental Reabsorption of Calcium and Sodium

Direct confirmation has been obtained, by glomerular puncture in the Munich-Wistar rat (7-9), that about 60% of the total plasma calcium is normally filtered across the glomerular membrane, as across artificial membranes such as cuprophane and cellophane. This filtered calcium presumably consists of free calcium ions, together with calcium complexes with anions such as citrate and phosphate (2). Estimates of the proportion of calcium in plasma ultrafiltrate which is complexed vary between 5 and 20%, and depend especially upon the method used to measure ionized calcium. There may be differences in tubular handling of free and complexed calcium; however, since methods are not available to determine the concentration of ionized calcium in small tubule fluid samples, there is no direct information concerning this possibility. Even if only 5 percent of filtered calcium is complexed, it is clear that some of this calcium must normally be reabsorbed since this exceeds the normal total urinary excretion of calcium which some 50 percent may normally be complexed (2).

In the accessible superficial proximal tubule some 60 percent of filtered calcium is reabsorbed. The ratio of calcium concentration in tubule fluid : plasma ultrafiltrate (TF/UF Ca) has been found in most studies to be slightly above 1.0, usually in the range 1.0 to 1.2. This would be compatible with passive calcium reabsorption secondary to sodium and water reabsorption, since recent data indicate a potential difference of about +2mV, lumen positive, in the late superficial proximal tubule (10). However, if reabsorbed calcium traverses the tubular epithelial cell cytosol rather than passing through intercellular channels, it must clearly be transported actively out of the cell at the basolateral cell surface, since the intracellular free calcium concentration is probably one thousand fold lower than that in the lumen or peritubular space (11), while the cell interior may have a potential of -60mV relative to the peritubular space and lumen. Little is known of the nature of this calcium transport process. Calcium activated ATPase has been shown to be concentrated in the basolateral membranes (12), and could provide the energy for calcium ejection from the cell; alternatively counter-transport of calcium against sodium, entering the cell down its electrochemical gradient, has been suggested (13). The mitochondria, which are concentrated near to the anteluminal border of the proximal tubule cell (14) and are rich in calcium may influence the active transport of calcium out of the cell (11). A substantial back-leak of calcium into the proximal tubule lumen, amounting to 3 or 4 times the net flux, has been demonstrated in microperfusion studies in the rat (15); such a back-leak would prevent the development of TF/UF calcium ratios appreciably below 1.0. Values slightly below 1.0 have been observed in saline and mannitol infusion (6, 16) and following phosphate (17) and bicarbonate (18) infusion. The ratio of calcium concentration in proximal tubule fluid to

that in the glomerulus or in plasma ultrafiltrate has been observed to rise following infusion of calcium (19,20,9), ferro-
cyanide (21) and sulphate (22). It is possible that each of these
manoeuvres increases the proportion of complexed calcium in the
glomerular filtrate, and that this fraction is less well absorbed
that ionized calcium. Recently very high proximal TF/UF calcium
ratios of 1.5 - 1.6 have been observed in acutely thyroparathyoid-
ectomized (TPTX) rats (23) and hamsters (24). In chronically
TPTX dogs, however, proximal TF/UF calcium ratio is not different
from controls (25). In these acutely TPTX animals, following
cyclic AMP infusion in the rat (23) or PTH infusion in the hamster
(24) proximal TF/UF calcium ratio fell significantly. It seems
unlikely that an excess of luminal complexed calcium accounts for
the high TF/UF calcium in acutely TPTX animals since absolute
luminal Ca and P concentrations are probably below normal in these
animals; the observations therefore suggest that acute withdrawal
of PTH may impair proximal tubular calcium transport. Furthermore,
at least under this circumstance, calcium does not rapidly diffuse
out of the lumen to equalise the concentration in lumen and peritubular space. Despite this apparent effect of PTH on proximal
calcium transport, recent data suggest that the effect of PTH upon
urinary calcium excretion is mainly due to an action in the terminal part of the nephron (24,25). Other factors which may selectively alter calcium excretion including thiazide diuretics (26),
metabolic acidosis (27), 25(OH)D_3 (28) and phosphate depletion
(29,30) have been shown not to dissociate sodium and calcium
transport significantly in the proximal tubule.

Although calcium reabsorption in the proximal tubule does not
precisely parallel that of sodium and water under all circumstances, the proximal tubule does not appear to be the site at
which the final excretion of calcium is normally determined.

Calcium transport has not been studied in the pars recta of
the proximal tubule, which is inaccessible to micropuncture. Calcium reabsorption may continue into this segment, and hence the
limited available data (6,31,32), which suggest that some 40% of
filtered calcium may reach the tip of Henle's loop, may imply some
addition of calcium to the tubule fluid along the descending limb,
as has recently been reported for magnesium (33). However, microperfusion data have been interpreted (15) as suggesting imperme-
ability of the nephron to calcium between the end of the proximal
and the early distal tubule. In any case punctured loops probably derive from a different (deep) nephron population from that
providing superficial micropuncture data. Two recent studies
have found TF/P sodium ratio at the hairpin turn to exceed TF/UF
calcium (31,32) suggesting that calcium may be preferentially removed, or sodium preferentially added, down the descending limb,
since at the late proximal puncture site the calcium ratio slightly
exceeds that of sodium. Furosemide was observed to equalise the
ratios at the hairpin turn (32).

Between the hairpin turn and the early distal tubule (Fig. 1), 20-30 percent of filtered calcium and sodium are reabsorbed; and TF/P sodium and TF/UF calcium ratios fall in parallel to 0.5 or less. Sodium transport is believed to be at least partly secondary to the potential grandient generated by active chloride transport (34,35); calcium transport may be similarly mediated wholly or in part. Preliminary perfusion studies on isolated loop segments (36) suggest however, that the flux ratio for calcium may be greater than can be accounted for by the positive intraluminal P.D. and an additional active transport process for calcium may therefore be present in the thick ascending limb. Furosemide, which blocks sodium reabsorption at this site (37), also blocks calcium transport (26). Recent data from the hamster (24) suggest that parathyroid hormone may selectively enhance calcium reabsorption in the ascending limb, since the fraction of filtered calcium reaching the early distal tubule falls significantly in TPTX hamsters after PTH. Furthermore, the presence of PTH activated adenyl cyclase has been demonstrated in the thick ascending limb of the rabbit (38). In the hamster, the selective enhancement by PTH of calcium reabsorption was less apparent at the late than the early distal tubule, suggesting that calcium reabsorption in the distal tubule itself might be relatively less dependent upon the presence of PTH (24).

A progressive fall in TF/UF calcium and a rise in TF/P inulin between early and late distal puncture sites has been observed in rat and hamster (6,24,39) indicating that active reabsorption of calcium occurs in this nephron segment. There have been few studies which have shown changes in calcium transport within the distal tubule itself in response to stimuli, but a recent report (39) suggests that chlorothiazide enhances calcium transport at this site at which sodium reabsorption is simultaneously inhibited. The study with PTH (24) reported above suggests that the distal convolutions may not be a major site of PTH enhancement of calcium transport. Furthermore, the unique and striking dissociation by thiazides of sodium and calcium reabsorption in the distal nephron is independent of the presence of parathyroid hormone (40), while in the TPTX dog, the differential effects of chlorothiazide and PTH upon Na and Ca transport are additive, consistent with different sites of action of these agents (41). Several studies in the dog have shown that specific effects on calcium reabsorption of chlorothiazide, PTH, metabolic acid-base changes, $25(OH)D_3$, acetazolamide, respiratory alkalosis and phosphate deficiency, which are not manifested at the late proximal tubule, are apparent at the superficial distal tubule (25-28, 18,42,30). Such studies in the dog, in which surface distal tubules are infrequent and the selective puncture of early and late distal tubules has not been accomplished, cannot precisely define the sites of the dissociating effects of these agents within the loop or distal tubule. Furthermore, although the comparison of distal tubule fluid and final

urine suggests that these agents continue to dissociate sodium and
calcium transport in the segment beyond the distal tubule, nephron
heterogeneity, with altered distribution of glomerular filtration
for example between superficial and deep nephrons, could also contribute to these observed effects. However, the data suggest, in
a preliminary way, that in the dog, acetazolamide, metabolic
alkalosis, PTH and 25(OH)D_3 may selectively enhance calcium transport in the final nephron segment, while chronic (but not acute)
metabolic acidosis, hypercalcaemia (19) and phosphate depletion may
impair calcium reabsorption at this site. In the rat, the major
effect of calcium infusion to inhibit calcium reabsorption appeared
to be mediated in or beyond the superficial distal tubule (20).

In recent studies (30) of dogs depleted of phosphate by means
of diet and aluminum hydroxide, which have high baseline calcium
excretions, we have observed an initial high distal TF/UF calcium
ratio, which fell sharply after PTH administration, along with a
fall in urinary calcium. These experiments confirm the previous
suggestion (43) that hypercalciuria in phosphate depletion is
related at least partly to the parathyroid suppression which accompanies this condition and may be the result of mild hypercalcaemia. This effect of PTH is at least partly mediated in or prior
to the superficial distal tubule, but beyond the late proximal
tubule. Intravenous phosphate infusion, sufficient to restore
normal plasma phosphate levels further reduced calcium excretion,
without a further fall in distal TF/UF calcium, suggesting an effect beyond the distal tubule.

In dogs with chronic (but not acute) metabolic acidosis (27)
hypercalciuria was associated with an increased delivery of calcium
to the distal (but not proximal) puncture site, indicating an impairment of calcium reabsorption in the loop or distal tubule.
Bicarbonate administration with correction of the acidosis, even
in TPTX animals, abruptly corrected the dissociation at the distal
tubule, while bicarbonate administration in the non-acidotic
intact or TPTX dog (44) selectively decreased calcium delivery to
the distal puncture site and the final urine, indicating an enhancing effect upon calcium reabsorption, at least partly mediated
before the distal puncture site.

Between late superficial distal puncture sites and the final
urine, up to 5% of the filtered load of calcium as well as sodium
may normally be reabsorbed, by an active transport process (since
the intraluminal P.D. is negative and urinary calcium concentration
may be lower than that of plasma ultrafiltrate), so this final
nephron segment clearly provides an important potential site for
final modulation of urinary composition (Fig. 1). Recent data in
the hamster (24) strongly suggest that this is the major site
at which PTH exerts its important effect to reduce urinary calcium
excretion. We have recently shown in clearance studies in the

hamster (45) that cAMP and dibutyryl cAMP infusions, like PTH,
selectively enhance tubular calcium reabsorption. It is therefore
likely that this PTH effect in the terminal nephron segment may be,
like the inhibitory effect upon phosphate reabsorption in the
proximal tubule, mediated via PTH stimulated adenyl cyclase (46).

In addition to the factors whose actions have been studied by
micropuncture methods, several other agents appear to dissociate
calcium and sodium transport in the nephron. Adrenal mineralo-
corticoids selectively enhance distal sodium reabsorption but
probably have little action on calcium reabsorption at that site
(47). $1,25(OH)_2D_3$, the probable final active metabolite of
vitamin D, uniquely synthesised in the renal cortex, was shown in
clearance studies in TPTX dogs to enhance calcium (as well as
sodium and phosphate) reabsorption (48). In preliminary studies
in the TPTX hamster, in which $25(OH)D_3$ had no significant effect
upon calcium excretion, $1,25(OH)_2D_3$ modestly increased fractional
calcium excretion despite a fall in plasma calcium concentration
(49). No effect was observed on calcium excretion in intact, non-
TPTX hamsters. Other factors which may have specific effects on
tubular calcium handling as discussed elsewhere (1) include growth
hormone, calcitonin, thyroid hormone, cardiac glycosides, glucose
ingestion, and magnesium infusion.

Possible Sites of Modulation of
Calcium Transport in the Nephron

Calcium Reabsorption

	Retarded	Enhanced
Proximal Tubule	Hypercalcaemia Acute TPTX Sulfate & Ferrocyanide	Bicarbonate Mannitol ? Saline ? Phosphate
Thick Ascending Limb	Furosemide (Calcium and Sodium)	PTH
Distal Convoluted Tubule		Thiazide
Loop and/or Distal Tubule	Chronic Metabolic Acidosis	Bicarbonate
Collecting Duct	Hypercalcaemia Phosphate Depletion	PTH

In summary, little is known concerning the cellular mechanisms
of calcium transport in each nephron segment, beyond the probability
that some form of active transport of calcium is present in the
proximal tubule, ascending limb, distal tubule and collecting system. Some agents which profoundly alter calcium excretion (PTH,
calcium infusion) are able to influence calcium transport independently of that of sodium and water in the proximal tubule. However,
these effects are probably not important in determining the final
excretion of calcium. The fine adjustment of urinary calcium excretion appears to be carried out in the late nephron segments,
where available data suggest that there may be at least two
functionally separate reabsorptive systems for calcium (which need
not be anatomically separate) at which controlling factors may
operate (see table). Chlorothiazide probably enhances calcium
transport within the distal convoluted tubule while parathyroid
hormone probably has this effect in the loop and the collecting
duct. The inhibitory effects of furosemide upon calcium reabsorption appear to be mediated in the thick ascending limb, while
those of hypercalcaemia and phosphate depletion may be mainly in the
terminal collecting system.

REFERENCES

1. Massry, S.G. and Coburn, J.W. The hormonal and non-hormonal control of renal excretion of calcium and magnesium. Nephron 10:66, 1973.

2. Walser, M. Divalent cations: Physiochemical state in glomerular filtrate and urine and renal excretion. In: Handbook of Physiology and Renal Physiology, ed. Berliner and Orloff, Chapter 18, p. 535, 1974.

3. Sutton, R.A.L. and Dirks, J.H. The renal excretion of calcium: A review of micropuncture data. Can. J. Physiol. and Pharmacol. 53:979, 1975.

4. Goldberg, M., Agus, Z.S. and Goldfarb, S. Renal handling of phosphate, calcium and magnesium. In: The Kidney, ed. Rector and Brenner, Chapter 10, p.344,

5. Walser, M. Calcium clearance as a function of sodium clearance in the dog. Am. J. Physiol. 200:1099, 1961.

6. Lassiter, W.E., Gottschalk, C.W. and Mylle, M. Micropuncture study of renal tubular reabsorption of calcium in normal rodents. Am. J. Physiol. 204:771, 1963.

7. Harris, C.A., Baer, P.G., Chirito, E. and Dirks, J.H. Composition of mammalian glomerular filtrate. Am. J. Physiol. 227:972, 1974.

8. LeGrimellec, C., Poujeol, P. and De Rouffignac, C. ^{3}H-Inulin and electrolyte concentrations in Bowman's capsule in rat kidney. Pflugers Arch. 354:117, 1975.

9. Harris, C.A., Sutton, R.A.L. and Dirks, J.H. Glomerular calcium and phosphate ultrafilterability: Effects of hypercalcaemia. Fed. Proc. 34,393, 1975.

10. Fromter, E. and Gersner, K. Free-flow potential profile along rat kidney proximal tubule. Pflugers Arch. 351:69, 1974.

11. Borle, A.B. Calcium metabolism at the cellular level. Fed. Proc. 32:1944, 1973.

12. Kinne, R., Kinne-Safran, E., Shlatz, L., et al. Polarity of the proximal tubule epithelial cell and the action of parathyroid hormone. Current Probl. Clin. Biochem. 4:218, 1975.

13. Ullrich, K.J. Abstracts of International Society of Nephrology
     Meeting, Florence, 1975.

14. Sjostrand, F.S., Rhodin, J. The ultrastructure of the pro-
     ximal convoluted tubules of mouse kidney as revealed by high
     resolution electron microscopy. Exp. Cell Res. 4:426, 1953.

15. Murayama, Y., Morel, F., and LeGrimellec, C. Phosphate,
     calcium and magnesium transfers in proximal tubules and
     loops of Henle, as measured by single nephron microperfusion
     experiments in the rat. Pflugers Arch. 33:1, 1972.

16. Duarte, C.G. and Watson, J.F. Calcium reabsorption in pro-
     ximal tubule of the dog nephron. Am. J. Physiol. 212:1355,
     1967.

17. LeGrimellec, C., Roinel, N., and Morel, F. Simultaneous Mg,
     Ca, P, K and Cl analysis in rat tubular fluid. IV. During
     acute phosphate plasma loading. Pflugers Arch. 346:189, 1974b.

18. Sutton, R.A.L., Wong, N.L.M., and Dirks, J.H. Renal tubular
     Na and Ca reabsorption: Dissociation by manoeuvres which
     increase bicarbonate excretion. Clin. Res. 24:413A, 1976.

19. Edwards, B.R., Sutton, R.A.L., and Dirks, J.H. Effect of
     calcium infusion on renal tubular reabsorption in the dog.
     Am. J. Physiol. 227:13, 1974.

20. LeGrimellec, C., Roinel, N., and Morel, F. Simultaneous
     Mg, Ca, P, K and Cl analysis in rat tubular fluid. III.
     During acute Ca plasma loading. Pflugers Arch. 346:171, 1974a.

21. LeGrimellec, C., Roinel, N., and Morel, F. Simultaneous Mg,
     Ca, P, K, Na and Cl analysis in rat tubular fluid. I. During
     perfusion of either inulin or ferrocyanide. Pflugers Arch.
     340:181, 1973.

22. Lechene, C., Abraham, E., and Warner, R. Effect of sulfate
     loading on ionic distribution along the rat nephron. Clin.
     Res. 23:432A, 1975.

23. Kuntziger, H., Amiel, C., Roinel, N., and Morel, F. Effects
     of parathyroidectomy and cyclic AMP on renal transport of
     phosphate, calcium and magnesium. Am. J. Physiol. 227:905,
     1974.

24. Harris, C.A., Burnatowska, M., Sutton, R.A.L., and Dirks, J.H.
     Evidence for parathyroid hormone enhancement of calcium and
     magnesium reabsorption in the terminal nephron segment of the
     hamster. Clin. Res. 24:401A, 1976.

25. Sutton, R.A.L., Wong, N.L.M., and Dirks, J.H. Effects of
     parathyroid hormone on sodium and calcium transport in the dog
     nephron. Clinical Science and Molecular Medicine, 1976. In
     the Press.

26. Edwards, B.R., Baer, P.G., Sutton, R.A.L., and Dirks, J.H.
     Micropuncture study of diuretic effects on sodium and calcium
     reabsorption in the dog nephron. J. Clin. Invest. 52:2418,
     1973.

27. Sutton, R.A.L., Wong, N.L.M., and Dirks, J.H. The hyper-
     calciuria of metabolic acidosis - a specific impairment of
     distal calcium reabsorption. Clin. Res. 23:434A, 1975.

28. Sutton, R.A.L., Wong, N.L.M., and Dirks, J.H. 25 hydroxychole-
     calciferol (25(OH)D$_3$) enhancement of distal tubular calcium
     reabsorption in the dog. Abstracts of 8th Annual Meeting of
     American Society of Nephrology, p. 8, 1975.

29. Goldfarb, S., Westby, G.R., Goldberg, M., and Agus, Z.S.
     Chronic phosphate depletion: Proximal tubule function and
     hypercalciuria. Clin. Res. 24:401A, 1976.

30. O'Callaghan, T., Quamme, G., Wong, N.L.M., Sutton, R.A.L., and
     Dirks, J.H. Micropuncture study of tubular calcium transport
     in the phosphate depleted dog. Unpublished.

31. De Rouffignac, C., Morel, F., Moss, N., and Roinel, N. Micro-
     puncture study of water and electrolyte movements along the
     loop of Henle in Psammomys with special reference to magnesium,
     calcium and phosphorus. Pflugers Arch. 334:309, 1973.

32. Jamison, R.L., Frey, N.R., and Lacy, F.B. Calcium reabsorption
     in the thin loop of Henle. Am. J. Physiol. 227:745, 1974.

33. Brunette, M.G., Vigneault, N., and Carriere, S. Micropuncture
     study of renal magnesium transport in magnesium loaded rats.
     Am. J. Physiol. 229:1695, 1975.

34. Rocha, A.S., and Kokko, J.P. Sodium, chloride and water
     transport in the medullary thick ascending limb of Henle.
     Evidence for active chloride transport. J. Clin. Invest. 52:
     612, 1973.

35. Burg, M., and Green, N. Function of thick ascending limb of
     Henle's loop. Am. J. Physiol. 224:659, 1973.

36. Rocha, A.S., and Magaldi, J.B. Calcium and phosphate transport in isolated segments of Henle's loop. Abstracts of Free Communications, VI International Congress of Nephrology, p. 209, 1975.

37. Burg, M., Stoner, L., Cardinal, J., and Green, N. Furosemide effects on isolated perfused renal tubules. Am. J. Physiol. 225:119, 1973.

38. Chabardes, D., Imbert, M., Cligne, A., Montegut, M., and Morel, F. PTH sensitive adenyl cyclase in different segments of the rabbit nephron. Pflugers Arch. 354:229, 1975.

39. Costanzo, L.S., and Windhager, E. Distal reabsorption of calcium: Effect of load and chlorothiazide (CTZ). Fed. Proc. 35:466, 1976.

40. Quamme, G.A., Wong, N.L.M., Sutton, R.A.L., and Dirks, J.H. The inter-relationship of chlorothiazide and parathyroid hormone: A micropuncture study. Am. J. Physiol. 229:200, 1975.

41. Costanzo, L.S., and Weiner, I.M. Relationship between clearances of Ca and Na: Effect of distal diuretics and PTH. Am. J. Physiol. 230:67, 1976.

42. Sutton, R.A.L., Wong. N.L.M., and Dirks, J.H. Micropuncture study of calcium transport in the dog nephron in acute respiratory alkalosis. Unpublished.

43. Coburn, J.W., and Massry, S.G. Changes in serum and urinary calcium during phosphate depletion: Studies on mechanisms. J. Clin. Invest. 49:1073, 1970.

44. Sutton, R.A.L., Wong, N.L.M., and Dirks, J.H. Micropuncture study of renal calcium transport in metabolic alkalosis in the TPTX dog. Unpublished.

45. Burnatowska, M., Harris, C.A., Sutton, R.A.L., and Dirks, J.H. Effects of PTH, cAMP and dibutyryl cAMP on the renal excretion of calcium in the hamster. Unpublished.

46. Agus, Z.S., Gardner, L.B., Beck, L.H., and Goldberg, M. Effects of parathyroid hormone on renal tubular reabsorption of calcium, sodium and phosphate. Am. J. Physiol. 224:1143, 1973.

47. Massry, S.G., Coburn, J.W., Chapman, L.W., and Kleeman, C.R. The effect of long-term desoxycorticosterone acetate administra-

tion on the renal excretion of calcium and magnesium. J. Lab.
Clin. Med. 71:212, 1968.

48. Puschett, J.B., Fernandez, P.C., Boyle, I.T., Gray, R.W.,
     Omdahl, J.L., and DeLuca, H.F. The acute renal tubular ef-
     fects of 1,25-dihydroxycholecalciferol (36781). Proc. Soc.
     Exp. Biol. Med. 141:379, 1972b.

49. Sutton, R.A.L., Burnatowska, M., Wong, N.L.M., and Dirks, J.H.
     Effects of vitamin D and parathyroid hormone on renal tubular
     calcium reabsorption. Abstracts of International Symposium
     on Urolithiasis Research, Davos, Switzerland, 1976.

ACKNOWLEDGEMENTS

Some of the work reported in this review was supported by
grants from the Canadian Medical Research Council, MA-5276 (RALS)
and MT-1915 (JHD), as well as the Quebec Medical Research Council
(RALS).

We also wish to acknowledge the collaboration of Drs. N.
Wong, G. Quamme, B. Edwards, P. Baer, C. Harris, and T. O'Callaghan
and Miss M. Burnatowska, in the experiments mentioned.

RENAL TUBULAR EFFECTS OF VITAMIN D AND ITS METABOLITES

Jules B. Puschett

Allegheny General Hospital and the University of

Pittsburgh School of Medicine, Pittsburgh, Pa.

Perhaps no other area of investigation has been less extensively studied or the subject of more controversy than that involving the effects of vitamin D on the renal tubular reabsorption
or phosphate and calcium. When my colleagues and I began a re-
examination of this matter several years ago, we asked ourselves
principally two questions: 1) Does the vitamin exert a direct effect
upon renal tubular electrolyte transport, and 2) If so, is this
effect one of enhancement or inhibition of reabsorption? In planning
our studies and after reviewing the data available at the time, we
noticed certain deficiencies in experimental design which appeared
to be responsible to a great extent for the conflicting results then
extant. These impediments to data interpretation and the steps taken
in our studies to remedy them can be summarized as follows:

1. First, because uncontrolled variations in the circulating
levels of parathyroid hormone and thyrocalcitonin can greatly
influence ionic excretion, we performed our studies on stable,
chronically thyroparathyroidectomized animals replaced with thyroid
hormone. 2. Second, since fluctuations in extracellular fluid calcium
concentration, per se, can directly influence phosphate reabsorption
(1), we maintained the serum calcium concentration within a narrow
range throughout the study. 3. To avoid any difficulty in separating
bone or gut effects of vitamin D from those on the kidney, we evaluated the vitamin's actions within 2-3 hours of the onset of administration. 4. Since alterations in renal hemodynamics and filtered
load can themselves alter excretion rate, we did not utilize for
study any animals with widely varying glomerular filtration rate or
renal plasma flow. 5. Because chronically hypoparathyroid animals
not receiving parathyroid extract almost uniformly excrete very
little phosphate, any further fall in the excretion of this ion

29

would be difficult or impossible to detect. Therefore, we volume-
expanded these dogs by 2.5-3% of body weight and supplied vasopressin
continuously throughout the experiment. The latter hormone was given
not merely to enhance phosphate excretion, but also to obviate any
effect of the vitamin on phosphate transport which was not related
to parathyroid hormone-mediated adenylate cyclase activity. 6. Considerable evidence has accrued documenting substantial differences
between the effects of physiological vs. pharmacological doses of the
vitamin (2). Therefore, we attempted to avoid supraphysiologic
amounts by employing biologically active metabolites of the vitamin.
7. Finally, it is well known that variations in the degree of vitamin
D depletion critically alter the experimental results of the vitamin's
administration (3). Accordingly, since we found it virtually impossible to maintain D-depleted TPTX dogs alive in any kind of a reasonable condition, we made no attempt to induce vitamin D deficiency
whatsoever.

Utilizing this study protocol, we found that sustained volume
expansion resulted in a mild continued rise in the percentage of
filtered phosphate excreted without any change in renal hemodynamics
or in serum ultrafilterable calcium concentration (4). We next performed a series of pilot studies with various amounts of vitamin D,
with the finding that at a dose of 10,000 IU (that is, approximately
250 μg), percentage phosphate excretion fell consistently, with a
mean decline of 39% from control levels (4). Again, there was no
consistent change in glomerular filtration rate, estimated as the
clearance of inulin, in serum ultrafilterable calcium concentration,
or in renal plasma flow. Because of the limited physiological significance which could be attached to the use of this massive dose of
the parent vitamin, we next studied the effect of 25-hydroxy vitamin
D_3 (or, 25-hydroxycholecalciferol, 25 HCC) in this experimental model.
The administration of as little as 25 units (that is, .625 μg) of
25 HCC resulted in a consistent reduction in phosphate excretion
(figure 1). In these studies, as in those with vitamin D_3, glomerular
factors and alterations in extracellular fluid calcium concentration
could be excluded as contributory to the changes observed in phosphate excretion (4).

A characteristic feature of the effect of vitamin D on the transport of calcium and phosphate in the gut is a time lag between its
administration and the manifestation of its biological activity.
This delayed response is thought to represent the time required for
metabolic conversion of vitamin D to its biologically active metabolites, and the transcription of DNA required for new protein formation. We were interested, therefore, to examine the time sequence
of the response of renal phosphate excretion to these agents. The
action of vitamin D_3 on renal tubular transport required 60-90 minutes
to become evident. 25 HCC acted faster than did vitamin D_3 with an
onset in 50-60 minutes, and the magnitude of the reduction in percentage phosphate excretion which it induced was greater than that obtained

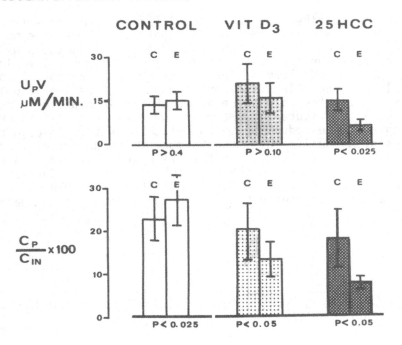

Figure 1. Comparison of the effects of vitamin D_3 and 25-hydroxy vitamin D_3 (25 HCC) on absolute phosphate excretion (U_pV) and the percentage of filtered phosphate excreted (C_p/C_{In} x 100) to the results obtained in control dogs.

with the parent vitamin. These findings are similar to those obtained by DeLuca and his colleagues who studied gut calcium transport utilizing these two agents. In their studies, performed in the rachitic chick, the metabolite induced a more rapid increase in calcium absorption and was more potent than vitamin D_3 (5).

We next examined the possibility that 25 HCC affected sodium and calcium excretion as well as that of phosphate. We found that, in a general way, the alterations in phosphate excretion were paralleled by those for both sodium and calcium, both for the control studies in which excretion either stayed the same or increased, and for the 25 HCC experiments in which reduced phosphate excretion was accompanied by a fall in urinary sodium and calcium.

To evaluate whether the renal tubular action of the metabolite
interacted in any way with that of parathyroid hormone, the metabolite
was infused in animals undergoing sustained mild volume expansion,
at a rate of 50-60 units/hr. for 1½-2 hours. Thereafter, various
dosages of parathyroid hormone were superimposed upon the action of
the metabolite. When PTH was given in amounts exceeding 30 units/
hr. for 1½-2 hrs., the hormone reversed the antiphosphaturia due
to the metabolite (figure 2). However, when PTH was administered
in lower dosage, the reduction in phosphate excretion induced by the
25 HCC persisted, unaltered by the hormone. The sequence of administration of these two agents was then reversed, yielding the results
depicted in figure 3. As in the previous studies, the dose of the
metabolite infused was kept at 50-60 units/hr. When PTH was administered in amounts exceeding 50 units/hr., addition of the metabolite

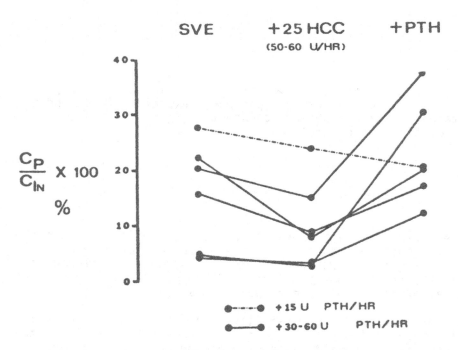

Figure 2. The effect on percentage phosphate excretion (ordinate)
of graded doses of parathyroid hormone (+ PTH) given intravenously
to TPTX dogs receiving 50-60 units of 25 HCC/hr., superimposed on
sustained volume expansion (SVE). Reproduced, with permission,
from Puschett, et al, J. Clin. Invest. 51: 373-385, 1972 (4).

did not alter the phosphaturia resulting from the action of the
hormone. However, when smaller amounts of PTH were employed, not
only did the metabolite prevent any further increase in phosphaturia,
but in fact an antiphosphaturia occurred (figure 3). Thus, when
given in appropriate dosage, PTH and 25 HCC could be demonstrated
to possess antagonistic effects on renal tubular phosphate transport (4).

Finally, to investigate the mechanism by which the reduction
in phosphate excretion due to the metabolite had been accomplished,
we examined the effect of 25 HCC on urinary cyclic AMP excretion.
Our findings indicate that the invariant fall in phosphate excretion
induced by the metabolite was not accompanied by a consistent
reduction in the excretion of the cyclic nucleotide (6). Thus, at
least in this experimental model, the action of the metabolite is

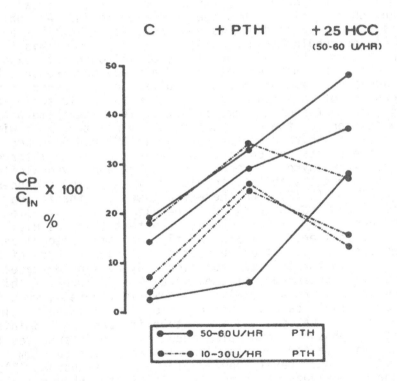

Figure 3. Percentage phosphate excretion (ordinate) in hydropenic,
TPTX dogs when 25 HCC (50-60 U/hr.) was infused into animals already
receiving PTH in dosages of from 10-60 u/hr. From Puschett, et al,
J. Clin. Invest. 51: 373-385, 1972 (4).

not mediated by the adenylate cyclase system.

Because of the interaction which we observed between the effects of parathyroid hormone and 25 HCC, we next investigated the inter-relationship between the actions of both cyclic AMP and thyrocalcit-onin, and that of the metabolite. When substantial doses of the dibutyryl derivative of cyclic AMP (50 mg/hr.) were given to TPTX dogs, fractional phosphate excretion increased markedly as is the case with parathyroid hormone. The addition of 25 HCC in the same dosage as that given previously (50-60 units/hr.) was then incapable of reversing this phosphaturia. Indeed, phosphate excretion continued to rise, just as was the case when the metabolite was infused into animals receiving large doses of parathyroid hormone. No consistent variations occurred in serum ultrafilterable calcium concentration. Likewise, renal hemodynamics did not contribute to the excretion results (7).

We come next to a consideration of the interaction of thyro-calcitonin and 25 HCC on renal phosphate transport. Whereas in the rat and man, thyrocalcitonin has been reported to induce a phos-phaturia (1,8-10), in the dog this hormone does not exhibit any direct effect on tubular transport (11). We confirmed this finding in our own studies. The infusion of thyrocalcitonin into expanded animals in which phosphate excretion had already been reduced by the prior administration of 25 HCC, resulted in no further change in the excretion of this ion. However, when thyrocalcitonin was given first, the antiphosphaturic effect of the metabolite was ob-viated, reminiscent of the situation in which pre-treatment with large doses of parathyroid hormone or cyclic AMP had been accom-plished. There exists now considerable evidence that all three of these agents---parathyroid hormone, cyclic AMP and thyrocalcitonin---may share in common the ability to elevate the cytosolic concen-tration of calcium (2,12). We therefore posed the thesis that all three agents inhibited the action of the vitamin D metabolite by raising intracellular calcium content. To test this postulate, we performed experiments in which exactly the same protocol as des-cribed previously was utilized, except that larger amounts of cal-cium were given in the infusion solution. By raising extracellular fluid calcium, we presumed that the intracellular level of this ion would likewise be increased (12). As shown in figure 4, when the serum ultrafilterable calcium concentration was elevated to almost double the previous values, and the metabolite was then administered, no reduction in phosphate excretion occurred. We interpreted these findings as evidence for the view that intracellular calcium is an important modulator of renal tubular electrolyte transport (7). Further, the data suggest that for the vitamin to enhance reabsorption, low levels of calcium must exist. Finally, it would appear that elevation of the calcium level precludes further transepithelial transport from occurring, thus acting as a "servo-control" mechanism.

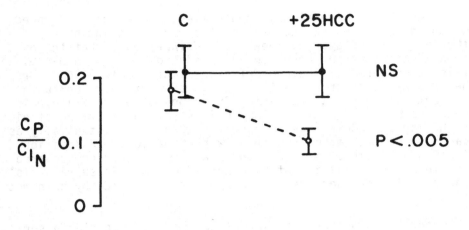

Figure 4. Comparison of the actions of 50-60 units of 25 HCC/hr. on
fractional phosphate excretion (ordinate) in the TPTX dog during
hypocalcemia (open circles) and hypercalcemia (closed circles).
The control data (C) in both groups were obtained during steady-
state modest saline expansion (2.5% body weight). SUF_{Ca}=serum
ultrafilterable calcium concentration.

In collaboration with Dr. DeLuca's group we studied the effects
of the 1,25-dihydroxylated derivative of vitamin D_3 on phosphate
excretion. Like 25 HCC, this metabolite invariably reduced both
absolute and percentage phosphate excretion without affecting either
glomerular filtration rate or renal plasma flow (13). There was a
fall in mean phosphate excretion of 40% from control levels, a value
no greater than that obtained with 25 HCC, although the administration
of 1,25 DHCC did further shorten the response time to about 30-40
minutes. These data suggested to us that 1,25 DHCC might not be the
tissue-active form of the vitamin in the kidney, as it appears to be
in the skeleton and gastrointestinal tract.

Subsequently, several well-controlled studies have appeared
in which the vitamin and its metabolites have been administered
to the rat. Drs. Costanzo, Sheehe and Weiner found that the excretion of calcium and phosphate were reduced in vitamin D-replete
animals as compared to their D-deficient litter mates (14). Drs.
Pechet and Hesse reported on the results of continuous perfusion
experiments in TPTX rats receiving infusions of both parathyroid
hormone and triiodithyronine. The administration of 0.1 µg of either
1,25 DHCC or 1 α HCC reduced phosphate excretion substantially as
compared to control animals over a 12 hour period. In addition,
a significant increase in serum phosphate concentration occurred.
Furthermore, the provision of parathyroid extract in supraphysiologic
dosage readily reversed the antiphosphaturia effected by both metabolites.

Recently, Popovtzer and his colleagues have reported a series
of acute clearance studies performed both in intact and acutely
parathyroidectomized rats (16,17). The acute administration of 25
HCC in a dose of 4 units/100 grams/hr. in intact animals resulted
in a 25% fall in fractional phosphate excretion within 40 minutes.
But when they gave the metabolite to acutely parathyroidectomized
rats, there were no alterations in phosphate excretion. However,
superimposition of the metabolite upon a constant infusion of a
small dose of parathyroid extract (1 unit/100 grams/hr.) resulted
in restoration of the antiphosphaturic action of the 25 HCC (16).
Continuous perfusion studies of D-depleted, non-expanded parathyroidectomized rats in my laboratory have yielded similar results (18).

Two further observations of importance have subsequently been
made by this group of workers. Both in intact rats and in PTX rats
perfused with parathyroid extract, the antiphosphaturia associated
with the administration of 25 HCC was accompanied by a fall in the
urinary excretion of cyclic AMP (17). These workers concluded from
these and the other studies described, that the metabolite was
dependent upon the presence of the hormone for its action on phosphate transport to become manifest, and they ascribed this effect
of the metabolite to suppressed cyclic AMP formation (16,17). An
additional finding of consequence by these workers is that the antiphosphaturic action of the dihydroxylated metabolite is likewise
dependent upon the presence of parathyroid hormone, just as appeared
to be the case for 25 HCC (16). These data could mean that 1,25 DHCC
must itself be further metabolized before it is effective in directly
altering renal tubular transport, and that PTH promotes this conversion as it does that from 25 HCC to 1,25 DHCC. Alternatively, the
"permissive" effect of PTH could be mediated through some other
mechanism entirely. When compared to our own data (4,13), these
observations in the rat confirm a direct renal tubular effect of
the metabolites of vitamin D on phosphate transport, but raise the
question as to why parathyroid hormone seems to be required for
this effect to become manifest in the rat (16), but not in the dog
(4,13).

Drs. Sutton, Dirks and their collaborators have recently
presented preliminary observations describing the effects of a somewhat larger dose of 25 HCC than we utilized (they gave 250 units as
a priming dose and 200/hr.), on electrolyte excretion in both intact
and thyroparathyroidectomized dogs (19). They noted a reduction in
calcium excretion in both groups of animals which effect they localized
to the distal nephron by micropuncture methods. However, an antiphosphaturia developed only in animals with intact glands, and tubular fluid phosphate determinations were not performed (19). Peraino,
et al, have presented some provisional findings regarding the effects
of 60 units of 25 HCC/hr. on electrolyte excretion in both acutely
thyroparathyroidectomized and intact bicarbonate-loaded dogs. The
results are similar to our own as regards calcium and sodium excretion. However, while phosphate excretion declined numerically
in their intact animals, this alteration did not reach statistical
significance (20).

To summarize thus far, the data available seem to answer in the
affirmative the question as to whether or not vitamin D, through the
biological activity of its metabolites, can directly influence electrolyte reabsorption. Doubt persists, however, as to whether or not
parathyroid hormone is required in some way to mediate the antiphosphaturic effect of the vitamin. While this problem cannot be
completely resolved at this time, let me speculate for you as to
its solution based upon recently available evidence. In the intact
dog, the vast majority of phosphate transport occurs in the proximal
nephron. However, we now know that removal of the parathyroid
glands in the dog unmasks a distal transport pathway for phosphate
of substantial proportions (21-23). In our hands (24), as well as
those of other workers (22,23), modest volume expansion (of the
order of 2.5-3% of body weight) in the TPTX dog results in a reduction in proximal phosphate reabsorption but no phosphaturia.
However, doses of parathyroid hormone which reduce proximal phosphate transport to the same extent as does mild volume expansion,
also inhibit distal phosphate reabsorption, resulting in incremental
phosphate excretion (23). In our dog studies, pharmacologic amounts
of vasopressin were infused (4,13). This substance causes a phosphaturia by inhibiting transport mainly in the distal nephron (25-27).
We propose, therefore, that the antiphosphaturic effect of the
vitamin D metabolites is demonstrable, in clearance studies, only
when both proximal and distal phosphate reabsorption have been
inhibited enough initially, so that a reduction in the excretion of
this ion can be detected in the final urine when the metabolites
are administered. Preliminary clearance results from our laboratory
support this hypothesis. However, definitive answers await the
completion of appropriate micropuncture studies, which are currently
underway.

In conclusion, we suggest that the data which have been developed in recent years strongly support the contention that vitamin D,

through the action of one or more of its metabolites, directly enhances renal tubular electrolyte transport. The question which now confronts us is the disclosure of the mechanism by which this effect of the vitamin is subserved.

This work was supported, in part, by National Institute of Health Grants AM 14708, AM 17575 and 5S01 RR 05709, by funds from the Health Research Services Foundation, Pittsburgh, Pa. and by institutional funds from the Allegheny General Hospital (884) and the Philadelphia Veterans Administration Hospital. During the tenure of a portion of this work, Dr. Puschett was a Clinical Investigator of the Veterans Administration.

REFERENCES

1. Rasmussen, H., Anast, C., and Arnaud, C.: Thyrocalcitonin, EGTA, and urinary electrolyte excretion. J. Clin. Invest. 46: 746-752, 1967.

2. Rasmussen, H., and Bordier, P.: In: The Physiological and Cellular Basis of Metabolic Bone Disease. Baltimore: Williams and Wilkins Co., 1974

3. Harrison, H.E. and Harrison, H.C.: The interaction of vitamin D and parathyroid hormone on calcium, phosphorous and magnesium homeostasis in the rat. Metabolism 13: 952-958, 1964.

4. Puschett, J.B., Moranz, J., and Kurnick, W.S.: Evidence for a direct action of cholecalciferol and 25-hydroxycholecalciferol on the renal transport of phosphate, sodium, and calcium. J. Clin. Invest. 51: 373-385, 1972.

5. Omdahl, J., Holick, M., Suda, T., Tanaka, Y., and DeLuca, H.F.: Biological activity of 1,25-dihydroxycholecalciferol. Biochemistry 10: 2935-2940, 1971.

6. Puschett, J.B., Beck, W., and Fernandez, P.C.: Role of calcium concentration in regulating renal transport effects of calcitonin, cyclic AMP and 25-hydroxy vitamin D. Clin. Res. 21: 703, 1973.

7. Puschett, J.B., Beck, W.S., Jr., Jelonek, A., and Fernandez, P.C.: Study of the renal tubular interactions of thyrocalcitonin, cyclic adenosine 3',5'-monophosphate, 25-hydroxycholecalciferol, and calcium ion. J. Clin. Invest. 53: 756-767, 1974.

8. Aldred, J.P., Kleszynski, R.R., and Bastian, J.W.: Effects of acute administration of porcine and salmon calcitonin on urine electrolyte excretion in rats. Proc. Soc. Exp. Biol. Med. 134: 1175-1180, 1970.

9. Bijvoet, O.L.M., van der Sluys Veer, J., deVries, H.R., and van Koppen, A.T.J.: Natriuretic effect of calcitonin in man. New Engl. J. Med. 284: 681-688, 1971.

10. Robinson, C.J., Martin, T.J., and MacIntyre, I.: Phosphaturic effect of thyrocalcitonin. Lancet 2: 83-84, 1966.

11. Pak, C.Y.C., Ruskin, B., and Casper, A.: Renal effects of porcine thyrocalcitonin in the dog. Endocrinology 87: 262-270, 1970.

12. Borle, A.B.: Calcium metabolism at the cellular level. Fed. Proc. 32: 1944-1950, 1973.

13. Puschett, J.B., Fernandez, P.C., Boyle, I.T., Gray, R.W., Omdahl, J.L., and DeLuca, H.F.: The acute renal tubular effects of 1,25-dihydroxycholecalciferol. Proc. Soc. Exp. Biol. Med. 141: 379-384, 1972.

14. Costanzo, L.S., Sheehe, P.R., and Weiner, I.M.: Renal actions of vitamin D in D-deficient rats. Am. J. Physiol. 226: 1490-1495, 1974.

15. Pechet, M.M. and Hesse, R.H.: Metabolic and clinical effects of pure crystalline 1 α 25-dihydroxyvitamin D_3. Studies of intestinal calcium transport, renal tubular function and bone metabolism. Am. J. Med. 57: 13-20, 1974.

16. Popovtzer, M.M., Robinette, J.B., DeLuca, H.F., and Holick, M.F.: The acute effect of 25-hydroxycholecalciferol on renal handling of phosphorous. Evidence for a parathyroid hormone-dependent mechanism. J. Clin. Invest. 53: 913-921, 1974.

17. Popovtzer, M.M. and Robinette, J.B.: Effect of 25 (OH) vitamin D_3 on urinary excretion of cyclic adenosine monophosphate. Am. J. Physiol. 229: 907-910, 1975.

18. Puschett, J.B., Beck, W.S., Jr., and Jelonek, A.: Parathyroid hormone and 25-hydroxy vitamin D_3: synergistic and antagonistic effects on renal phosphate transport. Science 190: 473-475, 1975.

19. Sutton, R.A.L., Wong, N.L.M., and Dirks, J.H.: 25 hydroxy vitamin D_3: enhancement of distal tubular calcium reabsorption in the dog. Abstracts of the 8th Annual Meeting of the American Society of Nephrology, Washington, D.C., November, 1975, p. 8.

20. Peraino, R., Ghaffary, E., Rouse, D., and Suki, W.N.: Effects of 25-hydroxy vitamin D_3 in the intact and acutely thyroparathyroid-ectomized dog. Clin. Res. 24: 460A, 1976.

21. Fernandez, P.C. and Puschett, J.B.: Proximal tubular actions of metolazone and chlorothiazide. Am. J. Physiol. 225: 954-961, 1973.

22. Beck, L.H. and Goldberg, M.: Mechanism of the blunted phosphaturia in saline-loaded thyroparathyroidectomized dogs. Kidney Int. 6: 18-23, 1974.

23. Knox, F.G. and LeChene, C.: Distal site of action of parathyroid hormone on phosphate reabsorption. Am. J. Physiol. 229: 1556-1560, 1975.

24. Puschett, J.B.: Site and mechanism of the phosphaturia due to volume expansion. Proc. of First Annual International Workshop on Phosphate, Paris, June 1975, Armour-Montagu (in press).

25. Kurtzman, N.A., Rogers, P.W., Boonjarern, S., and Arruda, J.A.L.: Effect of infusion of pharmacologic amounts of vasopressin on renal electrolyte excretion. Am. J. Physiol. 228: 890-894, 1975.

26. Antoniou, L.D., Burke, T.J., Robinson, R.R., and Clapp, J.R.: Vasopressin-related alterations of sodium reabsorption in the loop of Henle. Kidney Int. 3: 6-13, 1973.

27. Wen, S.F.: The effect of vasopressin on phosphate transport in the proximal tubule of the dog. J. Clin. Invest. 53: 660-664, 1974.

PHYLOGENY OF RENAL PHOSPHATE TRANSPORT IN THE VERTEBRATES

Olav L.M. Bijvoet and Pieter H. Reitsma

Department of Clinical Endocrinology and Metabolism
University Hospital, Leiden, the Netherlands

INTRODUCTION

Extracellular phosphate concentration can only remain constant when the input and the output from the extracellular space are equal. The main input is dietary, from the phosphate bound in food; the only output is through the kidney. This is the case not only in man but probably throughout the whole vertebrate subphylum[1]. In man the rate at which phosphate is filtered through the glomerular membrane at a normal plasma phosphate concentration is about 4500 mg/day. This is much more than the average 750 mg/day absorbed from the gut. Excessive loss of phosphate from the extracellular fluid is prevented by tubular reabsorption. These two renal operations, glomerular filtration and tubular reabsorption, largely determine the level and constancy of the plasma phosphate[2].

The reabsorption of phosphate, which for a great part is carried out in the proximal tubule, has generally been considered as the only significant element in tubular phosphate transport. This in contrast to tubular transport of other substances that may consist of combined reabsorptive and secretory processes occuring at various sites along the renal tubule. Recent data however suggests that tubular phosphate transport may occur at more than one site and that net tubular phosphate reabsorption may also be the result of combined reabsorptive and secretory processes[3]. Most of this information stems from studies in man, dog and rat. This is, of course, a sample of vertebrates and such selection may significantly bias our view of possible modes of phosphate transport. Indeed consideration of the few experimental data obtained in the non-mammalian vertebrates shows that tubular reabsorption is certainly not always the sole or even the most important element of tubular phosphate transport.

One may postulate that the direction of renal tubular transport
necessary to maintain plasma phosphate concentration around a
certain value may depend on whether the phosphate filtered through
the glomeruli is more than, or less than, phosphate absorbed from
the diet. The rate of glomerular phosphate filtration is equal to
the product of glomerular filtration rate (G.F.R.) and plasma
phosphate concentration. Phosphate output through the kidney is
equal to the filtered phosphate minus the reabsorbed phosphate or
plus the phosphate secreted into the tubules. To infer something
about the direction of tubular phosphate transport necessary to
maintain a constant extracellular phosphate concentration, one needs
therefore information about glomerular filtration rate, about the
plasma phosphate concentration and about the phosphate absorbed from
the diet. In the next sections we will consider what information is
available about these three factors in the various classes of
vertebrates (Table 1) and also review some of the direct studies of
renal phosphate transport made in the non-mammalian vertebrates.

TABLE 1.   EVOLUTION OF THE VERTEBRATES. Within brackets modern
           specimens of the various classes

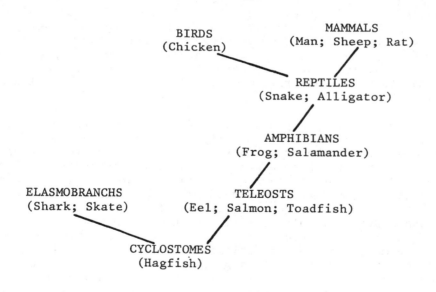

GLOMERULAR FILTRATION IN THE VERTEBRATES

Table 2 compares glomerular filtration rates of different classes of vertebrates. When this rate is expressed in ml per kg body weight per day, wide variations are apparent. The rate is lowest in the fishes as a group, but even amongst fishes it may vary from zero in aglomerular fishes living in sea water, to 200 ml per kg per day in fresh water fishes[4-8]. In man the average G.F.R. is about 20 times higher and the intermediate classes of vertebrates, the amphibians[9,10], reptiles[11,12] and birds[13,14], take an intermediate position. Glomerular development appears to be related to water excretion. It is now thought that the vertebrates evolved in fresh water[7]. A fresh water animal lives in a medium more dilute than its body fluids; in consequence water tends to enter the body by osmosis at any membranous surface. To prevent overhydration large amounts of water have to be eliminated. The early vertebrates had glomeruli sufficiently large to produce large amounts of urine. Descendants of the early vertebrates migrated to the sea. These animals were faced with a salt concentration in the environment that was higher than that of the body fluids. From modern marine fishes one may deduce an adaptation by excreting salts (but not phosphate) through their gills and by reducing glomerular filtration rate. Some of them even became aglomerular. A different adaptation is found in elasmobranchs, that by retention of urea elevate their osmolality to that of sea water. Despite the high osmolality of their environment, they retained a G.F.R. comparable to that of fishes living in fresh water. None of these animals possess a mechanism to make hyperosmolar urine like that of mammals.

Amphibians, the frog and necturus, live in fresh water and developed a liberal glomerular filtration rate, but the remaining land vertebrates, reptiles, birds and mammals, were faced with the same problem of water conservation and salt excretion as the marine fish. In reptiles and birds conservation of water was now accomplished by excretion of uric acid, which precipitates out of solution and leaves practically all the water osmotically free to be reabsorbed from the cloaca.

Mammals developed a different method of conserving water. With the amphibians, the primitive water-excreting function of the glomerulus had already been secondarily converted to a filtration-reabsorption system designed to filter large amounts of water and salt, and extracellular osmolality could be adjusted by regulation of tubular reabsorption. In addition the mammals developed a concentrating mechanism, morphologically characterized by the loop of Henle, which enable them to produce hyperosmolar urine. All these animals therefore possess a mechanism to reabsorb water, which enables them to filter huge quantities of extracellular fluid without the danger of water loss[14-16].

TABLE 2.   GLOMERULAR FILTRATION IN THE VERTEBRATES

CLASS	ENVIRONMENT	G.F.R. (ml/kg/day)
Cyclostomes	sea water	10
	fresh water	10
Elasmobranchs	sea water	25-100
Teleosts		
glomerular	fresh water	25-200
	sea water	5-15
aglomerular	sea water	0
Amphibians	fresh water	500
Reptiles	land	75-300
Birds	land	300-2000
Mammals	land	2000

Legends : G.F.R. = glomerular filtration rate;References in text.

One may summarize by saying that glomerular filtration rate varies widely throughout the different classes of vertebrates. The extremes are found amongst the fishes on the one hand and mammals on the other. Amongst fishes G.F.R. varies between 0 and 200 ml per kg body weight per day, depending on the salinity of their environment. The mammals may be exemplified by man, who has a glomerular filtration rate of the order of 2000 ml per kg body weight per day.

THE PHOSPHATE TURNOVER IN FISHES

Direct measurements of 24 hour excretion rates of phosphate have been made in the marine elasmobranchs. The rate of excretion varies from 1 to 2 mmol per kg body weight per day[9,17]. These data can not be generalized. One may, however, gain an impression of phosphate turnover in fishes by using available data about their food intake. Most fishes are carnivorous or feed on plankton. These forms of food contain around 13 mg of inorganic phosphorus per

gram of protein[18,19]. The protein requirement of fishes has been
estimated at the relatively high value of 25 to 50% of the diet
(dry weight). The feeding rate required to maintain their weight
is 2.5% of the body weight (dry weight per life weight)[20]. One can
derive that the protein requirement of fish must therefore be in
the order of 5 to 25 gr per kg per day. From the phosphate :
protein ratio in fish-food and plankton, one can then derive an
estimate of the phosphate intake, which is in the order of 60 to
300 mg per kg body weight per day, that is 2 to 10 mmoles per kg
per day. These are of course minimal figures. There is no data on
the efficiency of phosphate absorption, but 50% should certainly be
a very low figure and therefore one may consider 1 mmole per kg
body weight per day as a low estimate of phosphate turnover in
fish. This figure agrees with the direct measurement in elasmobranch
fishes mentioned earlier. It is about twice that found in man.

It is interesting to note that sea water and fresh water have a
low phosphate content. From this it has been posited that the main
problem in fish would be phosphate conservation[21]. It should however
be clear that phosphate turnover is independent of the phosphate
concentration of the environment since phosphate uptake is of
metabolic origin[8].

The 24 hour excretion rate of phosphate in man amounts to
about 30 mmoles per day and phosphate turnover, expressed per kg
body weight, is therefore in the order of 0.5 mmoles per kg body
weight per day. From the intermediate vertebrate classes one may
mention the reptiles. In these animals phosphate clearance values
were found to be three times as high as the creatinine clearance[11].
Since their glomerular filtration rate is around 300 ml per kg
body weight per day[11], the phosphate clearance should be in the
order of 1 liter per kg per day. It has been found[22] that they have
a serum phosphate of 1 mmole/l and their phosphate excretion rate
would therefore equal 1 mmole per kg per day, comparable to that
of the fishes.

THE PLASMA PHOSPHATE IN THE VERTEBRATES

Assuming that the ultrafiltrability of phosphate is the same
throughout the vertebrates, the rate of filtration of phosphate
will be found equal to the product of plasma phosphate concentration
and G.F.R. Table 3 lists observed plasma phosphate concentrations
in various species related to successive developmental phases of
vertebrate evolution. With some exceptions the plasma phosphate
varies around 3 mmoles/l in glomerular fishes[5,8,24-28] and is rather
higher from 4.5 to 8 mmoles/l, in aglomerular fishes[29,30]. In
reptiles[12,31,32], amphibians, birds and mammals, the plasma phosphate
is often below 2 mmoles/l and with a few exceptions around 1 mmole/l,
as it is in man[2].

TABLE 3.   PHOSPHATE TURNOVER IN THE VERTEBRATES

CLASS	INPUT	G.F.R.	x	[P]	FILTERED	S or R
	μmoles/kg/day	ml/kg/day		μmole/ml	μmoles/kg/day	
Cyclostomes	> 1000	10		< 2	< 20	S
Elasmobranchs	> 1000	< 100		< 3	< 300	S
Teleosts						
glomerular	> 1000	< 200		< 3	< 600	S
aglomerular	> 1000	0		< 8	0	S
Amphibians		500		≃ 1	500	R(S?)
Reptiles	≃ 1000	300		< 2	< 600	R;S
Birds		300-2000		< 1	300-2000	R;S
Mammals	500	2000		< 2	< 4000	R

Legends : G.F.R. = glomerular filtration rate; [P] = plasma
phosphate concentration; S = secretion; R = reabsorption.

TUBULAR PHOSPHATE TRANSPORT IN THE NON-MAMMALIAN VERTEBRATES

    The preceding data allow one to calculate what minimum G.F.R.
would be required in animals to filter phosphate at a rate which
is at least equal to the phosphate input into the extracellular
fluid (Table 3). If the filtration rate is above that value,
animals could do without phosphate secretion and should in
addition reabsorb some phosphate in the tubules. If G.F.R. is,
however, lower, the animals would not be able to maintain the serum
phosphate concentration without additional secretion of phosphate
into the tubular lumen.

    A low estimate of daily phosphate production in fish is, as
we have seen, 1 mmole of phosphate per kg body weight per day.
The plasma phosphate concentration of glomerular fish is 3 mmoles/1
or below that. Fish should therefore need a G.F.R. of at least
300 ml per kg per day to maintain their plasma phosphate at, or

below that value. This value is far more than the maximum G.F.R. found in these species. We may infer that fish cannot do without tubular phosphate secretion. The situation in amphibians and birds is borderline but reptiles have such a low G.F.R. that they probably also possess secretion. In mammals however tubular reabsorption of phosphate is clearly required to maintain plasma phosphate homeostasis. This kind of evidence is largely theoretical, but the deductions can be supported by direct measurements which will now be reviewed in sequence.

Hagfish are survivors of the oldest known group of vertebrates, the jawless fishes or *Cyclostomes*, and the most primitive of living vertebrates. In hagfish, in particular, osmotic and ionic regulation and related renal function have been examined with the intention of clarifying the still controversial question of a marine or fresh-water origin of the vertebrates. Data were reviewed by McInerney[35]. In these fish G.F.R. is not more than 10 ml per kg body weight per day and the serum phosphate 2 mmoles/l. McInerney states that tubular phosphate secretion has been demonstrated, but gives no direct figures. The skate and the spiny dogfish are representatives of the *Elasmobranchs*, the next oldest group of living vertebrates. In the dogfish[36] phosphate concentrations in the urine have been found to vary from zero to 79 mmoles/l, that is far above their serum phosphate concentration of less than 2 mmoles/l. The same has been found for the skate[26]. In these fish the urine production is not far less than the glomerular filtration rate and these data therefore suggest that their tubules do indeed secrete phosphate. The question was more recently reexamined by Wolbach[6]. He found in these fishes that renal phosphate excretion rate always exceeded glomerular filtration rate, sometimes even by a factor 10, during infusions of inorganic phosphate. This is firm evidence for phosphate secretion. The secretion was, unlike glucose reabsorption, phlorrhizin-insensitive, in contrast to phosphate transport in mammals. The secreted phosphate in these animals may be produced from an organic precursor, as suggested earlier by Marshall and Grafflin for the phosphate secretion in aglomerular teleosts[29]. This possibility has never been proved or disproved. Since phosphate clearance never exceeded PAH-clearance, the phosphate present in the blood perfusing the kidneys could account for all of the excreted phosphate. The third and last class of fishes are the *Teleosts*. Amongst these, the aglomerular teleosts living in sea water are particularly interesting because they depend entirely upon tubular secretion as a mechanism to excrete waste products in the urine. Two representatives are the monkfish (goosefish or angler fish) and the toadfish. Both fishes have urine containing phosphate with concentrations up to 18.3 mmoles/l, concentrations well above the concentration in blood. Free diffusion could therefore not explain the transtubular phosphate movement. Marshall and Grafflin found that raising the inorganic phosphate levels in Lophius-plasma did not increase phosphate excretion and suggested

that the excreted phosphate had an organic precursor[8,26]. Direct
studies of renal phosphate transport have also been made in
glomerular Teleosts, sculpin[8] and cod[26], either by comparison of
simultaneous xylose and phosphate clearances or by comparing
urinary phosphate concentrations with the plasma phosphate.
Allowing for some xylose and water reabsorption in these kidneys
the ratios were always so far in excess of xylose clearance (up to
50 in sculpin) or plasma phosphate (up to 15 in cod), that they
can only be explained by secretion.

There is no direct data showing the converse in fish, lower
urinary than plasma phosphate concentration, that would indicate
net tubular phosphate reabsorption. Two measurements by Homer Smith[24]
in elasmobranchs are a possible exception. Recently Dave[37] found
that starvation caused a 50% decrease of plasma phosphate
concentration in the eel. This suggests inadequate phosphate
conservation but does not confirm the absence of reabsorption.
Homer Smith[38] found that the phosphate expected from tissue
breakdown after estivation of lungfish is not excreted, in contrast
to potassium or nitrogen. He concluded that the phosphate may have
been conserved in an organic form.

In summary, fish do exhibit tubular phosphate secretion. This
is necessary for the maintenance of plasma phosphate at a
sufficiently low concentration. Organic precursors may or may not
play a role in the secretory mechanism.

In the next class of animals, the *Amphibians*, the situation
has somewhat changed. These animals have a liberal glomerular
filtration rate, in frog it is 500 ml per kg body weight per day,
and they may reabsorb up to 90% of the filtrate[9]. The rate of
filtration seems large enough to excrete more than the ingested
phosphate and indeed, both in the frog and in the salamander, net
reabsorption has clearly been demonstrated[10]. In the frog no
secretion of phosphate could be found but Walker and Hudson[39] who
perfused proximal tubules of the necturus with phosphate free fluid
found that the fluid might contain some phosphate at the end of
the perfusion. He could not, however, differentiate between
diffusion or secretion as a mechanism for the inward phosphate
flux.

The *Reptile* best studied in this respect is the snake and
there are some data on the alligator. G.F.R. in snakes is more
comparable to fishes than to amphibians in being low. Even though
the ancestors of the reptiles are considered to be of amphibian
origin, they seem not to have lost their ability to secrete
phosphate, as the amphibians have largely done. In intact animals
phosphate to inulin clearance ratios were found of 2.6, comparable
to a phosphate-creatinine clearance ratio of 3 found in the
alligator[12]. Like the amphibians the snake also has a mechanism

for tubular reabsorption of phosphate, because Clark and Dantzler
were able to show that the phosphate-creatinine clearance ratio
in snakes decreased from 2.6 to 0.3 (that is far below unity) after
parathyroidectomy[11,12].

     Phosphate reabsorption in the *Birds* has been studied
in chicken[13,14]. Birds have a relatively high glomerular filtration
rate and have a filtration-reabsorption system. The basal phosphate
excretion rate, in chicken, is however rather high, 0.2 to 2 mmoles
per kg per day and their plasma phosphate concentration is not
higher than 1 mmole/l. Indeed the filtered phosphate often equals
turnover, and net phosphate secretion, sensitive to parathyroid
hormone and probably insensitive to phlorrhizin has been
demonstrated. These animals are apparently also able to reabsorb
phosphate and the reabsorption mechanism is phlorrhizin-sensitive[13].
Levinsky found that the secretory mechanism was not responsive,
within wide limits, to the phosphate concentration of the blood[14].
The possibility of organic precursors of the secreted phosphate
seems not to have been examined.

TUBULAR PHOSPHATE TRANSPORT IN THE MAMMALIAN VERTEBRATE: CONCLUSIONS

     One needs not review here the situation in *Mammals*. It is well
known that in this class net reabsorption by the tubules plays a
great role in the regulation of plasma phosphate. Observations in
sheep, man and dog indicate that fluid and phosphate reabsorption
in the proximal tubule may be proportional and that a threshold
phosphate concentration exists below which most filtered phosphate
is conserved, and above which most is excreted[2,40,41]. The value
of this threshold concentration may greatly influence the plasma
phosphate concentration. Marshall and Smith[15] long ago stressed
that the development of a filtration-reabsorption system for water
was a major event in the vertebrate evolution. It is rather
surprising to see how fundamental this change has worked out with
respect to phosphate. Phosphate secretion, normal in fishes, is
very difficult or well nigh impossible to demonstrate in mammals
and certainly does not assist in maintaining a normal plasma
phosphate when renal failure decreases phosphate filtration to or
below phosphate intake. It would be interesting to know if animals
in whom phosphate secretion has been demonstrated would be able to
maintain a normal plasma phosphate concentration when their G.F.R.
is artificially reduced. Recent studies have nevertheless indicated
the possibility in mammals of an inward transport of phosphate
across the tubule walls, be it active or passive. At this point it
is interesting to recall a communication of Falbriard[42] who during
stopped-flow demonstrated distal influx of peritubular radioactive
phosphate, that was not influenced by parathyroid hormone or by
the concentration of inorganic phosphate in plasma. It will be
recalled that studies in non-mammalian vertebrates raised the
possibility that secreted phosphate in fishes may be derived from

organic percursors. Surprisingly Taugner and von Bubnoff were able
to demonstrate tubular secretion of phosphate in the cat[43], and
possibly in the dog[44], when they infused them with organic phosphate
esters. Similar studies have not been repeated in these or other
animals.

All vertebrates during embryonic life and all adult vertebrates
other than the mammalia possess a renal-portal system, draining the
posterior part of the body and delivering blood to peritubular
capillaries. From these it is ultimately collected into the efferent
renal veins. Phylogenetically this system is one of the most
fundamental features of the renal circulation in the vertebrates.
In the aglomerular fishes the only blood supply to the kidney is
venous in nature and is in large part derived from the portal vein.
There is an association between the presence of a renal portal vein
and the preponderance of tubular secretion over reabsorption.
Levinsky and Davidson[14] could, however, not find an effect on
phosphate secretion when they infused chicken-leg-veins with
phosphate, whereas infusion of the wing-veins had such an effect.
Yet parathyroid extract, when injected unilaterally in the portal
system had an unilateral effect[14] and the extract has been shown
to affect secretion rather than phosphate reabsorption in chicken[13].
The question, whether having a renal-portal system and possessing
tubular phosphate secretion, are related facts or not, is therefore
yet undecided.

These data on renal phosphate transport in the various classes
of vertebrates support the general conclusions of Marshall and
Smith that the type of tubular transport depends on glomerular
development and glomerular development should be related to water
excretion. In the mammals, and to some extent in all four-footed
vertebrates, the primitive water-excreting function of the glomerulus
has been secondarily diverted to a filtration-reabsorption system
designed to excrete waste with active retention in the body of
optimal quantities of solutes and water.

REFERENCES

1. Smith, H.W. : The absorption and excretion of water and salts
   by marine teleosts, Amer. J. Physiol., 93, 480-505, 1930.
2. Bijvoet, O.L.M. : The importance of the kidneys in phosphate
   homeostasis, in : Proceedings of the first International
   Workshop on Phosphate, Armour, 1975.
3. Proceedings of the first International Workshop on Phosphate,
   Armour, passim.
4. Fänge, R. : Structure and function of the excretory organs of
   myxinoids, in : The biology of the myxine, Brodal, A. and
   Fänge, R. Eds., Universitetsforlaget, Oslo, Ch. VIII, 516-529,
   1963.

5. Clarke, R.W. and Smith, H.W. : Absorption and excretion of water and salts by the elasmobranch fishes, J. Cell. Comp. Physiol., 1, 131–143, 1932.

6. Wolbach, R.A. : Phlorizin and renal phosphate secretion in the spinydogfish Squalus acanthias, Amer. J. Physiol. 219, 886–888, 1970.

7. Smith, H. : From fish to philisopher. The natural history library, Anchor books, Doubleday and Co. Inc., Garden City, New York, passim, 1961.

8. Grafflin, A.L. : Renal function in marine teleosts, Biol. Bull. 71, 360–374, 1936.

9. Forster, B.P. : The nature of the glucose reabsorptive process in the frog renal tubule, J. Cell. Comp. Physiol. 20, 55–69, 1942.

10. Hogben, C.A.M. and Bollman, J.L. : Excretion of phosphate by isolated frog kidney, Amer. J. Physiol. 164, 662–669, 1951.

11. Hernandez, T. and Coulson, R.A. : Renal clearance in the alligator. Fed. Proc. 15, 91, 1956.

12. Clark, N.B. and Dantzler, W.H. : Renal tubular transport of calcium and phosphate in snakes : role of parathyroid hormone, Amer. J. Physiol. 223, 1455–1464, 1972.

13. Ferguson, R.K. and Wolbach, R.A. : Effects of glucose, phlorizin, and parathyroid extract on renal phosphate transport in chickens, Amer. J. Physiol. 212, 1123–1130, 1967.

14. Levinsky, N.G. and Davidson, D.G. : Renal action of parathyroid extract in the chicken, Amer. J. Physiol. 191, 530–536, 1957.

15. Marshall, E.K. and Smith, H.W. : The glomerular development of the vertebrate kidney in relation to habitat, Biol. Bull. 59, 135–153, 1930.

16. Smith, H.W. : Water regulation and its evolution in the fishes, Quart. Rev. Biol. 7, 1–26, 1932.

17. Pitts, R.F. : Urinary composition in marine fish, J. Cell. Comp. Physiol. 4, 389–395, 1933–34.

18. Documenta Geigy Wissenschaftliche Tabellen, J.R. Geigy, Basle, 1960.

19. Clarke, G.L. and Bishop, D.W. : The nutritional value of marine zooplankton with a consideration of its use as an emergency food, Ecology 29, 54–71, 1948.

20. Cowey, C.B. and Sargent, J.R. : Fish nutrition, Adv. Mar. Biol. 10, 382–492, 1972.

21. MacIntyre, I., Colston, K.W., Evans, I.M.A. et al. : Regulation of vitamin D : an evolutionary view, Clin. Endocrinol. 5 suppl., 855–955, 1976.

22. Coulson, R.A., Hernandez, T. and Brazda, F.G. : Biochemical studies on the alligator. Proc. Soc. Exp. Biol. Med. 73, 203–206, 1950.

23. Robertson, J.D. : Osmoregulation and ionic composition of cells and tissues, in : The biology of the myxine, Brodal, A. and Fänge, R. Eds., Universitetsforlaget, Oslo, ch. VII, 503–515, 1963.

24. Smith, H.W. : The absorption and excretion of water and salts by the elasmobranch fishes, Amer. J. Physiol. 98, 279-310, 1931.

25. Urist, M.R., Uyeno, S., King, E., Okada, M and Applegate, S. : Calcium and phosphorus in the skeleton and blood of the lungfish Lepidosiren paradoxa. With comment on humoral factors in calcium homeostasis in the osteichthyes, Comp. Biochem. Physiol. 42A, 393-408, 1972.

26. Marshall, E.K. and Grafflin, A.L. : The structure and function of the kidney of Lophius piscatorius, Bull. Johns Hopkins Hosp. 43, 205-234, 1928.

27. Chan, D.K.O. and Chester Jones,I. : Regulation and distribution of plasma calcium and inorganic phosphate in the european eel (Anguilla anguilla L.), J. Endocrinol. 42, 109-117, 1968.

28. Pang, P.K.T. : The relationship between corpuscles of Stannius and serum electrolyte regulation in Killifish, Fundulus heteroclitus, J. Exp. Zool. 178, 1-8, 1971.

29. Marshall, E.K. and Grafflin, A.L. : Excretion of inorganic phosphate by the aglomerular kidney, Proc. Soc. Exp. Biol. Med. 31, 44-46, 1933.

30. Forster, R.P. and Berglund, F. : Osmotic diuresis and its effect on total electrolyte distribution in plasma and urine of the aglomerular teleost, Lophius americanus, J. Gen. Physiol. 39, 349-359, 1956.

31. Clark, N.B. : Experimental and histological studies of the parathyroid glands of fresh-water turtles, Gen. Comp. Endocrinol. 5, 297-312, 1965.

32. Clark, N.B., Pang, P.K.T. and Dix, M.W. : Parathyroid glands and calcium and phosphate regulation in the Lizard, Anolis carolensis, Gen. Comp. Endocrinol. 12, 614-618, 1969.

33. Walker, A.M. : Quantitative studies of the composition of glomerular urine, J. Biol. Chem. 101, 239-254, 1933.

34. Cortelyou, J.R., Quipse, P.A. and McWhinnie, D.J., Parathyroid extract effects on phosphorus metabolism in Rana pipiens, Gen. Comp. Endocrinol. 9, 76-92, 1967.

35. McInerney, J.E. : Renal sodium reabsorption in the hagfish, Eptatretus Stouti, Comp. Biochem. Physiol. 49A, 273-280, 1974.

36. Clarke, R.W. and Smith, H.W. : Absorption and excretion of water and salts by the elasmobranch fishes. J. Cell. Comp. Physiol. 1, 131-143, 1932.

37. Dave, G., Johansson-Sjöbeck, M.L., Larsson, Å., Lewanda, K. and Lidman, U. : Metabolic and hematological effects of starvation in the european eel, Anguilla anguilla L., Comp. Biochem. Physiol. 52A, 423-430, 1975.

38. Smith, H.W. : Metabolism of the lung-fish, Protopterus aethiopicus, J. Biol. Chem. 88, 97-130, 1930.

39. Walker, A.M. and Hudson, Ch.J. : The role of the tubule in the excretion of inorganic phosphates by the amphibian kidney, Amer. J. Physiol. 118, 167-173, 1937.

40. Tomas, F.M. : Renal response to intravenous phosphate infusion in the sheep, Aust. J. Biol. Sci. 28, 511-520, 1975.

41. Hellman, D.H., Baird, H.R. and Bartter, F.C. : Relationship of maximal tubular phosphate reabsorption to filtration rate in the dog, Amer. J. Physiol. 207, 89-96, 1964.

42. Falbriard, A., Vassali, P. and Schaller, G. : Préparation de l'animal non anesthésié à des recherches rénales (en particulier à la diurèse interrompue), J. Urol. Néphrol. 68, 128-132, 1962.

43. Taugner, R., von Bubnoff, M. and Braun, W. : Gibt es eine tubuläre Phosphatsekretion? Ueber die Ausscheidung von anorganischem und organischem Phosphat bei der Katze, Pflügers Arch. 258, 133-148, 1953,

44. Schmid, E., von Bubnoff, M. and Taugner, R. : Zur Nierenausscheidung von organischem und anorganischem Phosphat beim Hund, Naunyn Schmiedeberg Arch. Exp. Pharmacol. 228, 207-208, 1956.

45. Smith, H.W. : The kidney. Oxford University Press, New York, 1951.

TRANSEPITHELIAL TRANSPORT OF PHOSPHATE ANION IN KIDNEY.   POTENTIAL MECHANISMS FOR   HYPOPHOSPHATEMIA

C.R. Scriver, T.E. Stacey, H.S. Tenenhouse and
W.A. MacDonald
Medical Research Council Genetics Group
McGill University-Montreal Children's Hosp.
Research Inst., 2300 Tupper St.
Montreal, Quebec H3H 1P3

The kidney is an important determinant of endogenous Pi pools in the mammal. Pi is filtered with plasma water and the major fraction of the filtered load is then reabsorbed by the tubule; a variable remainder is excreted (1-3). Many endogenous factors including PTH, Ca^{2+} and pH influence the process of net reabsorption, or reclamation, and it is now apparent that transepithelial transport of Pi in mammalian kidney is more complex than was anticipated from the classic observations of Pi reclamation (4,5). Accordingly, we will consider the phenomenon of transepithelial transport which underlies net reabsorption, and the evidence for heterogeneity between nephrons, and within nephrons, in the response to regulatory events which influence Pi transport. We believe these findings, and evidence concerning a carrier (or channel) for anion transport in membranes will be relevant to the ultimate interpretation of XLH, a genetic form of hypophosphatemia in which negative reabsorption of Pi occurs, and HBD, a newly recognized trait in which an equivalent hypophosphatemia is associated with less renal loss of Pi and less severe bone disease.

Abbreviations: Pi, phosphate anion ($H_2PO_4^-$ and HPO_4^{2-}); P, inorganic phosphorus; PTH, parathyroid hormone; GFR, glomerular filtration rate; FPi, filtered Pi; TRPi, tubular reabsorption of Pi; TmPi, maximum rate of TRP_i; TRPT, theoretical renal phosphorus threshold; FEPi, fractional excretion of Pi; PCT, proximal convoluted tubule; DCT, distal convoluted tubule; XLH, X-linked hypophosphatemia; HBD, hypophosphatemic bone disease.

RENAL REABSORPTION OF Pi IN MAN

Under normal circumstances interindividual variation
in plasma phosphorus, [P], is observed in the normal
range (below 4 mg/dl ($<$1.29 mM) in the adult and above
4 mg/dl in the child). Intraindividual circadian variation also occurs which is partly a reflection of variation in net tubular reclamation of Pi. Plasma Pi is
almost completely ultrafilterable and at pH 7.4 the ratio
of $H_2PO_4^-$:HPO_4^{2-} is 19:81 in glomerular filtrate. However,
FEPi in bladder urine is $<$0.2 of FPi under normal endogenous conditions suggesting that regulation of TRPi may
influence plasma [P]. The early literature reports progressive saturation of TRPi as plasma [P] and FPi increase until TmPi is achieved (6); there is interindividual variation in TmPi (normal value: 130±20 (mean±SD)
mg/min·100 ml glomerular filtrate). The actual mechanisms
underlying the phenomena of TRPi, FEPi and TmPi in human
kidney have yet to be delineated.

In recent years there has been renewed interest to
define, as precisely as possible, the parameters of TRPi
and TmPi in man (7-10). A standardized infusion method
to produce a linear rise in plasma [P] has been used to
measure GFR (9); under these conditions exposure of the
tubule to a range of [Pi] yields data pertaining to TRPi,
TmPi and the derived TRPT (or TmPi/GFR) (Fig. 1). A
nomogram has also been developed to calculate TRPT from
single plasma measurements and short-term urine collections without infusion protocols (11). Such data can,
in turn, be used to evaluate clinical events which influence plasma [P] and TRPi (Fig. 1); for example, TRPT
is elevated in children and adolescents relative to the
adult, while it is depressed in primary and secondary
hyperparathyroidism (10); diphosphonates in long-term
low doses raise TRPT (12). *However, such observations
tell us only that certain events modulate net transepithelial fluxes of Pi and plasma [P]; we are not informed
as to the mechanism involved.*

TRANSEPITHELIAL TRANSPORT OF Pi

Epithelial cells determine Pi transport in the nephron. They are asymmetrical, possessing luminal and
basilar poles which have different morphology and function. The luminal pole faces the ultrafiltrate where
Pi is topologically *outside* the body; the basilar pole
is in contact with peritubular interstitial fluid *inside*
the body (Fig. 2). The luminal membranes of PCT, pars

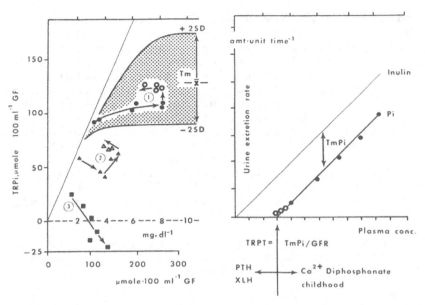

Figure 1. Left: Effect of Pi infusion (closed symbols) and Pi + Ca^{2+} (open symbols) on TRPi in man. (1) Normal subject; normal range (shaded); (2) HBD subject; (3) XLH subject exhibiting negative reabsorption. Right: Alternate method of plotting [Pi]-dependent TmPi showing TRPT value and effect of various events on TRPT.

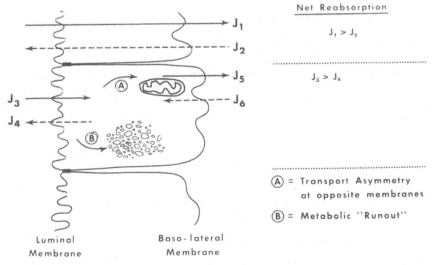

Figure 2. Transepithelial transport of Pi showing various fluxes (J_1 to J_6); paracellular fluxes are impeded by tight junctions. See text for details.

recta and DCT are enlarged with microvilli (brush border),
while the basolateral membranes possess infoldings which
embrace mitochondria. This structural asymmetry is presumably associated with a functional asymmetry (13,14).
Vectorial and transepithelial movement of solute is an
important function achieved by the tubule, which serves
as a more or less continuous permeability barrier because
of tight junctions between epithelial cells at their luminal pole (15). Accordingly Pi traverses two sets of
plasma membranes, one at the luminal and the other at the
basolateral surface, rather than moving by a paracellular
route, to reach peritubular fluid during reclamative
transport from ultrafiltrate (Fig. 2). Net transcellular
transport of Pi is normally against an electrochemical
gradient in PCT.

During net tubular reabsorption, the Pi flux inward
(J_1) exceeds its outward flux (J_2) (Fig. 2). Each flux
must follow the general equation

$$J = k \cdot Pi* \tag{1}$$

where k is the rate coefficient, not necessarily independent of Pi*, the activity of anion. If the two species
of Pi anion (mono- and divalent) move in parallel, and
if they do not have identical activities and rate coefficients, equation 1 resolves into the components

$$J_a = k_a \cdot H_2PO_4^- \quad \text{and} \quad J_b = k_b \cdot HPO_4^{2-} \tag{2}$$

During net reabsorption from ultrafiltrate the
fluxes J_3 (influx) and J_4 (efflux or backflux) (Fig. 2)
at the luminal membrane are most pertinent, in which
case the relationship is: $J_3 > J_4$. We must now consider
how the cell is likely to achieve asymmetry of fluxes at
the luminal membrane and across the cell during net reabsorption of Pi.

Carrier-mediated transport for several anions exists
in many epithelia, however, the best-described case is in
the erythrocyte membrane (16,17). If Pi fluxes have carrier-mediated components in renal membranes, luminal influx (J_3, Fig. 2) is described by the modified equation

$$J_3 = J_{in} = \frac{Jmax_{in} \cdot [Pi]_e}{Km_{in} + [Pi]_e} + k_D \cdot Pi_e^* \tag{3}$$

which combines the Michaelis-Menten term for concentra-

tion-dependent transport and a linear term for passive
permeability (18); the latter can be expanded according
to equation 2. The corresponding equation for efflux
(J_{eff}) or backflux of intracellular Pi is

$$J_4 = J_{eff} = \frac{Jmax_{eff} \cdot [Pi]_i}{Km_{eff} + [Pi]_i} + k_D \cdot Pi_i^* \quad (4)$$

It is important to know something about the proportions of Pi permeating by passive diffusion and by carrier in the nephron. If passive diffusion of lipid-in-
soluble anion is quantitatively important, one would
expect restriction to diffusion in the membrane to be
greater for larger molecules (19). Membrane permeability
to Pi diminishes at alkaline pH (20,21). Gel filtration
on Sephadex G-15 reveals that HPO_4^{2-}, which is the dominant species above pH 6.82, is larger than $H_2PO_4^-$ (Fig. 3).
Accordingly, lower Pi flux at more alkaline pH could be
related to the lower proportion of the smaller and hence
faster diffusant species. Whereas intracellular pH is
acid (about 7.25) relative to the luminal pH of early
PCT (about 7.4), it is less acid relative to later PCT
which has a luminal pH of 6.7-6.8 (22). Accordingly, at
the luminal membrane, net backflux would be favored in
early PCT but net influx would be favored in later PCT
at comparable [P] on opposite sides of the membrane.

Measurement of intracellular [P] in renal cortex
(23) suggests that net uptake of Pi from filtrate occurs
against a chemical gradient. However, this is not necessarily so, if cellular Pi is compartmentalized so that
cytoplasmic Pi is low. *Unfortunately, data pertaining
to the compartmentalization and topology of Pi in
tubular cells are very limited at present.*

How then is an asymmetry of Pi fluxes at the
luminal membrane achieved? Two possibilities exist:
     i) The effective cytoplasmic [Pi] is kept lower than
that which would be at equilibrium with luminal [Pi].
     ii) Km_{eff} exceeds Km_{in} in the Michaelis-Menten term.

We know nothing about the relative values for Km_{in}
and Km_{eff} on the postulated anion carrier (or channel)
at the luminal membrane and can say nothing here about
this alternative. We are left to speculate about the
remaining and important alternative namely a process
which lowers the effective concentration (or activity)
of Pi in cytoplasm at the luminal pole. Two mechanisms

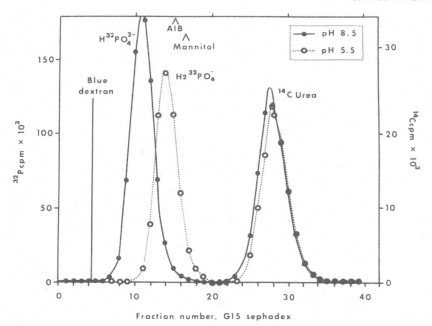

<u>Figure 3</u>. Sephadex elution profile of Pi anion. HPO_4^{2-} predominates over $H_2PO_4^-$ at pH 8.5 and is a larger anion; α-aminoisobutyrate (AIB) and other markers are shown.

for "run-out" from this topological pool can be postulated. <u>Metabolic run-out</u> is the first in which Pi dis-
posal occurs by incorporation into organic pools; for
this event to be successful there must be net efflux of
combined phosphate to the peritubular space. <u>Membrane
run-out</u> is the second potential mechanism. In this case,
the net efflux of Pi at the basolateral membrane ($J_5 > J_6$)
required for net transepithelial transport ($J_1 > J_2$) must
arise by asymmetry of that membrane's carrier. *Unfortunately there are no data which describe the respective
characteristics of Pi permeability in isolated luminal
and basolateral membranes.*

        Borle (24,25) has proposed a 3-compartment model in
which the mitochondria play a major role in the transepithelial transport of Ca^{2+}; Pi could be an attendant
anion. However, if this mechanism is functionally important in net transepithelial transport, Pi leaving the
mitochondrial pool must reach the peritubular space without entering the cytoplasmic pool to which the luminal
membrane is exposed. As it happens, mitochondria at the

basilar pole apparently restrict the intracellular diffusion and distribution of Ca^{2+} in salivary gland epithelium
(26); the influence of Pi on Ca^{2+} diffusion has not been
investigated.

*These speculations serve two purposes here: they
raise issues requiring investigation; and they indicate
that Pi backflux from epithelial cells could be a normal
physiological event susceptible to modulation and which
may significantly influence FEPi.*

IN VIVO HANDLING OF Pi BY MAMMALIAN NEPHRONS

We have selected some recent studies to illustrate
the problem that exists in the interpretation of mechanisms of Pi transport and regulation thereof. We believe
these studies indicate that modulation of luminal influx,
and of backflux, can occur as independent events to control FEPi and hence plasma [P].

<u>Fluxes</u>: Boudry et al (27) measured whole-kidney Pi
clearance in the rat at endogenous plasma [P] and after
elevating plasma [P] by intravenous infusion over 30-
180 min. in intact and TPTx (48 hr) animals. At elevated
[Pi] and with time, net TRPi fell and FEPi increased
significantly in the intact and TPTX rat. This "unortho-
dox" response to Pi loading has also been observed by
others (28,29). Under the conditions of these experiments, flux J_6 (Fig. 2), from peritubular space to cell,
must increase; accordingly intracellular [Pi] and ultimately flux J_4 will be influenced and might account for
the decrease in net transepithelial reabsorption (flux J_1)

Micropuncture studies were also performed (27) at
endogenous or elevated plasma [P]. Chemical [P] was determined in plasma (Pl) and tubular fluid (TF) of PCT and
DCT from superficial nephrons and in urine from the ipse-
lateral ureter. The $(TF/Pl)_p$ ratio in PCT was 0.77 under
endogenous conditions indicating reabsorption of Pi in
excess of water in this segment; the ratio was 1.28 in
the Pi-loaded rats. However it is remarkable that the
chemical ratio is constant all along the PCT in such experiments. Microinjection experiments (30) show that a
unidirectional inward flux of ^{33}Pi occurs all along the
perfused PCT. Therefore, the constant chemical $(TF/Pl)_p$
ratio suggests either that Pi backflux to the lumen occurs
to keep the ratio constant; or that Pi and H_2O move inward at exactly equal rates under various conditions along
the later PCT. The finding of disproportionately elevated FEPi in PCT at raised plasma [P], and also presumably at elevated cellular [P], strongly suggests
increased backflux if leakage at the micropuncture site

is eliminated. Backflux equivalent to 17% of net flux
at the endogenous state has, in fact, been calculated
in the rat (31).

During microperfusion of PCT with ^{32}P and carrier
Pi at elevated or endogenous [P], there is evidence either
for net reabsorption ($J_3 > J_4$) or net backflux ($J_4 > J_3$) of
Pi, depending on the physiological conditions (27). Measurement of specific activity along the nephron reveals
a dilution during transit down the nephron; the longer
the perfused segment of tubule, the greater is the dilution. Leakage of Pi from cells at the puncture site is
unlikely to account for these findings; again they indicate Pi backflux from tubular cells to lumen.
  *It seems apparent that while net reabsorption pre-
dominates along the total nephron under normal endogenous
conditions, there is bidirectional flux of Pi; under
circumstances in which cellular and peritubular [P] are
likely to be elevated, backflux can become important.*

Intersegmental, intranephron heterogeneity, and
internephron heterogeneity, also characterize Pi transport. Ureteral FEPi is significantly lower than DCT
FEPi (27,32) indicating net reabsorption in a distal segment of the nephron. However ureteral FEPi data are obtained from mixed populations of deep and superfician nephrons, while DCT FEPi data reflect superficial nephrons.
Microinjection studies with ^{33}Pi (30) show clearly that
distal segments of superficial nephrons do not reclaim
Pi. Accordingly internephron heterogeneity in Pi handling
between deep and superficial nephrons must exist. *Heterogeneity of Pi transport along the nephron may reflect different physiological environments acting on Pi anion; but
it may also indicate non-uniform distribution of regulating factors or of cellular and membrane components (gene
products) mediating Pi fluxes.*

Effect of Various Agents on Pi transport. Microinjection
studies in superficial rat nephrons (30) reveal that PTH
diminishes the absorptive flux of ^{33}Pi along the PCT, but
largely in the early segment. A similar localized effect
of PTH in PCT has also been identified in isolated perfused segments of rabbit PCT (33). This highly region-
alized intrinsic response is at some variance with the
finding of a brisk adenyl cyclase response to PTH throughout PCT and to a lesser extent in pars recta (34). In
fact, PTH increases FEPi to above 1.0 in Pi-loaded rats,
in early PCT and to a lesser extent in late PCT and pars
recta (27). PTH-dependent cAMP formation throughout PCT,

and the in vivo PCT response to PTH in Pi handling, are thus concordant when intracellular Pi is probably elevated throughout PCT. The same microinjection studies (30) found DCT and distal segments of superficial nephrons insensitive to PTH, whereas mixed nephron studies (27) reveal PTH responsiveness in a segment of nephron beyond the DCT. This in vivo evidence for internephron heterogeneity in the distal nephron response to PTH is reconciled with the in vitro evidence that surface and deep DCT segments differ in their adenyl cyclase response to PTH (35).

Enhanced backflux of Pi (flux J_4) appears to accompany the PTH response, particularly in early PCT (27), but the mechanism of the effect in the different segments of the nephron is not known. In the context of transepithelial transport, PTH could act to modify either intracellular Pi activity; the permeability coefficient for backflux by cellular or paracellular paths, or the Km_{eff} of anion carrier in the membrane.

Calcium ion (Ca^{2+}) has a direct modifying effect on TRPi independent of its effect on PTH (36). TmPi in man is raised within minutes after raising serum calcium by intravenous infusion (Fig. 1); and Ca^{2+} abruptly decreases FE_{Pi} (which can exceed 1.0) in XLH, without change in ultrafilterability of Pi (37). These PTH-independent effects could again be related to changes in intracellular Pi activity, the permeability coefficient, or Km_{eff}; Ca^{2+} can indeed modify membrane permeability (38), perhaps by an effect on microtubule/microfilament assemblies.

If Pi is the major anion accompanying Ca^{2+} flux in renal epithelium, and if significant amounts of Pi are stored as a Ca-Pi complex in mitochondria, PTH might increase intracellular Pi activity transiently, and Ca^{2+} would have the opposite effect according to the Borle model (24,25). That is to say, effects on Pi activity influencing both the Michaelis and linear terms of equation 4 could be postulated. A test of the hypothesis awaits methods to locate and measure intracellular Pi activity; currently available membrane electrodes or electron probes do not have this capability.

The effect of ambient pH on TRPi must also be considered, particularly if PTH exerts a major effect on H^+ in responsive cells (39). Acid intraluminal pH (6.05-6.83) enhances, while alkaline intraluminal pH (7.50-7.80) retards unidirectional Pi absorption in PCT (40). Net efflux of Pi can occur in alkaline tubular fluid without

change in water reabsorption. The fast reabsorption of
Pi in early PCT might therefore be explained in part by
an important change during transit in the relative proportions of the anion species in the lumen, with the pH
change favoring the more permeable and smaller $H_2PO_4^-$.
PTH impairs Pi reabsorption when $H_2PO_4^-$ predominates, but
has little effect when HPO_4^{2-} is the major species (40).
Direct measurements with antimony electrodes reveal that
PTH causes alkalization of PCT fluid apparently by blocking H^+ secretion, an effect evident only when the tubular
lumen is acid. Accordingly, while PTH could enhance backflux (J_4) through an intracellular effect on Pi activity
in PCT, it can also reduce Pi influx (J_3) through its effect on the luminal anion species. The effects of PTH on
DCT handling of Pi in relation to pH are still unknown.

As if there was not sufficient ambiguity in the interpretation of PTH and Ca^{2+} effects on transepithelial
transport of Pi, there are other findings to compound the
problem. For example, phlorizin (1-3), diphosphonates
(12) and profound dietary depletion of Pi (41) all enhance
TRPi. It is difficult to anticipate how these findings
can be interpreted without considering the topology of
intracellular Pi and asymmetrical transport.

MUTATION AS A PROBE OF Pi TRANSPORT

The inborn errors of membrane transport are useful
probes of membrane and cellular transport mechanisms in
man (14,42). XLH and HBD are specific disorders of Pi
transport in which the transport of other solutes is
apparently unaffected. Therefore one anticipates that
single-gene products are affected in these two traits.
High FEPi in both must reflect a decrease of net inward
flux secondary to any of the aforementioned mechanisms.
It is unlikely that altered paracellular transport is an
important component in XLH or HBD. *Any mechanism account-
ing for impaired Pi transport in XLH and HBD must acco-
modate the hypophosphatemia.*

Specific Pi transport proteins have been identified
in genetic studies of bacterial plasma membranes (43,44).
An anion exchange system has also been identified by chemical methods in mammalian red cell membranes (16,17).
Monovalent anion exchange is more specific and many times
more rapid than divalent anion exchange in erythrocyte
membranes, and high activation energies ($\sim$30 kcal/mole)
characterize both. The erythrocyte anion exchange protein
is about 95,000 daltons. The reactive site is located on

a pronase-resistant portion of the protein (65,000 daltons), it possesses three positive charges and it is exposed at the external face of the plasma membrane. It has been suggested that the protein acts as a permeation channel through the lipid and that local conformational change permits anion exchange across the membrane. Studies of anion exchange have largely concerned Cl^- and SO_4^{2-}; less work has been done on the role of the protein in Pi transport and no studies of its presence in the various renal membranes have been published to our knowledge. We have studied Pi exchange in erythrocytes of XLH subjects and found no abnormality (21). This finding merely indicates either that the Pi carrier is not affected in XLH or that the Pi exchange mechanisms in kidney and erythrocyte are not identical, a situation for which there is adequate precedent with other substances (e.g. glucose) (14).

XLH and HBD are severe forms of hypophosphatemia. In affected XLH males, there is florid bone disease and dwarfing; oral Pi treatment stimulates linear growth and the rickets show considerable healing (43). The renal lesion (Fig. 1) is characterized by markedly decreased TRP_i in the absence of PTH excess; negative TRP_i values occur under Pi loading (37). HBD is characterized by an equivalent degree of hypophosphatemia but endogenous TRP_i is greater in HBD than in XLH ($75 \pm 7.3 \mu$moles/100 ml GF vs 31 ± 12.8 (mean, SD) in XLH at plasma [P], 0.6-1 mM; $p < 0.01$); however, TmPi is clearly reduced in HBD (Fig.1). Pi excretion is not stimulated by PTH in XLH males (37), whereas it is modestly but belatedly stimulated in HBD (unpub. obs.). Ca^{2+} infusion stimulates TRP_i in both conditions (Fig. 1 and ref. 37).

The bone disease which accompanies HBD is modest compared to XLH, and dwarfing is less, at the equivalent day-to-day plasma [P]. *Interpretation of this difference hinges on an explanation for the different FEPi and yet similar endogenous plasma [P] in the two diseases.* It is evident that other factors must contribute to regulation of plasma [P]. Total extracellular fluid [P] in the normal adult male is about 400 mg; the bone pool is about 1000 fold larger, while intracellular [P] in soft tissues is about 700 mg. These pools equilibrate with dietary Pi (diet intake - fecal loss = about 500 mg/day) and with urinary loss (about 500 mg per day). One must conclude that equilibration between dietary Pi (which is similar in XLH and HBD), bone [P] (which is apparently different in the two diseases), and blood [P] (which is the same), is different in XLH and HBD; the origins of these differences

are evidently reflected in kidney where the abnormal
mechanisms affecting TRPi are clearly different.

     A unique opportunity to identify the abnormal Pi flux
in XLH kidney may be available in an animal model. An
X-linked mutation (Hyp) causing hypophosphatemia and increased FEPi has been identified in the mouse (44). Hypophosphatemia appears soon after birth and before weaning
in affected males (Hyp/Y); rickets and dwarfing follow.
There is no evidence for hyperparathyroidism and the renal lesion is highly selective for Pi. Intracellular [P]
in kidney cortex is similar in Hyp/Y and normal +/Y litter
mates (46±1.0 ng/mg prot. and 46±1.1 ng/mg protein, mean
and SEM respectively). Since plasma [P] is low in Hyp/Y
(3.3±0.2 mg/dl vs 6.9±0.4 mg/dl in +/Y), renal [P] in
Hyp/Y is abnormally high relative to plasma. If intracellular Pi has access to backflux in Hyp/Y kidney, impairment of net TRP_i would result and under appropriate
conditions negative TRP_i might occur. The cause of high
intracellular [P] in Hyp/Y kidney has not yet been identified.

                          EPILOGUE

     Net reabsorption of Pi from filtrate involves trans-
epithelial transport against an electrochemical gradient
in the tubule, various segments of which play different
roles in this process; internephron heterogeneity also
exists. Although there is an apparent TmPi in the mammal,
the rate-limiting step is not known and indeed may vary
with tubular site and prevailing conditions. Net reabsorption requires only that Pi influx shall exceed backflux at the luminal pole of epithelium; how this asymmetry
of fluxes is maintained and modulated is still a subject
of speculation.

     It is clear that reabsorbed Pi must be removed from
the cytoplasmic pool at the luminal pole, by metabolism
or transport if a net flux is to be maintained. Even if
sequestration occurs, eventual net efflux at the basolateral membrane must occur to avoid an equilibrium with
the recipient compartment which would dissipate its effect.

     The mechanism of modulation of Pi reabsorption by
PTH, Ca^{2+}, Vitamin D or any other agents shown to affect
renal Pi handling, such as the conditions XLH and HBD, remains unclear. Their effect, both direct and secondary,
on intracellular pools, on metabolism, on the properties
both passive and specific of each set of membranes involved, and on other factors such as pH and activity of

other ions must all be rigorously studied before a reasonable hypothesis can be formulated. In other words, the study of Pi transport in health and disease is apparently just beginning.

ACKNOWLEDGEMENT

This work was supported by the Medical Research Councils of Canada and the UK.

REFERENCES

1. Knox, F.G., Schneider, E.G., Willis, L.R., Strandhoy, J.W. and Ott, C.E. Site and control of phosphate reabsorption by the kidney. Kidney Int. 3:347,1973.
2. Massry, S.G., Friedler, R.M. and Coburn, J.W. Excretion of phosphate and calcium. Physiology of their renal handling and relation to clinical medicine. Arch. Intern. Med. 131:828, 1973.
3. Goldberg, M., Agus, Z.S. and Goldfarb, S. Renal handling of phosphate, calcium and magnesium. In Brenner, B.M. and Rector, F.C. Jr., The Kidney, Vol. I, 344, W.B. Saunders, Phila. 1976.
4. Pitts, R.F. The excretion of urine in the dog. Am. J. Physiol. 106:1, 1933.
5. Pitts, R.F. and Alexander, R.S. The renal reabsorptive mechanism for inorganic phosphate in normal and acidotic dogs. Am. J. Physiol. 142:648, 1944.
6. Smith, H.W. The Kidney. Structure and function in health and disease. p. 113, Oxford Univ. Press, New York, 1958.
7. Bijvoet, O.L.M. Relation of plasma phosphate concentration to renal tubular reabsorption of phosphate. Clin. Sci. 37:23, 1969.
8. Bijvoet, O.L.M., Morgan, D.B. and Fourman, P. The assessment of phosphate reabsorption. Clin. Chim. Acta 26:15, 1969.
9. Stamp, T.C.B., Stacey, T.E. and Rose, G.A. Comparison of glomerular filtration rate measurements using inulin, ^{51}CrEDTA and a phosphate infusion technique. Clin. Chim. Acta 30:351, 1970.
10. Stamp, T.E.B. and Stacey, T.E. Evaluation of theoretical renal phosphorus threshold as an index of renal phosphorus handling. Clin. Sci. 39:505, 1970.
11. Walton, R.J. and Bijvoet, O.L.M. Nomogram for derivation of renal threshold phosphate concentration. Lancet 2:309, 1975.
12. Walton, R.J., Russell, R.G.G. and Smith, R.

Changes in the renal and extrarenal handling of phosphate induced by disodium editronate (EHDP) in man. Clin. Sci. and Molec. Med. 49:45, 1975.

13. Kinne, R.K.H. Polarity of the renal proximal tubular cell. Function and enzyme pattern of the isolated plasma membranes. Med. Clin. N. Am. 59:615, 1975.

14. Scriver, C.R., Chesney, R.W. and McInnes, R.R. Genetic aspects of renal tubular transport. Diversity and topology of carriers, Kidney Int. 9:149, 1976.

15. Diamond, J.M. Tight and leaky junctions of epithelia: A perspective on kisses in the dark. Fed. Proc. 33:2220, 1974.

16. Sachs, J.R., Knauf, P.A. and Dunham, P.B. Transport through red cell membranes. In Surgenor, D.M. The Red Blood Cell Vol. 2, p. 613, 2nd edit. Academic Press, New York, 1975.

17. Rothstein, A., Cabantchik, Z.I. and Knauf, P. Mechanism of anion transport in red blood cells and role of membrane proteins. Fed. Proc. 35:3, 1976.

18. Jacquez, J.A. One-way fluxes of α-aminoisobutyric acid in Ehrlich ascites tumor cells. Trans effects and effects of sodium and potassium. J.Gen. Physiol.65:57,1975

19. Lieb, W.R. and Stein, W.D. Implications of two different types of diffusion for biological membranes. Nature 234:220, 1971.

20. Deuticke, B. Anion permeability of the red blood cell. Naturwissenschaften 57:172, 1970.

21. Tenenhouse, H.S. and Scriver, C.R. Orthophosphate transport in the erythrocyte of normal subjects and of patients with X-linked hypophosphatemia. J. Clin. Invest. 55:644, 1975.

22. Viera, F.L. and Malnic, G. Hydrogen ion secretion by rat renal cortical tubules as studied by an antimony microelectrode. Am. J. Physiol. 214:710, 1968.

23. Strickler, J.C., Thompson, D.D., Klose, R.M. and Giebisch, G. Micropuncture study of inorganic phosphate excretion in the rat. J. Clin. Invest. 43:1596, 1964.

24. Borle, A.B. Calcium metabolism at the cellular level. Fed. Proc. 32:1944, 1973.

25. Borle, A.B. Calcium and phosphate metabolism. Ann. Rev. Physiol. 36:361, 1974.

26. Rose, B. and Loewenstein, W.R. Calcium ion distribution in cytoplasm visualized by Aequorin: Diffusion in cytosol restricted by energized sequestering. Science 190:1204, 1975.

27. Boudry, J.-F., Troehler, U., Touabi, M., Fleisch,H. and Bonjour, J.-F. Secretion of inorganic phosphate in the rat nephron. Clin. Sci. Mol. Med. 48:475, 1975.

28. Frick, A. Reabsorption of inorganic phosphate

in the rat kidney. I. Saturation of transport mechanism. II. Suppression of fractional phosphate reabsorption due to expansion of extracellular fluid volume. Pflügers Arch. 304:351, 1968.

29. Engle, J.E. and Steele, T.H. Renal phosphate reabsorption in the rat: effect of inhibitors. Kidney Int. 8:98, 1975.

30. Brunette, M.G., Taleb, L. and Carriere, S. Effect of parathyroid hormone on phosphate reabsorption along the nephron of the rat. Am.J. Physiol. 225:1076, 1973.

31. Murayama, Y., Morel, F. and LeGrimellac, C. Phosphate, calcium and magnesium transfers in proximal tubules and loops of Henle, as measured by single nephron microperfusion experiments in the rat. Pflügers Arch. 338:1, 1972

32. Amiel, C., Kuntziger, H.E. and Richet, G. Micropuncture study of handling of phosphate by proximal and distal nephron in normal and parathyroidectomized rat. Evidence for distal reabsorption. Pflügers Arch. 317:93, 1970.

33. Hamburger, R.J., Lawson, N.L. and Schwartz, J.H. Response to parathyroid hormone in defined segments of proximal tubule. Am. J. Physiol. 230:286, 1976.

34. Chabardès, D., Imbert, M. Clique, A., Montegut, M. and Morel, F. PTH sensitive adenyl cyclase activity in different segments of the rabbit nephron. Pflügers Arch. 354:229, 1975.

35. Morel, F., Chabardès, D., Imbert, M., Montegut, M. and Clique, A. Functional segmentation of the rabbit distal tubule by microdetermination of hormone-dependent adenylate cyclase activity. Kidney Int. 9:264, 1976.

36. Cuche, J.L., Ott, C.E., Marchand, G.R., Diaz-Buxo, J.A. and Knox, F.G. Intrarenal role of calcium in phosphate handling. Am. J. Physiol. 230:790, 1976.

37. Glorieux, F. and Scriver, C.R. X-linked hypophosphatemia: Loss of a PTH-sensitive component of phosphate transport. Science 175:997, 1972.

38. Baker, P.F. Transport and metabolism of calcium ions in nerve. Prog. In Biophys. and Mol. Biol. Butter, J.A.V. and Noble V. eds. 24:179, 1972.

39. Rasmussen, H. Ionic and hormonal control of calcium homeostasis. Am. J. Med. 50:567, 1972.

40. Bank, N., Aynedjian, H.S. and Weinstein, S.W. A microperfusion study of phosphate reabsorption by the rat proximal renal tubule. Effect of parathyroid hormone. J. Clin. Invest. 54:1040, 1974.

41. Steele, T.H. and DeLuca, H.F. Influence of dietary phosphorus on renal phosphate reabsorption in the parathyroidectomized rat. J. Clin. Invest. 57:867, 1976.

42. Scriver, C.R. and Hechtman, P. Human genetics of

membrane transport with emphasis on amino acids. Adv. in
Hum. Gen. 1:211, 1970.
   43. Glorieux, F.H., Scriver, C.R., Reade, T.M.,
Goldman, H. and Roseborough, A. Use of phosphate and
vitamin D to prevent dwarfism and rickets in X-linked
hypophosphatemia. New Eng. J. Med. 287:481, 1972.
   44. Eicher, E.M., Southard, J.L., Scriver, C.R. and
Glorieux, F.H. Hypophosphatemia: Mouse model for human
familial hypophosphatemic (vitamin D-resistant) rickets.
Proc. Nat. Acad. Sci. In press, 1976.

RENAL ADENYLATE CYCLASE, CALCITONIN RECEPTORS AND PHOSPHATE

EXCRETION IN RATS IMMUNIZED AGAINST TUBULAR BASEMENT MEMBRANES

N. LOREAU, J.P. COSYNS, C. LEPREUX, R. ARDAILLOU

I. N. S. E. R. M. 64, Tenon hospital

4, rue de la Chine, 75020 Paris, France

Specific receptors for calcitonin (CT) (1,2) and CT-sensitive adenylate cyclase (3,4) have been clearly demonstrated in cellular membranes purified from rat kidney cortex. We tried to obtain an experimental model in the rat devoid of CT receptors in order to correlate the absence of binding and adenylate cyclase stimulation in vitro with physiological disorders in vivo. This model was obtained after active immunization of Brown Norway rats with heterologous tubular basement membrane (TBM). The immunological and pathological study of this experimental nephritis has been already performed by Lehman, Wilson and Dixon (5).

Methods - Male Brown Norway rats were injected subcutaneously with bovine TBM mixed with complete Freund's adjuvant. Bordetella pertussis vaccine also was injected intradermly. Control rats only received Freund's adjuvant and B. pertussis vaccine. Seven control and seven immunized rats were sacrificed 9, 12, 21, 35 and 40 days after immunization and their kidneys removed. Presence of anti-TBM antibodies along TBM in the immunized rats was controlled using immunofluorescence techniques.

Tubular membranes were purified from the renal cortex according to Fitzpatrick et al. (6). Binding of ^{125}I salmon CT to these membranes was measured as previously described (2). Adenylate cyclase activity was assayed under basal conditions, in the presence of fluoride (10^{-2} M) and in the presence of salmon CT or 1-34 bovine PTH (10^{-6} M) as detailed in a previous study (4). Membranes from control rats were also incubated in the presence of IgG obtained from the serum of either immunized or control rabbits. Plasma of immunized rabbits contained a high titer of anti-TBM antibodies.

Blood and urine samples were collected just before sacrifice
of the rat and fractional clearance of phosphate calculated from
creatinine and phosphorus determinations.

Results – Interstitial nephritis developed in immunized rats
and direct immunofluorescence of kidneys revealed linear deposits
of IgG along TBM of renal tubules. Binding of ^{125}I CT to the
membranes purified from immunized rats was markedly decreased.
In time-course studies the level of the plateau was less than
15 % of that observed with the membranes from control rats.
Number of sites and apparent dissociation constant (K_D) were
calculated from the Scatchard's transformation of the data obtained in binding experiments at equilibrium. The number of sites
was approximately 50 % less and the K_D value four times greater
with the preparation from immunized rats. Degradation of ^{125}I CT
was similar in both preparations. Adenylate cyclase activity under
basal conditions was not significantly different whereas stimulation in the presence of CT or of PTH was completely abolished
in the experimental group. Some degree of stimulation by fluoride
persisted, but much lower than in the control group. The same
results concerning CT binding and adenylate cyclase activity were
observed within each group whatever the date of sacrifice of the
rats.

^{125}I CT binding also was clearly decreased when control
membranes were preincubated with anti-TBM IgG. At equilibrium,
binding was approximately 30 % less. In the same conditions, there
was no change in basal adenylate cyclase activity but a marked
decrease in CT-or PTH-sensitive activity.

All immunized rats had elevated plasma creatinine concentration (11.6 ±0.98 mg/l) compared to controls (5.66 ± 0.16 mg/l).
The fractional excretion of phosphate was much higher in immunized (27.2 ± 4.5 %) than in control (6.0 ± 1.0 %) rats. There was
no difference within each group whatever the date of sacrifice.

Discussion – The decrease in CT receptors and the suppression
of CT and PTH stimulation of adenylate cyclase activity is likely
to be due both to the presence itself of anti-TBM antibodies along
TBM and to the interstitial nephritis secondary to the deposition
of these antibodies. The binding of ^{125}I CT to control membranes
was smaller following incubation with anti-TBM IgG ; however, the
decrease in binding was less than that observed using membranes
from immunized rats.

Immunized rats developed an interstitial nephritis with
moderate renal failure. Increase in the fractional excretion of
phosphate was observed although there was no stimulation of renal
adenylate cyclase by PTH or CT. Thus, in this particular model of
renal failure, phosphorus excretion can increase independently of
any effect of these hormones on the adenylate cyclase system.

REFERENCES

1. Marx, S.J., Woodard, C.J., Aurbach, G.D., Glossmann, H., and
    Keutmann, H.T. Renal receptors for calcitonin: binding and
    degradation of hormone. J. Biol. Chem. 248:4797, 1973.

2. Sraer, J., Ardaillou, R. Renal receptors of salmon calcitonin.
    In Endocrinology 1973, Proc. Int. Symp. 4th, p. 170, Heinemann
    Medical Books, London, 1974.

3. Marx, S.J., Woodard, C.J., Aurbach, G.D. Calcitonin receptors
    of kidney and bone. Science 178:199, 1972.

4. Loreau, N., Lepreux, C., Ardaillou, R. Calcitonin-sensitive
    adenylate cyclase in rat tubular membranes. Biochem. J. 150:
    305, 1975.

5. Lehman, D.J., Wilson, C.B., Dixon, F.J. Interstitial nephritis
    in rats immunized with heterologous tubular basement membrane.
    Kidney Int. 5:187, 1974.

6. Fitzpatrick, D.F., Davenport, G.R., Forte, L., Landon, E.J.,
    Characterization of plasma membrane protein in mammalian
    kidney. J. Biol. Chem. 241:3561, 1969.

RENAL TUBULAR HANDLING OF 3',5'- cAMP IN NORMAL AND PARATHYROIDEC-
TOMIZED RATS

H. KUNTZIGER, H.L. CAILLA, C. AMIEL, AND M.A. DELAAGE

INSERM U.64, HOPITAL TENON, PARIS, and CBBM, CNRS,

MARSEILLE, FRANCE

Urinary excretion exceeding filtered load indicates net tubular addition of 3',5'- cAMP in normal mammals. Tubular addition of
the nucleotide depends on parathyroid hormone. This study investigated :
1. the nephron segment where 3',5'- cAMP addition occurs,
2. a possible reabsorptive transport participating in net overall
renal handling,
3. the localization of the altered tubular transport induced by
parathyroidectomy (PTX).

Normal animals (NRL) were compared to acute (APTX) and to
chronic (CPTX) PTX. 17 nephrons were micropunctured in NRL and
APTX, 16 in CPTX. For each nephron, fluid from both its early
distal and its late proximal tubular segments was collected.
Plasma, urine and tubular fluid (^{3}H) Inuline and ^{32}P radiophosphate were measured as described (1). Endogenous 3',5'- cAMP was
measured in these fluids by radio-immunoassay (2).

Results are summarized in Table 1. Urinary fractional excretion of 3',5'- cAMP was higher in NRL than in APTX ($p < 0.01$) and
in CPTX ($p < 0.05$). In NRL, net addition of 3',5'- cAMP, of the
same magnitude as filtered load, occured in the proximal tubule.
In APTX, proximal addition was decreased ($p < 0.05$). In CPTX,
addition was also decreased but less than in APTX and not significantly different from NRL.

Filtered 3',5'- cAMP delivered to early distal tubule was
higher in NRL than in APTX ($p < 0.02$) and in CPTX ($p < 0.01$). The increased difference, between NRL and PTX, in 3',5'-cAMP delivery to
early distal, as compared to late proximal tubule, might be explained by an increased loop reabsorption of the nucleotide in PTX.

75

Table 1. FRACTION OF FILTERED 3',5'- cAMP DELIVERED, X 100
        (N = 5 in each group, mean $\pm$ SEM)

	END PROXIMAL TUBULE	EARLY DISTAL TUBULE	LEFT KIDNEY URINE
NRL	197.7 $\pm$ 18.0	186.1 $\pm$ 15.0	178.2 $\pm$ 20.3
APTX	125.0 $\pm$ 25.0	108.4 $\pm$ 19.1	96.4 $\pm$ 7.6
CPTX	148.0 $\pm$ 19.3	119.6 $\pm$ 13.5	108.8 $\pm$ 16.0

It is concluded that the proximal tubular, parathyroid hormone dependent, net addition of 3',5'- cAMP is responsible for its urinary excretion exceeding filtered load. Net reabsorption might occur in the loop and might be enhanced in PTX.

References

1. Amiel, C., Kuntziger, H., and Richet, G. : Micropuncture study handling of phosphate by proximal and distal nephron in normal and parathyroidectomized rat. Evidence for distal reabsorption. Pflügers Arch. 317 : 93, 1970.

2. Cailla, H.L., Racine-Weisbuch, M.S., and Delaage, M.A. : Adenosine 3',5'- cyclic monophosphate assay at 10^{-15} Mole level. Anal. Biochem. 56 : 394, 1973.

EFFECTS OF GLUCOSE ON INTESTINAL AND RENAL HANDLING OF CALCIUM

L.MONNIER, C. SANY, H. COLLET, J. MIROUZE

Department of Endocrinology and Metabolism

St-Eloi Hospital.34059-MONTPELLIER Cedex (F)

For a number of years , it has been demonstrated that some sugars increase the calcium absorption by intestinal segments isolated from different species of animals (I,2). In order to evaluate the mechanism of these phenomena, we studied the intestinal absorptive and renal tubular reabsorptive capacities for calcium when a large amount of glucose is transported from the luminal to the serosal pole of these 2 epithelia . High glucose flow across intestinal and renal tubular cells were obtained by giving an oral glucose load to patients with an overt diabetes mellitus.

MATERIALS AND METHODS

Ten male diabetic patients treated with insulin (9 cases) or oral antidiabetic agents (I case) received a diet providing 800 mg of calcium and 2000 calories per day. All patients were hospitalized during 2 periods of IO days separated by a 4-month-interval. During each period the intestinal absorption rate of radiocalcium (IACa) and the urinary excretion rate of calcium(UVCa) wererespectively determined on days 4 and 7. During the first period IACa was measured at 8a.m after an overnight fast and UVCa was obtained by urine collection from 8 a.m to II a.m after a breakfast providing 280 mg of calcium . The procedure was similar during the second period except that each subject received at 8 a.m on days 4 and 7 an oral glucose tolerance test(OGTT

with 40 gm of glucose/m2 of body surface. The glucose
was diluted with tridistilled water in order to obtain
a I5 gm per cent solution. During each period, all patients had a satisfactory 24-hour control.
The intestinal absorption rate of radiocalcium was determined by using a double radiotracer technique (3,4)
At 8 a.m after an overnight fast, 5 μCi of ^{45}Ca Cl$_2$
(Saclay France)were injected intravenously as a single
bolus through an indwelling catheter. Simultaneously,
each subject received orally 20 μCi of ^{47}Ca Cl$_2$ (Amersham,UK) with I5 mg of non radioactive calcium as calcium chloride diluted in 200 ml of tridistilled water.
Blood samples were withdrawn I5,30,60,90,I20,I50,I80
and 480 minutes after the two radiotracers had been given to the patients. Known aliquots of administered
radioactivities were respectively diluted to 200 and
50 ml for oral and I.V. doses. Serum and diluted oral
doses were assayed for ^{47}Ca radioactivity from 5 ml
samples counted in a Packard γ ray spectrometer. After
8 weeks of storage to allow for ^{47}Ca decay , 2 ml of
serum and of diluted ^{45}Ca doses were mixed to I5 ml of
Instagel(Packard) and were counted in a liquid scintil-
lation spectrometer (SL 30 Intertechnique). The oral
and intravenous radiotracer concentrations were expressed as a percentage of the total dose per litre of
plasma (%TD/l). The values were plotted vs. time on a
semilogarithmic paper. The pattern of transfer of oral
calcium from gut lumen to plasma i.e. the transit time
curve of radiocalcium was calculated from the time courses of oral and intravenous plasma activities, by
using a mathematical procedure of inverse convolution.
This calculation consisted in a numerical sequence ap-
proximation on I5 minute -intervals and was obtained
with the aid of a PPD8E computer. The transit time values were expressed as a percentage of oral dose absorbed per minute(%TD/min.)
Four parameters were obtained from transit time curves:
(a) the total fractional absorption rate(TFACa) expressed as percentage of total oral dose (%TD) and calculated from the area under the transit time curve,(b) the
maximal absorption rate (%TD/min) (c) the time of maximal absorption (min),(d) the mean transit time across the
intestinal barrier (min). Furthermore, the time course of
the cumulative fractional absorption rate (%TD) was
obtained from the calculation at different times of the
area under the transit time curve.
The urinary excretion rate of calcium (UVCa) was measured
over a 3 hour period of time. After the bladder had
been emptied at 8 a.m. the urine was collected until
11 a.m. The complexometric procedure was used for

determination of calcium concentration in urine. The results were corrected by the glomerular filtration rate (GFR) determined by using a constant infusion technique of Iothalamate ^{125}I (5).

RESULTS

Values of intestinal calcium absorption were compared in diabetic patients and in 9 control subjects. Results are shown on table I. After an OGTT we observed a significant increase in TFA Ca from 68 % TD ± 4.8 to 82.4 ± 4.I (P < 0.05) and in mean transit time from 60.I min ± I3.3 to III.4 ± I5.5 (P < 0.05).No difference was found between TFACa in control subjects and in diabetics without an OGTT.

Table I:Values of the parameters of the intestinal calcium absorption. All results are given as mean±SEM

	Control subjects n=9	Diabetics without OGTT n=IO	Diabetics with OGTT n=IO
TFACa (% TD)	63.4±2.9	68.0±4.8	82.4±4.I
		← P < 0.05 →	
Maximal absorption rate (%TD/min)	I.08±0.I5	I.I9±0.20	0.87±0.I5
Time of maximal absorption (min)	3I.4±7.9	40.7±I2.2	44.2±9.0
Mean transit time (min)	48.2±7.5	60.I±I3.3	III.4±I5.5
		← P < 0.05 →	

The time courses of cumulative absorption rates showed that a significant increase in intestinal calcium absorption was only observed after the 3rd hour (fig.Ia). Furthermore during the first 30 minutes, the transit time curves of radiocalcium across the intestinal wall were quite identical with or without OGTT. The maximal absorption was reached at 30 minutes and was not significantly different whether an OGTT was given or not. After the maximum had been obtained, values of absorp tion rates per minute were significantly higher with an OGTT (fig.Ib). In 8 patients with normal kidney func-

L. MONNIER ET AL.

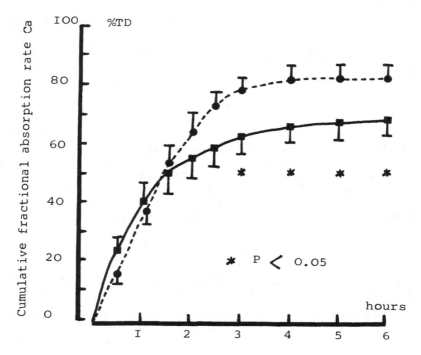

Fig. Ia: Time courses of cumulative fractional absorption rate of radiocalcium in IO diabetic patients
without OGTT (—■—) and with an OGTT (-●-)

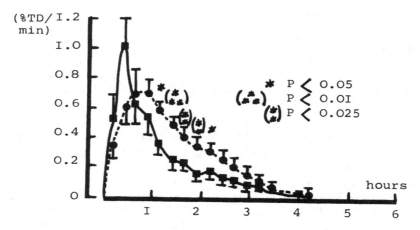

Fig. Ib: Transit time curves of radiocalcium
in IO diabetic patients without (-■-)
                                  with   (-●-) OGTT

tions, the urinary excretion rates of calcium expressed
as the UVCa/GFR ratio dropped significantly from
I.70 µg/ml± 0.23 to I.30 ± 0.I9 after an OGTT (P $<$ 0.05).
Furthermore, for these latter patients, an inverse corre
lation was found between the changes in TFACa and in the
UVCa/GFR ratio : r= 0.82, P $<$ 0.0I (fig 2).

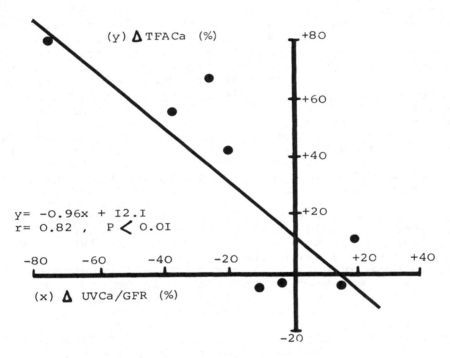

fig.2: Relationship between changes in TFACa (y) and
       in UVCa/GFR ratio (x) in 8 diabetic patients
       with normal kidney functions.

DISCUSSION.

According to these results, it can be concluded that
glucose transport from the luminal to the serosal pole
of the intestinal and renal tubular cells produces an
increase in the absorptive capacities for calcium. Moreover, the inverse relationship found between changes
in TFACa and in UVCa/GFR seems to indicate that the behavior of intestinal and tubular cells is similar for
calcium transfer when a high glucose concentration is
obtained at the luminal pole. These observations are
in agreement with the fact that similarities exist in

transport of sugars across intestinal and tubular epi-
thelia(6,7). On the other hand, increased uptake of calcium under the influence of glucose is not limited to
intestinal and tubular cells since this phenomenon has
been previously demonstrated in vitro for B-cells of
Langerhans islets (8).
An important question concerns the site of the increased transport of calcium under the influence of a high
glucose flow. If one consider the transport of sugars,
it has been previously demonstrated that some carbohydra
tes such as glucose are actively transported by a Na+
dependent carrier, located in the brush border of the
cell membrane (9,IO). On the contrary, it is well known
that the transport of some other sugars such as fructose
depends on a passive diffusion. Despite these differences
some authors have observed that both groups of sugars increase the intestinal absorption rate of calcium (II).
Furthermore, in our study, we did not find any significant difference in the intestinal transport of calcium
during the earliest period of absorption i.e. during
the cell membrane transport. For all these reasons, it
seems likely that sugars have no action on calcium
transfer across the brush border. Thus we suggest that
glucose increases the transfer of calcium through the
cell cytoplasm. This would be an explanation for the
significant difference observed during the latest period
of absorption i.e after the Ist hour.
Although some authors (I2) have previously assumed the
existence of a common carrier for calcium and glucose
in the intestinal cells, there is no evidence for this
hypothesis. It seems more probable that calcium is required for enzymatic reactions induced by presence of
glucose in the cytoplasm of intestinal and renal tubular
cells. This hypothesis is apparently supported by the
fact that in vitro experiments have demonstrated the
critical role of Ca^{2+} in the maintenance of cellular
function, e.g. insulin secretion for B cells in Langerhans islets (8).
The results concerning the effects of glucose on the u-
rinary excretion of calcium in diabetic patients are in
apparent disagreement with those found by Lennon et al.
in control subjects (I3). These authors reported that
ingestion of glucose produces an increase in urinary ex
cretion of calcium. These findings were related to an
elevation of organic acids in urine. The disagreement
with our results might be due to differences between
experimental procedures i.e between glucose concentrations reached in the lumen of renal tubules. In diabetic patients the amount of glucose delivered to tubular
cells is largely higher than in normal subjects. Thus,

in diabetics, it is suggested that the lowering effect of organic acids on the renal tubular reabsorptive capacity for calcium is negligible compared to the large enchancement of calcium reabsorption produced by the high glucose flow.

REFERENCES.

I-FOURNIER P., DUPUIS Y., DIGAUD A., FOURNIER A.: Contribution à l'étude du mode d'action des oses sur l'absorption et la rétention du calcium. C.R.Acad.Sci. Paris, 275: 85,1973.

2- FOURNIER P., DIGAUD A., DUPUIS Y., FOURNIER A. : Relations entre la présence de pentoses endogènes dans l'intestin et l'effet des glucides sur l'absorption du calcium. C.R. Acad. Sci. Paris, 276: I58I, 1973.

3- BIRGE S.G., PECK W.A., BERMAN M., WHEDON G.D.: Study of calcium absorption in man: A kinetic analysis and physiological model. J. Clin. Invest. 48: I705, I969.

4- MIROUZE J., MONNIER L.: Etude critique des techniques d'absorption du radiocalcium J. Urol. Nephrol. 8I: 92I, I975.

5-MIROUZE J., MONNIER L., OLIVIER C.: Study of renal functions by repeated constant infusion of radiotracers before and after initiation of therapy in hypertension or in diabetes mellitus. Pathol. Biol. 23: 599, I975.

6-ULLRICH K.J.: Renal tubular mechanisms of organic solute transport. Kidney Int. 9: I34, I976.

7- CRANE R.K.: Hypothesis for mechanism of intestinal active transport of sugars . Fed. Proc. 2I: 89I, I962.

8-MALAISSE W.J., DEVIS G., HERCHUELZ A., SENER A., SOMERS G.: Calcium antagonists and islet function.Diabète et Metabolisme 2: I, 1976.

9- BARNETT J.G., RALPH A., MUNDAY K.A:Structural requirements for active intestinal transport. Biochem. J. II8 : 843, I970.

IO- NEADE R.J., WISEMAN G.:Active transport of L glucose by isolated small intestine of the dietary restricted rat. J. Physiol. I98: 60I, 1968.

II- FOURNIER P., DUPUIS Y., FONTAINE N., SEVETTE A.M.:
Specificité moléculaire et activités des glucides sur
l'absorption du calcium. J. Physiol. 66:473, 1973.

I2-FOURNIER P., DUPUIS Y., FOURNIER A.: Relations entre
l'activité de divers glucides sur les échanges calci-
ques et leur aptitude à former des complexes. C.R.Acad.
Sci. Paris, 275 : I79I, 1972.

I3- LENNON E.J., PIERING W.F.: A comparison of the effects of glucose ingestion and NH4 Cl acidosis on urinary calcium and magnesium excretion in man. J. Clin.
Invest. 49 : I458, I970.

RENAL ACTIONS OF 25-HYDROXYVITAMIN D$_3$

R.A. Peraino, E. Ghaffary, D. Rouse, W.N. Suki

Baylor College of Medicine

Texas Medical Center, Houston, Texas

The kidney is uniquely involved in the maintenance of body calcium, magnesium, phosphorus, and acid-base balance, both as an endocrine secretory and a target organ. In this light, the kidney reabsorbs calcium and phosphorus more avidly under the stimulus of 25-hydroxycholecalciferol (1-4) while it effects conversion of this compound to the metabolite 1,25-dihydroxycholecalciferol, which is more active on gut (5,6). Controversy exists, however, as to the necessity for parathyroid hormone (PTH) to facilitate the renal actions of 25-hydroxycholecalciferol (1-4,7,8). The present studies were undertaken therefore to examine the affect of 25-hydroxycholecalciferol, henceforth referred to as 25-HCC, on the renal handling of calcium, magnesium and phosphate in the intact and acutely thyroparathyroidectomized dog. Since the absorption of phosphate in the latter preparation is virtually complete, bicarbonate infusion was used to increase its excretion.

METHODS

Mongrel dogs of either sex, maintained on a regular diet containing adequate amounts of calcium, phosphorus, and vitamins, were prepared as shown in Figure 1. Following induction of pentothal anesthesia and institution of tracheal respiration, both femoral arteries and veins were cannulated through groin incisions for infusion, blood sampling, and to monitor arterial pressure. Both ureters were cannulated through suprapubic incision and the left renal vein cannulated through a flank incision for determination of renal blood flow with the Wolf formula using inulin as the marker. Seventeen animals were acutely thyroparathyroid-ectomized on the morning of the study, by methods previously

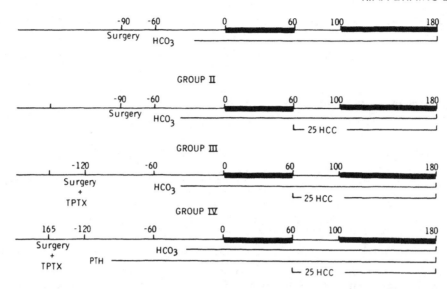

Figure 1

described (9), allowing at least two hours for the decline of
circulating levels of endogenous parathyroid hormone. All animals
then received an intravenous infusion of inulin for determination
of glomerular filtration rate, and of 0.7M sodium bicarbonate at a
rate sufficient to stabilize the plasma bicarbonate concentration
above 30 mM/L. Four groups were studied:

GROUP I. Four intact dogs were bicarbonate loaded as above,
and urine samples of 20 minutes duration each with mid-period blood
specimens were collected for 180 minutes.

GROUP II. Eight intact dogs were prepared as above.
Following stabilization of the plasma bicarbonate concentration,
4 control urine collections of 10-15 minutes duration each, with
mid-period blood samples, were obtained. 25-HCC, dissolved in
propylene glycol was then infused intravenously at 60 units/hr
and a further six collections of 20 minutes duration each
obtained.

GROUP III. Eight acutely thyroparathyroidectomized (TPTX)
dogs were studied as in Group II.

GROUP IV. Nine acute TPTX dogs were given an IV infusion of
purified PTH, 0.1 U/Kg load and 0.1 U/Kg/hr, for 2 hours prior to
control collections; 25-HCC was then superimposed upon the steady
state infusion of PTH. Otherwise the protocol was as stated for
Group II. Analysis of data by paired-t test compared the last
four periods (final 80 minutes), with the four control periods for
each group.

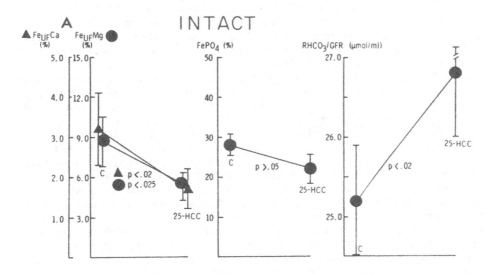

Figure 2A

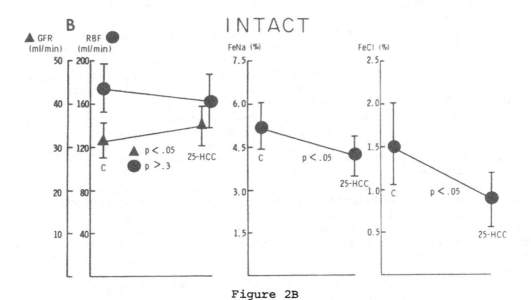

Figure 2B

RESULTS

GROUP I. Bicarbonate infusion to maintain a constant plasma bicarbonate concentration in intact dogs for a duration similar to the other three study groups, except for increasing fractional phosphate excretion slightly but significantly from 30.3% to 36.6%, (p>.05), exerted no remarkable effects on the renal handling of calcium or magnesium, or on GFR.

GROUP II. The effects of 25-HCC in the intact dogs are shown in Figure 2, A and B. Glomerular filtration rate rose slightly, but significantly, from 31.4 to 34.9 ml/min, (p<.05), while renal blood flow declined insignificantly from 175 to 163 ml/min (p>.3). Filtration fraction rose significantly from 0.31 to 0.36 (p<.05). The fractional excretions of sodium and chloride fell significantly from 5.2 to 4.2% (p<.05) and from 1.5 to 0.9% (p<.05), respectively. The fractional excretion of ultrafilterable calcium declined significantly from 3.2 to 1.7% (p<.02) and of ultrafilterable magnesium from 8.7 to 5.3% (p<.025). The excretion of phosphorus, however, fell insignificantly from 28.1% of the filtered load to 22.1% (p>..05), while bicarbonate absorption increased significantly from 25.2 to 26.8 micromoles/ml GFR (p<.02). Plasma phosphorus, ultrafilterable calcium and magnesium, and bicarbonate did not change following the administration of 25-HCC.

GROUP III. Figure 3, A and B, illustrates the effect of 25-HCC in the TPTX dogs. Glomerular filtration rate rose insignificantly from 32.9 to 35.5 ml/min (p>.05). Renal blood flow also declined insignificantly from 143 to 118 ml/min, (p>.1), while filtration fraction again rose significantly from 0.36 to 0.43 during 25-HCC infusion (p<.05). The fractional excretion of sodium and of chloride fell significantly during 25-HCC infusion from 5.7 to 4.8% (p<.05), and from 1.8 to 0.9% (p<.005), respectively. Ultrafilterable calcium excretion decreased from 3.7 to 2.3% of the filtered load (p<.005), and magnesium fell from 12.9 to 8.8% of the filtered load (p<.001), both significant decrements. The fractional excretion of phosphorus also declined from 11.4 to 10.4% during the infusion of 25-HCC, but this was not a significant change (p>.05). Unlike Group II, bicarbonate reabsorption was unchanged after 25-HCC. Plasma ultrafilterable calcium concentration fell significantly during the infusion of 25-HCC from 5.7 to 5.2 mg/deciliter, but the filtered load of ultrafilterable calcium was unchanged at 1.8 mg/min. Plasma phosphorus and ultrafilterable magnesium concentrations were unchanged, while plasma bicarbonate concentration fell slightly, but significantly, from 33.6 to 32.7 mM/L after 25-HCC (p<.025).

GROUP IV. The results of the administration of 25-HCC to bicarbonate-infused acute TPTX dogs receiving an infusion of PTH is illustrated in Figure 4, A and B. Glomerular filtration rate rose significantly from 29.0 to 32.9 ml/min (p<.01), while renal

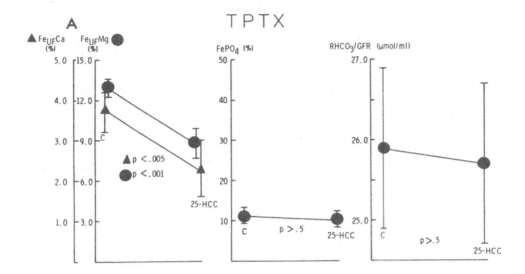

Figure 3A

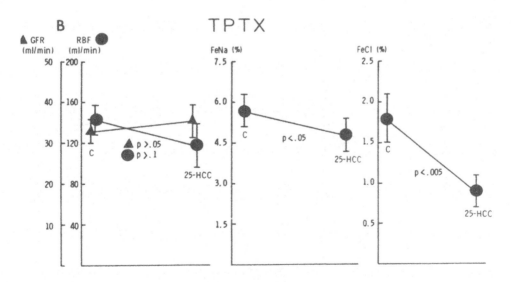

Figure 3B

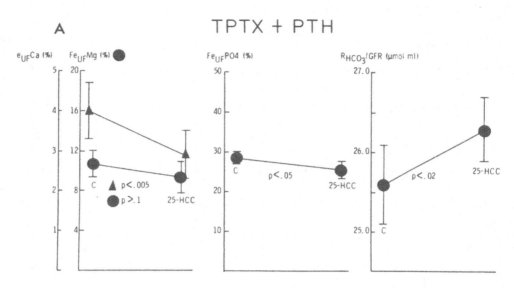

Figure 4A

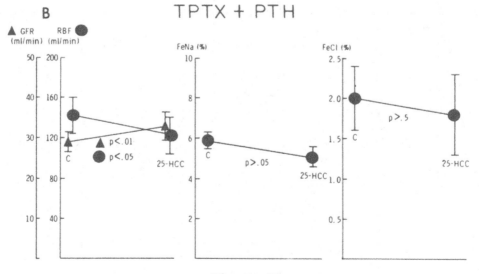

Figure 4B

blood flow fell from 142 to 123 ml/min (p<.05), and filtration fraction increased from 0.31 to 0.40 (p<.005). The fractional excretions of sodium and chloride declined from 5.9 to 5.1% and from 2.0 to 1.8%, respectively, but the decrements were not significant (p>.05 and p>.5, respectively). Fractional ultrafilterable calcium excretion fell from 4.0 to 2.9% (p<.005), and ultrafilterable magnesium excretion declined in 8 of 9 studies from 10.7% of the filtered load to 9.4% (p>.1). Fractional ultrafilterable phosphate excretion in contrast to Groups II and III, fell significantly from 28.6 to 25.6% (p<.05). Like Group II, bicarbonate absorption also increased significantly from 25.6 to 26.3 µmol/ml GFR (p<.02). Plasma ultrafilterable calcium concentration decreased significantly during 25-HCC infusion from 5.2 to 4.8 mg/100 ml (p<.01), but the filtered load of ultrafilterable calcium did not fall (1.49 vs 1.57 mg/100 ml). Plasma bicarbonate and ultrafilterable magnesium and phosphate concentrations were unchanged.

DISCUSSION

The results of the present studies clearly demonstrate that 25-hydroxycholecalciferol augments the renal reabsorption of calcium, in agreement with other investigators (1,3). This effect appears to be independent of the level of circulating parathyroid hormone since it is exerted both in intact alkalotic dogs presumed to have elevated levels of the hormone and in TPTX dogs which should have only low levels. Although plasma ultrafilterable calcium concentration fell during the infusion of 25-HCC in Groups II and IV, this does not account for the enhanced reabsorption because the filtered load of ultrafilterable calcium remained unchanged.

In addition to enhancing calcium absorption, 25-HCC also increased the absorption of magnesium in 24 of 25 studies, a heretofore unreported action of this metabolite of vitamin D.

At the dosage used in our studies, 25-HCC failed to augment the renal reabsorption of phosphate in either the intact or acute TPTX dog, in disagreement with other investigators (2,3). Because circulating levels of endogenous PTH are elevated in alkalotic intact animals (10), and high levels of PTH antagonize the action of 25-HCC (1,8), we studied the effect of 25-HCC in alkalotic acute TPTX dogs receiving a low-dose infusion of PTH (Group IV). In these experiments, 25-HCC enhanced the absorption of phosphate. Thus PTH is required to demonstrate the effect of 25-HCC on renal phosphate handling, suggesting opposing actions of the hormone and vitamin D metabolite.

    In our study, the renal absorption of bicarbonate was enhanced
by 25-hydroxycholecalciferol in the intact and acute TPTX dogs
receiving PTH, but not in acute TPTX animals alone. Thus it
appears that 25-HCC most likely antagonizes the effect of parathyroid hormone to depress renal reabsorption of bicarbonate. This
may be accomplished either by inhibiting PTH secretion, or by
antagonizing its action via inhibition of adenylate cyclase
activation, or by inhibition of the effect of cyclic AMP on the
renal tubule. Our observation that 25-HCC enhanced bicarbonate
absorption in TPTX dogs receiving exogenous PTH argues against the
first possibility but does not allow clear resolution of the latter
two alternatives.

    Finally, 25-HCC induced similar hemodynamic changes in all
groups studied: a rise in GFR, fall in renal blood flow, and
consequently a significant increase of filtration fraction. Since
hemodynamic changes of this kind are known to enhance sodium
absorption, such could be the case with respect to calcium,
magnesium, phosphate and bicarbonate.

REFERENCES

1. Puschett, J.B., Moranz, J., and Kurnick, W.S.: Evidence for a
    direct action of cholecalciferol and 25-hydroxycholecalciferol
    on the renal transport of phosphate, sodium and calcium.
    J. Clin. Invest. 51:373-385, 1972.

2. Popovtzer, M.M., Robinette, J.B., DeLuca, H.F., and Holick, M.
    F.: The acute effect of 25-hydroxycholecalciferol on renal
    handling of phosphorus. Evidence for a parathyroid hormone
    dependent mechanism. J. Clin. Invest. 53:913-921, 1974.

3. Sutton, R.A.L., Wong, N.L.M., and Dirks, J.H.: 25 hydroxy
    vitamin D₃ {25(OH)D₃}: Enhancement of distal tubular calcium
    reabsorption in the dog. Am. Soc. Neph., 1975, p. 8.

4. Costanzo, L.S., Sheehe, P.R., and Weiner, I.M.: Renal actions
    of vitamin D in D-deficient rats. Am. J. Physiol. 226:1490-
    1495, 1974.

5. Fraser, D.R., and Kodicek, E.: Unique biosynthesis by kidney
    of a biologically active vitamin D metabolite. Nature (London)
    228:764-766, 1970.

6. Holick, M.F., Schnoes, H.K., DeLuca, H.F., Suda, T., and
    Cousins, R.J.: Isolation and identification of 1,25-dihy-
    droxycholecalciferol. A metabolite of vitamin D active in
    intestine. Biochem. 10(14):2799-2804, 1971.

7. Puschett, J.B., Beck, W.S., Jr., Jelonek, A., Fernandez, P.:
    Study of the renal tubular interactions of thyrocalcitonin,
    cyclic adenosine 3', 5'-monophosphate, 25-hydroxycholecal-
    ciferol, and calcium ion. J. Clin. Invest. 53:756-767, 1974.

8. Puschett, J.B., Beck, W.S., Jelonek, A.: Parathyroid hormone
    and 25 hydroxy vitamin D₃: Synergistic and antagonistic
    effects on renal phosphate transport. Science 190:473-475,
    1975.

9. Suki, W.N., Martinez-Maldonado, M., Rouse, D., et al: Effect
    of expansion of extracellular fluid volume on renal phosphate
    handling. J. Clin. Invest. 48:1888-1894, 1969.

10. Mercado, A., Slatopolsky, E., and Klahr, S.: On the mechanism
    responsible for the phosphaturia of bicarbonate administration.
    J. Clin. Invest. 56(6)1386-1395, 1975.

HYPERCALCIURIA AFTER DIPHENYLHYDANTOIN

A Study of Calcium Metabolism in Rats

A. Heidland, F. Viebke, E. Heidbreder

Nephrolog. Abteilung der Medizin. Univ.-Klinik

Josef-Schneider-Str. 2, Wurzburg, Germany

Like phenobarbital (1), hydantoin causes a disturbance of calcium metabolism (2,3). Diphenylhydantoin inhibits calcium transport in the rat intestine in vitro without affecting calcium binding protein activity (4).

Hormonal factors, especially vitamin D metabolites, may play an important role as mediator of these metabolic changes caused by hydantoin. The pathogenetic mechanism, however, is not fully understood as yet. The aim of this study was to investigate the renal effects of diphenylhydantoin under balance study conditions. In addition, the effect of diphenylhydantoin on bone collagen metabolism was investigated by measuring urinary hydroxyproline excretion.

Materials and Methods

Male Wistar rats (WU strain, Fa. Ivanovas, Kissleg, W. Germany) weighing 190-210 g at the beginning of the experiment, were placed into metabolic cages (Acme Metal Products, Cincinnati, Ohio). Balance studies were performed under conditions of constant temperature (24±1 C) and humidity (60±3%) in a room which was lighted from 8 a.m. to 9 p.m.

The rats were maintained on a specific feeding schedule. The animals received half of their daily portion of synthetic diet at 9:30 a.m. and the other half at 9:30 p.m. This synthetic diet, as described by Hartroft and Eisenstein (5), and modified by Mohring and Mohring (6), was prepared as a paste by mixing two parts of a powder with one part of demineralized water (w/w). The rats had been trained to consume the bulk of diet within 2.5 hr by withdrawal of the food cups after this time. Thereafter, the food cups were dried, weighed, and the amount of diet consumed by each rat was calculated. After one week of adaptation to metabolic cages and

feeding schedule, the rats were adjusted to the 24-hr balance
program for 21 days. Initially after four days (adaptive phase),
and later one, after 21 days (balance phase) blood was taken from
each animal for the measurement of serum calcium, magnesium, phosphate, sodium, potassium, urea-N and alkaline phosphatase. In the
balance phase, 8 rats were offered 25 mg Diphenylhydantoin-Na
(Epanutin, Parke Davis & Co) per kg daily. Eight animals served as
controls. The collected 24-hr urine and faeces were diluted to a
definite volume, and sodium and potassium concentrations of each
sample were determined with a flame photometer (Eppendorf); calcium
and magnesium were determined by atomic absorption spectrophotometry (Beckman), inorganic phosphate with a commercial method
(Merck, Darmstadt, Fiske and Subbarow, (7), total hydroxyproline
in urine with the method of Firschein and Shill (8).

Balance data were calculated for 24-hr periods. The daily
intake of electrolytes was calculated from the difference between
the food offered and the food left over. The rate of intestinal
absorption was estimated by subtraction of faecal electrolyte loss
from the electrolyte intake.

Results

Serum concentrations of divalent ions were identical in the
experimental and the control groups and stayed within the normal
range throughout the study.

Urinary excretion of Ca was markedly increased by diphenylhydantoin, while in the control group urinary excretion of Ca
stayed low throughout the experimental period, a significant rise
in urinary Ca was seen by the second day. The excretion of this
ion was doubled after 6 days and exceeded the control values by
fourfold on the 15th day (Figure 1).

Intestinal net absorption of calcium was not affected by
diphenylhydantoin. Specifically, an inhibitory effect of this
drug could not be observed. This finding is in contrast to the
in vitro observation that calcium transport in the upper intestine, as studied by the sack method, is decreased by diphenylhydantoin (4). The difference between the in vitro and our in vivo
findings may point to compensatory hyperabsorption in the distal
parts of the intestine. Such hyperabsorption would result in unchanged net absorption.

The fraction of Ca ingested which was excreted in the urine
was rather low (about 2%). This fraction was isgnificantly increased by treatment with diphenylhydantoin (Figure 2). Urinary
excretion of other electrolytes (magnesium, sodium and potassium)
was not influenced by the drug. The excretion of inorganic phosphorus was slightly, but insignificantly elevated on the sixth and
twelfth day; on other days it did not differ from the controls.

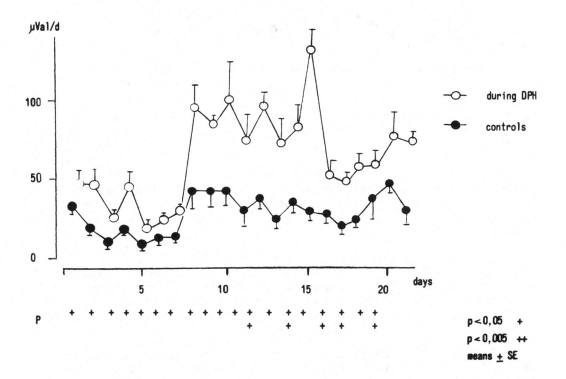

Fig 1. Renal excretion of calcium after application of diphenylhydantoin.

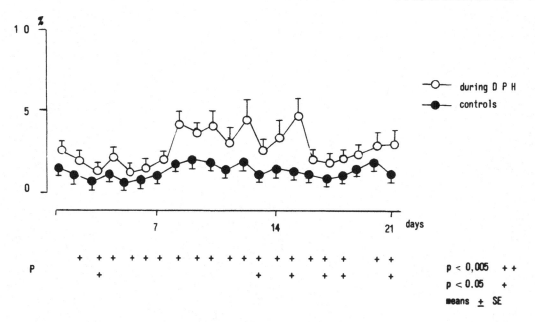

Fig 2.   Fractional calcium excretion in urine (as a percentage
          of the respective intake).

        Urinary excretion of total hydroxyproline (Figure 3) was normal
in the first week, but increased significantly thereafter and
remained on a high level to the end of the balance study.

Discussion

        The finding of hypercalciuria in experimental animals after
administration of diphenylhydantoin is surprising in view of the
known effects of diphenylhydantoin on calcium metabolism in
patients. After long-term treatment (the time factor must be emphasized) with this drug, osteoid accumulates in the skeleton;
this is associated with hypocalcemia, hypocalciuria and hyperphosphaturia (3).

        The 25-hydroxy-vitamin D_3 levels in serum of epileptics are
low after diphenylhydantoin (3,9). The derangement of vitamin D_3
metabolism appears to be a key factor in the pathogenesis of the
abnormalities of calcium metabolism. Diphenylhydantoin increases
the 25-hydroxylation of vitamin D_3 (10). Subsequent inactivation
steps of this metabolite are also enhanced. The accelerated turnover of 25-hydroxy-vitamin D_3 decreases the available stores of
vitamin D and of its active metabolites (11).

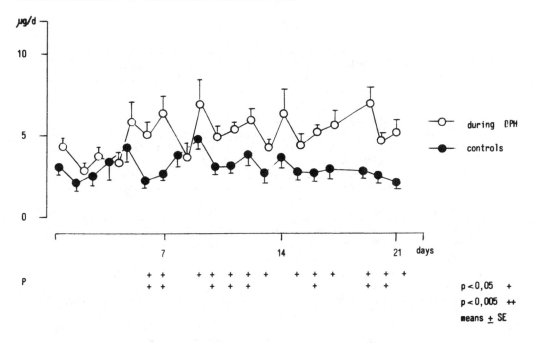

Fig 3.   Renal excretion of total hydroxyproline.

As demonstrated by Puschett et al (12), 25-hydroxy-vitamin D3 itself causes significant depression of renal phosphate excretion, accompanied by decline in sodium and calcium excretion. It is unknown whether 25-hydroxy-vitamin D3 deficiency produces an opposite renal excretion pattern similar to the one seen in our study.

Boullon and co-workers (3) found high parathyroid hormone levels in the serum of epileptic patients treated with diphenylhydantoin. Probably secondary hyperparathyroidism is an important factor for the characteristic electrolyte pattern in the serum and urine of these patients.

Diphenylhydantoin is known to influence the function of numerous organs directly by mechanisms which do not involve vitamin D or PTH. Therefore, the above results might point to a direct action of this drug on the kidney. However, direct proof for such an action would require the use of an isolated kidney preparation. Alternatively, hypercalciuria in the experimental animals might result from increased net bone resorption.

After a few days of treatment with diphenylhydantoin, hydroxyproline excretion in the urine increased. This finding documents and abnormality of bone cell metabolism which could be due to a direct effect of diphenylhydantoin on bone collagen turnover.

REFERENCES

1. Latham, A.N., Millbank, L., Richens, A., and Rose D.J.:
    Liver enzyme induction by anticonfulsant drugs, and its
    relationship to disturbed calcium and folic acid metabolism.

2. Schmid, F.: Osteopathien bei antiepileptischer Dauerbehand-
    lung. Fortschr. Med. 9:381, 1967.

3. Bouillon, R., Reynaert, J., Claes, J.H., Lissens, W., and
    de Moor, P.: The effect of anticonfulsant therapy on serum
    levels of 25-hydroxy-vitamin D, calcium and parathyroid
    hormone. J. Clin. Endocrinol. Metab. 41:1130, 1975.

4. Casparty, W.F.: Inhibition of intestinal calcium transport
    by diphenylhydantoin in rat duodenum. Naunyn-Schmiedeberg's
    Arch. Pharmac. 274:146, 1972.

5. Hartroft, P.M., and Eisenstein, A.B.: Alterations in the
    adrenal cortex of the rat induced by sodium deficiency:
    correlation of histological changes with steroid hormone
    secretion. Endocrinology 60:641, 1956.

6. Mohring, J., and Mohring, B.: Re-evaluation of DOCA escape
    phenomenon. Amer. J. Physiol. 223:1237, 1972.

7. Fiske, C.H., and Subbarow, Y.: Coloimetric determination of
    phosphorus. J. Biol. Chem. 66:375, 1925.

8. Firschein, H.E., and Shill, J.P.: The determination of total
    hydroxyproline in urine and bone extracts. Analyt. Bioche-
    mist. 14:296, 1966.

9. Hahn, T.J., Hendin, B.A., Sharp, C.R., and Haddad, J.G., Jr.:
    Effect of chronic anticonvulsant therapy on serum 25-hydroxy-
    calciferol levels in adults. New Engl. J. Med. 287:900, 1972.

10. Hahn, T.J., Birge, S.J., Sharp, C.R., and Avioli, L.V.:
    Phenobarbital-induced alterations in vitamin D metabolism.
    J. Clin. Invest. 51:741, 1972.

11. Dent, C.E., Richens, A., Rowe, D.J.F., and Stamb, T.C.B.:
    Osteomalacia with long-term anticonvulsant therapy in epilepsy.
    Brit. Med. J. 4:73, 1970.

12. Puschett, J.B., Moranz, J., and Kurnick, W.S.: Evidence for
    a direct action of cholecalciferol and 25-hydroxycholecalci-
    ferol on the renal transport of phosphate, sodium and calcium.
    J. Clin. Invest. 51:373, 1972.

RENAL PHOSPHATE TRANSPORT IN THE PHOSPHATE-DEPLETED DOGS

Sung-Feng Wen, James W. Boynar, Jr. and Robert W. Stoll

Department of Medicine, University of Wisconsin Center

for Health Sciences, Madison, Wisconsin 53706, U.S.A.

INTRODUCTION

Renal transport of phosphate is known to be regulated by such factors as filtered load of phosphate[1], parathyroid hormone[2], and extracellular volume[3]. The effect of dietary intake of phosphate, however, is less well understood. In order to investigate the effect of phosphate depletion on renal phosphate transport, clearance and micropuncture studies were performed in dogs on low phosphate diet to examine the responses to extracellular volume expansion(VE) and parathyroid hormone(PTH).

METHODS

Twenty dogs were placed on low phosphate diet containing less than 3 mmoles of phosphate per day plus administration of aluminum hydroxide gel 100 ml per day and results were compared with 15 normal dogs (N) containing approximately 100 mmoles of phosphate per day. The studies were carried out during hydropenia (H) and after volume expansion to 10% of body weight with Ringer's infusion or administration of highly purified PTH 150 U/hr. The phosphate-depleted animals were divided into short depletion of 17-41 days (S) and long depletion of 53-110 days (L). The animals were prepared for micropuncture as previously described[4], and tubule fluid samples were analyzed for phosphate by modification of the microclorimetric method[5] and for inulin by fluorometric method[6].

101

RESULTS AND DISCUSSION

The clearance and micropuncture data of both normal and phosphate-depleted dogs are summarized in the following table.

Summary of Clearance and Micropuncture Data

Exptl Groups		GFR ml/min	UF_{PO4} mmol/L	FE_{PO4} %	FE_{NA} %	SNGFR nl/min	$\left(\dfrac{TF}{P}\right)_{IN}$	$\left(\dfrac{TF}{UF}\right)_{PO4}$	RF_{PO4} %
N(6)	H	33.4	2.25	5.23	0.86	66.5	1.71	0.72	42
	VE	34.9	2.08	27.80‡	5.47‡	69.8	1.27‡	0.81‡	64‡
N+PX(9)	H	32.3	2.12	3.67	0.94	67.4	1.63	0.63	39
	VE	35.8	1.99	11.79†	7.11‡	73.4	1.31‡	0.80‡	60‡
S(5)	H	25.3	1.30	0.18	0.81	48.5	1.50	0.37	26
	VE	26.6	1.34	6.53†	7.78‡	50.0	1.32†	0.64†	51†
S+PX(5)	H	17.7	1.37	0.11	0.44	42.2	1.52	0.45	32
	VE	18.7	1.39	0.29†	5.85†	41.9	1.27†	0.71‡	58‡
L(5)	H	18.7	1.31	0.17	0.66	49.4	1.59	0.13	9
	VE	18.7	1.32	0.27‡	5.99‡	49.5	1.28‡	0.33†	26†
L(5)	VE	20.2	0.74	0.49	5.22	51.6	1.31	0.29	22
	PTH	18.8†	1.12‡	0.39	5.99	46.9	1.24	0.31	25

GFR = Glomerular filtration rate; UF = Plasma ultrafiltrate; FE = Fractional excretion; SN = Single nephron; TF = Tubule fluid; P = Plasma; RF = Remaining fraction in proximal tubule; PX = Acute thyroparathyroidectomy; †P < 0.05; ‡P < 0.01; Number in parentheses denotes that of animals.

Volume expansion in the normal dogs with intact parathyroids led to a dramatic increase in fractional phosphate excretion as well as reduction in fractional proximal tubule phosphate reabsorption. This phosphaturic response was significantly blunted in the acutely thyroparathyroidectomized normal dogs even though the proximal tubule response was similar to the intact dogs. In short phosphate-depletion groups, mean proximal TF/UF phosphate was lower than that of the normal groups but the proximal tubule response to volume expansion was comparable. However, the phosphaturic response was blunted in the intact parathyroid group and was virtually abolished with acute thyroparathyroidectomy. In long phosphate-depletion groups, mean proximal TF/UF phosphate was extremely low, and no significant phosphaturia occurred after volume expansion or administration of parathyroid hormone even with intact parathyroids. The difference in the phosphaturic response between short and long phosphate-depletion groups did not correlate with UF phosphate levels but rather with the duration of phosphate depletion. Other workers have also reported that some factor other than plasma phosphate must be responsible for the alteration in tubule handling of phosphate in phosphate depletion[7-9]. These observations suggest that intracellular content of inorganic phosphate may be important in regulating renal transport of phosphate.

REFERENCES

1. Pitts R.F: Physiology of the Kidney and Body Fluids. Year Book Med. Pub., Chicago, 3rd edition, 1974, p.78.
2. Albright F: The parathyroids - physiology and therapeutics. J.A.M.A. 117:527-533, 1941.
3. Massry S.G., Coburn J.W. and Kleeman C.R: The influence of extracellular volume expansion on renal phosphate reabsorption in the dog. J. Clin. Invest. 48:1237-1245, 1969.
4. Wen S.F: Micropuncture studies of phosphate transport in the proximal tubule of the dog. The relationship to sodium reabsorption. J. Clin. Invest. 53:143-153, 1974.
5. Chen P.S., Jr., Toribara T.Y. and Warner H: Microdetermination of phosphorus. Anal. Biochem. 28:1756-1758, 1956.
6. Vurek G.G. and Pegram S.E: Fluorometric method for determination of nanogram quantities of inulin. Anal. Biochem. 16:409-419, 1966.
7. Van Stone J.C. and Hano J: Phosphate excretion in the parathyroidectomized rat receiving parathyroid hormone. Metab. Clin. Exp. 21:849-854, 1972.
8. Tröhler U., Bonjour J.P. and Fleisch H: Inorganic phosphate homeostasis. Renal adaptation to the dietary intake in intact and thyroparathyroidectomized rats. J. Clin. Invest. 57:264-273, 1976.
9. Steele T.H. and DeLuca H.F: Influence of dietary phosphorus on renal phosphate reabsorption in the parathyroidectomized rat. J. Clin. Invest. 57:867-874, 1976.

DISSOCIATED REABSORPTION OF PHOSPHATE AND BICARBONATE IN THE POST-OBSTRUCTED DOG KIDNEY

C.K. Crumb, G. Barbour, R. Patterson, W.N. Suki, and
E.J. Weinman
V.A. Hospital, Little Rock, Arkansas and
V.A. Hospital and Baylor College of Medicine,
Houston, Texas

A parallel relationship exists between the absorption of phosphate and bicarbonate in the normal kidney(Table I). A number of maneuvers which inhibit phosphate absorption also inhibit absorption of bicarbonate such as volume expansion (1-3), parathyroid extract (2), parathyroid hormone (1), cAMP (4) and hypocalcemia (5). On the other hand, those maneuvers which enhance phosphate absorption also enhance bicarbonate absorption such as renal hypoperfusion (6), aortic constriction (7), parathyroidectomy (2), hypercalcemia (2) and vitamin D (8). The nature of the parallelism between phosphate and bicarbonate absorption is not known but it may be the result of a relation between the absorption of each of these anions to the

Table I. Comparison of the maneuvers which inhibit or enhance the absorption of phosphate and bicarbonate

Inhibited by:	Enhanced by:
Volume Expansion	Renal Hypoperfusion
Parathyroid Extract (PTE)	Aortic Constriction
Parathyroid Hormone(PTH)	Parathyroidectomy
cAMP	Hypercalcemia
Hypocalcemia	Vitamin D

absorption of sodium and water in the proximal tubule, since many of the maneuvers discussed above alter sodium absorption in a parallel fashion.

In the post-obstructed kidney a dissociation between phosphate and sodium has been reported (9,10). The absorption of phosphate is greatly enhanced and that of sodium is depressed. Furthermore, the post-obstructed kidney exhibits a blunted response to exogenous PTE (9). This unresponsiveness may be due to a damaged tubule, a parathyroid hormone unresponsive tubule, decrease in the parathyroid hormone responsive portion of phosphate absorption (11) or a decrease in the filtered load of phosphate per functioning nephron.

To examine the role of the filtered phosphate load and determine whether the parallelism between phosphate and bicarbonate holds in the post-obstructed kidney model studies were performed on eleven anesthetized and ventilated dogs(Figure I). An acute thyroparathyroidectomy (TPTX) was performed at least two and one half hours prior to the control period. A 0.7 molar solution of sodium bicarbonate was infused at a rate designed to raise the serum bicarbonate above threshold and maintain it between 30 and 36 mmol/liter. After two hours of equilibration, four 15-minute control collections of urine and blood were made. At this point, 100 units of purified parathyroid extract was given intravenously followed by a steady infusion of five units/minute for the duration of the experiment (2). After equilibration for 30 minutes, four 15-minute experimental collections were made. Two groups of animals were studied(Table II). Group I, referred to as the post-obstructed kidney group, consisted of six dogs studied three hours after the release of a unilateral ureteral ligature that had been in place for three to six days. Group II, referred to as the embolized kidney group, consisted of five dogs studied four to seven days after 0.45 micron microspheres had been injected into the renal artery of one kidney. The rationale for

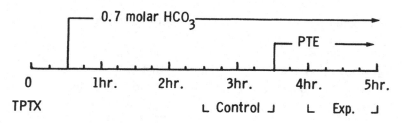

Fig. I.   Experimental design: TPTX = thyroparathyroidectomy,
          PTE = purified parathyroid extract.

Table II. Preparation of the experimental models

SNGFR

Group I: Post-Obstructed Kidney (P O Kidney) Group
n=6

Unilateral Ureteral Ligation 3-6 Days   ↓
Ligation Removed 3 Hrs Before Control Period

Group II: Embolized Kidney (E Kidney) Group   n=5

Microspheres Injected Into One Kidney   Normal or ↑
4-7 Days Before Experiment

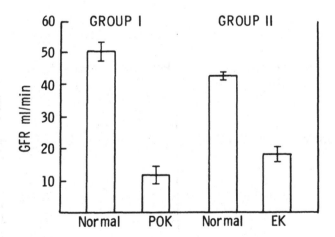

Fig. II. Comparison of the glomerular filtration rate (GFR) in the
normal, post-obstructed (PO), and the embolized (E) kidney. All values are means ± S.E.M.

these two groups is to compare the post-obstructed kidney which has
a decreased single nephron glomerular filtration rate (SNGFR) (12)
and therefore a decreased filtered load of phosphate per nephron,
to a group with a normal single nephron glomerular filtration rate
and therefore a normal filtered load of phosphate per nephron.

There was no difference in the serum bicarbonate, phosphate,
ultrafilterable calcium, potassium or hematocrit between groups or
from control to experimental periods. The glomerular filtration
rates in the two groups are depicted in Figure II. As can be seen
the glomerular filtration rate in the normal kidneys of both groups
is comparable and the glomerular filtration rate in the post-
obstructed kidney and the embolized kidney are greatly reduced when
compared to the normal. The absorption of phosphate in the normal
and post-obstructed kidney and the effect of parathyroid extract on
it is depicted in Figure III. Note that the percent reabsorption
of phosphate (%TRP) in the post-obstructed kidney was significantly
higher 96.8 ± 0.3% than in the normal kidney 89.5 ± 1.0% (p<0.05),
and as shown previously (9), administration of parathyroid extract
decreased the %TRP to a lesser degree from 96.8 ± 0.3% to 91.7 ±
0.4% in the post-obstructed kidney than in the normal kidney which
was from 89.5 ± 1.0% to 74.9 ± 1.1%. The results of similar studies

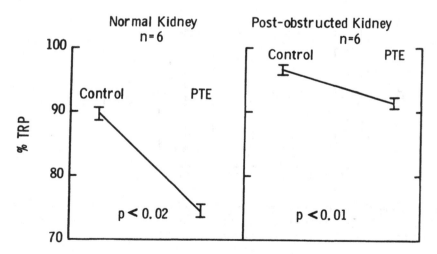

Fig. III.   Comparison of the effects of PTE on percent tubular
            reabsorption of phosphate (% TRP) in the normal and
            post-obstructed kidney.

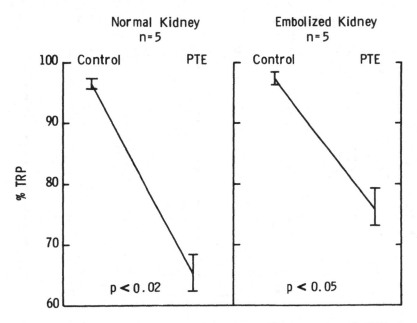

Fig. IV.   Comparison of the effects of PTE on the % TRP in the
normal and embolized kidney.

in the embolized kidney model are shown in Figure IV.   In contrast
to the post-obstructed kidney model the %TRP was the same in the
two kidneys during the control period and parathyroid extract greatly depressed the %TRP in both the normal from $97.3 \pm 0.4\%$ to $65.0 \pm$
3.0% (p<0.02) and the embolized kidneys from $98.2 \pm 0.2\%$ to $77.3 \pm$
3.1% (p<0.05).   The data on bicarbonate absorption ($RHCO_3$) in the
post-obstructed kidney model are shown in Figure V.   As for phosphate, the bicarbonate absorption in the post-obstructed kidney in
the control period was higher 28.1 ± 0.3 mmol/liter than in the
normal kidney 25.7 ± 0.5 mmol/liter (p<0.025).   Unlike phosphate,
however, the administration of parathyroid extract significantly
depressed $RHCO_3$ to the same level in the normal 22.2 ± 0.8 mmol/
liter as in the post-obstructed kidney 22.6 ± 0.7 mmol/liter.

The data in the embolized kidney model are shown in Figure VI.
In this model the $RHCO_3$ was slightly but insignificantly higher than
the normal kidney and the administration of parathyroid extract
resulted in a similar decline in the normal from 26.8 ± 1.7 to 23.4

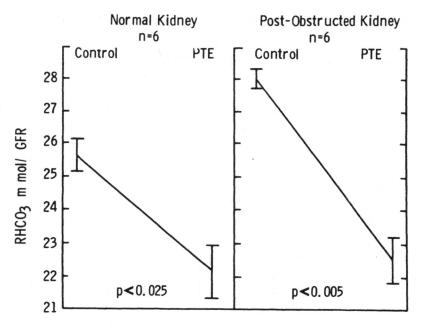

Fig. V.   Comparison of the effects of PTE on bicarbonate absorption
(RHCO$_3$) in the normal and post-obstructed kidney.

± 1.4 mmol/liter (p<0.05) as in the embolized kidney which was from
28.0 ± 1.7 to 22.8 ± 0.6 mmol/liter (p<0.05).

The results of these studies support the suggestion that a reduced filtered load of phosphate per nephron accounts for the blunted
phosphaturic effect of parathyroid extract in the post-obstructed
kidney. In this model, where the SNGFR is decreased and therefore
the filtered load of phosphate per nephron is decreased, the parathyroid extract has a blunted effect on phosphate. However, in the
embolized kidney, in which the whole kidney filtered phosphate load
is decreased but the SNGFR and the filtered load of phosphate per
nephron is normal parathyroid extract exhibited its accustomed inhibitory effect.

Of great interest in this study is the dissociation between the
behavior of phosphate and that of bicarbonate in response to para-

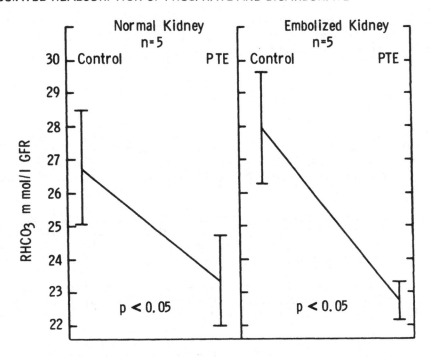

Fig. VI. Comparison of the effects of PTE on $RHCO_3$ in the normal
and embolized kidney.

thyroid extract in the post-obstructed kidney. The dissociation
suggests that the relationship between phosphate and bicarbonate is
fortuitous and not the result of coupling of one to the other. Alternatively, it is possible that the absorption of bicarbonate is
more closely associated to sodium than is phosphate. This is compatible with the observation that whereas phosphate absorption in the
post-obstructed kidney is enhanced, that of sodium is depressed.

In summary: 1) Parathyroid extract depresses phosphate absorption normally in the embolized kidney (normal SNGFR) but not the
post-obstructed kidney (reduced SNGFR) supporting the proposed importance of the reduced filtered load of phosphate per nephron. 2)
Both bicarbonate absorption and %TRP are enhanced in the post-
obstructed kidney. 3) Parathyroid extract inhibits absorption of
bicarbonate without markedly inhibiting phosphate absorption in the
post-obstructed kidney suggesting a dissociation between the transport on these two anions.

This work was supported in part by institutional support of the Little Rock Veterans Administration Hospital and the Houston Veterans Administration Hospital.

References

1. Diaz-Buxo, J.A., Ott, C.E., Cuche, J.L., Marchand, G.R., Wilson, D.M., and Knox, F.G.: Effects of extracellular fluid volume contraction and expansion on the bicarbonaturia of parathyroid hormone. Kidney Int. 8:105, 1975.

2. Crumb, C.K., Martinez-Maldonado, M., Eknoyan, G., and Suki, W.N.: Effects of volume expansion, purified parathyroid extract and calcium on renal bicarbonate absorption in the dog. J. Clin. Invest. 54:1287, 1974.

3. Purkerson, M.L., Lubowitz, H., White, R.W., and Bricker, N.S.: On the influence of extracellular fluid volume expansion on bicarbonate reabsorption in the rat. J. Clin. Invest. 48:1754, 1969.

4. Karlinsky, M.L., Sager, D.S., Kurtzman, N.A., and Pillay, V.K.G.: Effect of parathyroid hormone and cyclic adenosine monophosphate on renal bicarbonate reabsorption. Amer. J. Physiol. 227:1226, 1974.

5. Farrel, S.: Baylor College of Medicine, personal communication.

6. Popovtzer, M.M., Massry, S.G., Villamil, M., and Kleeman, C.R.: Renal handling of phosphorus in oliguric and nonoliguric mercury-induced acute renal failure in rats. J. Clin. Invest. 50:2347, 1971.

7. Puschett, J.B., Agus, Z.S., Senesky, D., and Goldberg, M.: Effects of saline loading and aortic obstruction on proximal phosphate transport. Amer. J. Physiol. 223:851, 1972.

8. Peraino, R.A., Ghaffary, E., Rouse, D., and Suki, W.N.: Renal actions of 25-hydroxyvitamin D_3. Baylor College of Medicine, (submitted for publication).

9. Purkerson, M.L., Rolf, D.B., Chase, L.R., Slatopolsky, E., and Klahr, S.: Tubular reabsorption of phosphate after release of complete ureteral obstruction in the rat. Kidney Int. 5:326, 1974.

10. Better, O.S., Tuma, S., Kedar, S., Chaimowitz, C.: Enhanced tubular reabsorption of phosphate. Arch. Intern. Med. 135: 245, 1975.

11. Glorieux, F., and Scriver, C.R.: Loss of a parathyroid hormone sensitive component of phosphate transport in x-linked hypophosphatemia. Science 175:997, 1972.

12. Harris, R.H., and Yarger, W.E.: Renal function after release of unilateral ureteral obstruction in rats. Amer. J. Physiol. 227:806, 1974.

PARATHYROID HORMONE-INDUCED INHIBITION OF BICARBONATE-DEPENDENT

FLUID ABSORPTION IN THE PROXIMAL RENAL TUBULE OF THE RABBIT

Vincent W. Dennis

Division of Nephrology
Duke University Medical Center
Durham, North Carolina 27710

Although phosphaturia is the most characteristic renal effect of parathyroid hormone, PTH may also affect the renal handling of sodium, bicarbonate, calcium, glucose and amino acids (1). The relationship between these changes and the alterations in phosphate transport is unclear but information on this point may be useful in determining the mechanisms whereby PTH affects such a broad range of renal function.

In the course of our investigations of phosphate transport in isolated segments of the rabbit nephron (2,3), we confirmed the observations of others (4,5) that one of the most prominent effects of PTH on the proximal convoluted tubule is the inhibition of fluid absorption. The following studies were designed to examine the mechanism of this effect.

METHODS

Isolated and perfused segments of the proximal convoluted tubule of the rabbit kidney were studied at 37°C according to the methods described by Burg (6) and as modified in our laboratory (7). All segments were perfused with an ultrafiltrate of the same rabbit serum used as the bathing medium. This rabbit serum was either normal rabbit serum or low bicarbonate rabbit serum prepared by a method adapted from that described by Cardinal et al (8). Fluid absorption was measured using ^{125}I-iothalamate. Bovine parathyroid hormone (458 U/mg) was obtained from Calbiochem, San Diego, CA. Chloride concentrations in the collected fluids were measured electrocoulometrically (9).

RESULTS

During perfusion of isolated segments of the proximal convoluted tubule with ultrafiltrate of normal rabbit serum, the fluid absorption rate averaged 1.14 $\pm$ 0.09 nl/mm·min (15 tubules) and was reduced to 0.68 $\pm$ 0.08 nl/mm·min after adding PTH to the bath to a final concentration of 1 U/ml. However PTH had no measurable effect on fluid absorption when added to the perfusion fluid only (Table I) suggesting that the receptor site for this effect may be at the antiluminal surface.

As seen in Fig 1, simultaneous with the PTH-induced reduction in fluid absorption, the chloride concentration in the collected fluid was also reduced. Since the increase in intraluminal chloride concentration that occurs in the proximal tubule as a result of isotonic fluid absorption has been widely attributed to the preferential absorption of bicarbonate over chloride, these data suggested that PTH affected bicarbonate absorption more so than chloride absorption. This assessment is supported further by the observation (Fig 1) that PTH had no measurable effect on net chloride fluxes.

Table I

Fluid Absorption Rate (nl/mm·min)

	C	E	C
Lumen (8)	1.03	0.77	0.88
	0.17	0.25	0.19
P		NS	NS
Bath (15)	1.14	0.68	0.90
	0.09	0.08	0.12
P		<0.005	<0.01
Bath & Lumen (5)	1.10	0.48	1.02
	0.28	0.11	0.10
P		<0.01	<0.01

Numbers in parenthesis refer to the number of segments studied C denotes the control periods during which tubules were perfused with isosmolal ultrafiltrate of the rabbit serum used as the bathing medium. E denotes the experimental periods during which PTH was added to the luminal fluid, the bath or to both fluids to a final concentration of 1 unit ml^{-1}.

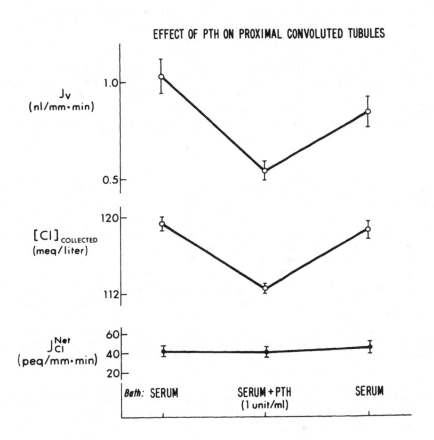

Figure 1. Effects of bovine parathyroid hormone on fluid absorption, intraluminal chloride concentration and net chloride flux in 16 proximal convoluted tubules. Each tubule was perfused with an ultrafiltrate of the same normal rabbit serum used as the bath.

Since these data indicated that bicarbonate was involved in the PTH-induced reduction in proximal fluid absorption, additional studies were performed using low bicarbonate ultrafiltrate as perfusion fluid and low bicarbonate rabbit serum as bath. The pH of the bath was maintained at 7.4 by gassing with oxygen rather than a mixture of oxygen and carbon dioxide. Under these conditions, during the control period in the absence of added PTH, the fluid absorption rate for six tubules averaged 0.84 ± 0.05 nl/mm·min which is significantly lower than the control value observed during perfusion with fluids containing normal levels of bicarbonate (1.14 ± 0.09 nl/mm·min; $P<0.005$). Moreover, in the absence of bicarbonate, the addition of PTH to the bath resulted in no further change in fluid absorption with an average experimental value of 0.81 ± 0.05 nl/mm·min. Thus, bicarbonate appears to be a necessary cofactor in the reduction of proximal fluid absorption by PTH.

DISCUSSION

Inhibition of proximal fluid absorption is one of the most constant and most quantitatively significant effects of PTH observed during micropuncture studies in the rat (10) and in the dog (4,5). The present studies suggest that the basis for this effect may be inhibition of bicarbonate transport, a possibility consistent with the observations of Hellman et al (11) that the acute administration of PTH results in increased bicarbonate excretion. These investigators also noted that the PTH-induced increase in bicarbonate excretion may precede or occur in the absence of increased phosphate excretion. The significance of this effect of PTH resides not only in partially explaining the hyperchloremic acidosis occasionally observed in patients with hyperparathyroidism but also in suggesting the possibility that some of the reduced solute reabsorption observed in response to PTH may be mediated by the reduction in bulk flow occurring across the leaky proximal tubular epithelium. In this regard, PTH would be acting in a manner not unlike extracellular fluid volume expansion in decreasing the fractional reabsorption of solute-containing fluid in a limited area of the nephron with the organ-level effects being determined by the availability of downstream reabsorptive events. In addition to this reduction in bulk, the effects of PTH may also result in changes in transepithelial electrical potential difference since the lumen-positive potential difference in the later portions of the proximal tubule has been interpreted as being a chloride diffusion potential (12). As such, the intensity of this force would be affected by any factor which lowers the intraluminal chloride concentration as occurred in the present studies. Although speculative, these and similar considerations may be useful in postulating testable hypotheses to explain the variety of renal effects of PTH.

REFERENCES

1. Aurbach, G.D., and Heath, D. A.: Parathyroid hormone and calcitonin regulation of renal function. Kidney Internat. 6: 331, 1974.

2. Dennis, V.W., Woodhall, P.B., and Robinson, R.R.: Characteristics of phosphate transport in the isolated proximal tubule. Am. J. Physiol. 231:979, 1976

3. Dennis, V.W., Bello-Reuss, E., and Robinson, R.R.: Responsiveness of phosphate transport to parathyroid hormone in three segments of the rabbit nephron. (Submitted for publication)

4. Agus, Z.S., Gardner, L.B., Beck, L. H., and Goldberg, M.: Effects of parathyroid hormone on renal tubular reabsorption of calcium, sodium, and phosphate. Am. J. Physiol. 224: 1143, 1973.

5. Schneider, E.G.: Effect of parathyroid hormone secretion on sodium reabsorption by the proximal tubule. Am. J. Physiol. 229: 1170, 1975.

6. Burg, M., Grantham, J., Abramow, M., and Orloff, J.: Preparation and study of fragments of single rabbit nephrons. Am. J. Physiol. 210: 1293, 1966.

7. Dennis, V. W.: Influence of bicarbonate on parathyroid hormone-induced changes in fluid absorption by the proximal tubule. Kidney Internat. 10:373, 1976.

8. Cardinal, J., Lutz, M.D., Burg, M.B., and Orloff, J.: Lack of relationship of potential difference to fluid absorption in the proximal renal tubule. Kidney Internat. 7: 94, 1975.

9. Ramsay, J.A., Brown, R.H.J., and Croghan, P.C.: Electrometric titration of chloride in small volumes. J. Exp. Biol. 32: 822, 1955.

10. Amiel, C., Kuntziger, H., and Richet, G.: Micropuncture study of handling of phosphate by proximal and distal nephron in normal and parathyroidectomized rat. Evidence for distal reabsorption. Pfluegers Arch. 317: 93, 1970.

11. Hellman, D.E., Au, W.Y.M., Bartter, F.C.: Evidence for a direct effect of parathyroid hormone on urinary acidification. Am. J. Physiol. 209: 643, 1965.

12. Barratt, L., Rector, F.C., Kokko, J.P., and Seldin, D.W.:
    Factors governing the transepithelial potential difference
    across the proximal tubule of the rat kidney. J. Clin. Invest.
    53: 454, 1974.

RENAL HANDLING OF SODIUM, WATER AND DIVALENT IONS

IN PATIENTS WITH PRIMARY BILIARY CIRRHOSIS

J. Rochman, C. Chaimovitz, S. Eidelman, O.S. Better

Rambam Univ. Hospital & Technicon School of Medicine

Haifa, Israel

ABSTRACT

1) Fluid retention and ascites are rarely seen in patients
with primary biliary cirrhosis (PBC). In an attempt to clarify this
clinical observation, renal handling of sodium, water and divalent
ions was studied during extracellular volume expansion (ECVE) and
maximal suppression of antidiuretic hormone (ADH) secretion in 5
patients with PBC and 9 normal subjects.

2) Mean fractional excretion of sodium, water, phosphate and
calculated fractional distal delivery of sodium were significantly
greater in patients with PBC as compared with normal controls.
Fractional C_{H2O} for given fractional urine flow was similar in
patients with PBC and normals.

3) The data suggest that patients with PBC have a greater
diminution of proximal tubular reabsorption of sodium in response to
ECVE than controls. This augmented elimination of salt during ECVE
in patients with PBC may explain the rarity of ascites and edema in
this type of cirrhosis.

INTRODUCTION

Renal salt and water retention with the formation of ascites
and edema is common in patients with Laennec's cirrhosis. In contrast, in patients with primary biliary cirrhosis (PBC) edema and
ascites are rare and may appear only late in the course of the
disease (1). Whereas renal handling of salt and water have been
extensively studied in patients with Laennec's cirrhosis (2-5),
and dogs with chronic liver damage (6), little is known on the
kidney function in patidnts with PBC. The purpose of this investigation was to study some tubular functions in patients with PBC

in an attempt to explain the rarity of fluid retention in PBC.

METHODS

Studies were performed in five patients with PBC and in nine normal volunteers. The nature and the purpose of the study were thoroughly explained to all test subjects, and their consent for participation was obtained. The diagnosis of biliary cirrhosis was established in our patients on clinical grounds and substantiated in each patient by characteristic histologic appearance in liver biopsy and the presence of antimitochondrial antibodies in their plasma. Pertinent clinical details are summarized in Table 1.

On the morning of the expeirment each subject received an oral water load of 20 ml per Kg body weight, and a sustained water diuresis was maintained by oral replacement equal to the urine flow. A steady rate of urine flow and urinary osmolality below 75 were used as the criterion of adequate suppression of antidiuretic hormone.

Following the establishment of the water diuresis, volume expansion was achieved with 2500 ml of isotonic saline/1.73 m^2 of body surface area infused intravenously at a rate of 15 ml per minute. Urine collections were obtained by voiding at intervals of 15 minutes and venous samples were drawn with minimal stasis at the midpoint of each clearance period. Urine volumes were replaced by oral water ingestion in order to attain maximal suppression of ADH during the saline load. Subjects were recumbent during the study and were allowed to sit only for voiding.

After an appropriate priming dose, a sustaining infusion of inulin and paraaminohippurate (PAH) in normal saline was given by constant infusion pump. The GFR and renal plasma flow were measured by inulin and PAH clearance, respectively. All blood and urine samples were analyzed for inulin, PAH, sodium, calcium, phosphate, magnesium and osmolality by methods previously described from our laboratory (7). The clearance of calcium and magnesium were calculated by assuming diffusible serum calcium of 60% of total serum calcium and diffusible serum magnesium of 75% of total serum magnesium (8). Levels of 25-hydroxycholecalciferol in plasma was determined in patients V.S., K.D., and M.Z., by the method described by Edelstein et al (9).

RESULTS

Table 2 contains a summary of the clearance data from all the experiments. The data respresent mean results obtained from the last three clearance periods at the end of the saline load. The clearance of inulin and PAH were comparable in both patients and controls. Since mean urinary osmolality was similar in both groups, it is reasonable to assume that antidiuretic hormone was similarly suppressed in all test subjects.

Rejection of fluid out of the proximal tubule, V/GFR x 100, averaged 28.8±3.9 (±SD) in PBC patients, a value which is

Table 1:   Clinical and laboratory findings in patients with PBC.

Subject	Bilirubin (mg/dℓ)	SGOT	Alkaline phosphatase*	Albumin (g/dℓ)	Choles-terol (mg/dℓ)	Antimito-chondrial Antibodies	Esopha-geal Varices	Ascites
V.S.	12	140	7.9	4.7	500	Positive	Yes	No
K.D.	1.5	46	10.5	4.3	438	Positive	No	No
M.Z.	3.8	144	23.4	4.1	480	Positive	Yes	No
A.I.	1.2	42	6.8	4.0	324	Positive	Yes	No
K.M.	1.5	45	7,I	4.4	275	Positive	Yes	No

* Bessy-Lowry units (normal up to 2.3 units).

TABLE 2.   SUMMARY OF CLEARANCE DATA DURING VOLUME EXPANSION IN PBC PATIENTS AND IN CONTROLS

SUBJECT	V ml/min	U_{osm} mOsm/kgH$_2$O	C_{in} ml/min	C_{pah}	V ml/min	CH_2O	C_{Na}	C_{PO4} ml/min/100ml GFR	C_{Ca}	C_{Mg}
P B C										
V.S.	22	97	80	502	27.5	19.1	8.8	30.1	8.8	15.6
K.D.	23.6	91	92	467	25.7	17.2	6.6	33.9	8.4	10.3
M.Z.	25.4	105	74	474	34.3	25.3	11.6	50.6	8.4	21.5
A.I.	33	96	105	1024	31.4	21.6	9.4	27.6	6.9	17.3
K.M.	25	80	100	473	25	15.3	7.3	25.4	10.3	19.1
MEAN	25.8	94	90.2	498	28.8	19.7	8.7	33.5	8.6	16.8
± S.D.	4.2	9.2	13.1	346	3.9	3.9	1.9	10.1	1.2	4.2
CONTROLS										
C.A.	27.8	98	114	702	24.4	16	4.8	19.6	9.9	23.4
E.H.	20.9	103	94	733	22.2	14.3	6.5	18.4	15.6	28.7
B.H.	42	98	197	895	21.3	14.3	6.2	13.8	10.8	19.
A.A.	31.9	77	136	758	23.5	17.4	4.4	19.5	11.8	40
K.I.	20.7	61	91	623	22.7	17.9	3.7	11.7	7.6	13.1
C.Z.	22.6	83	115	529	19.7	14.1	3.7	14.7	4	7.1
L.A.	19.9	78	119	851	16.7	12.1	2.7	21.1	8.7	26.1
S.M.	21.7	60	100	510	21.7	16.9	2.5	14.9	11.4	27.7
H.J.	27.5	70	146	647	18.8	14.2	3.6	16.7	9.4	9.4
MEAN	26.1	81	123	694	21.2	15.2	4.2	16.7	8.9	21.6
± S.S.	7.2	16	33	132	2.4	1.9	1.4	3.1	4.3	10.5
P	NS	NS	NS	NS	<0.001	<0.02	<0.001	<0.001	NS	NS

NOTE: V = Urinary flow; U_{som} = urine osmolality; C_{in} = clearance of inulin; C_{PAH} = clearance of p-aminohippurate; $CH2O$ = free water clearance; C_{Na} = clearance of sodium; C_{PO4} = clearance of phosphate; C_{Ca} = clearance of calcium; C_{Mg} = clearance of magnesium

significantly higher than 21.2±2.4 in the controls (p<0.001). The
fraction of filtered sodium excreted in the urine (FeNa) by the
PBC patients, 8.7±1.9, was significantly higher (p<0.001) than that
of the controls, 4.2±1.4. Fractional phosphate excretion (FePo4)
was 33.5±10.1 and 16.7±3.1 in the patients and controls, respectively (p<0.001). Whereas a larger natriuresis and phosphaturia
was seen in the PBC patients as compared with controls, mean fractional excretion of calcium and magnesium were not statistically
different in both groups. Since mean plasma concentration of
Na = 138±2.5 mEq/l, P = 3.4±0.4 mg/100 ml, Ca = 9.8±0.5 mg/100 ml,
and Mg = 1.8±0.2 mg/100 ml in the normal subjects were not statistically different from the values seen in the PBC patients (Na =
139±4.4 mEq/l, P = 3.2±0.5 mg/100 ml, Ca = 9.3±0.7 mg/100 ml, and
Mg = 1.8±0.4 mg/100 ml, the variations in the urinary excretion of
these ions in controls and patients cannot be merely explained by
differences in the filtered load of such solutes.

In Fig 1 free water clearance was plotted versus distal
delivery of sodium was estimated by the urinary flow. There is no
difference between PBC patients and controls in the generation of
free water clearance for given rates of distal delivery of sodium.
In Fig 2, clearance of calcium was plotted as a function of clearance
of sodium. It is apparent that clearance of calcium at any given
value of clearance of sodium is higher in PBC patients than in
controls. The slopes of the regression lines related calcium and
sodium clearances was significantly different (p<0.001). Plasma
level of 25-hydroxycholeclaciferol was 8.16 and 8.2 ng/ml in
patients V.S., K.D., and M.Z., respectively (average normal level
in Israeli subjects = 30 ng/ml).

DISCUSSION

Our results show that patients with PBC respond to extracellular
volume expansion (ECVE) with augmented urinary excretion of sodium,
water and phosphate as compared with healthy controls. Mean urinary
calcium and magnesium excretion were not statistically different
between patients with PBC and controls.

The augmented natriuretic response to ECVE in patients with
PBC may explain the rarity of fluid retention in this variety of
cirrhosis (1,10). Moreover, our study may provide information
about the possible localization of this functional change along
the nephron. Since the generation of free water for given rates of
distal delivery was simialr in the patients with PBC and controls,
the augmented rejection of sodium in response to ECVE appears to
be in the proximal nephron in patients with PBC. Furthermore,
phosphate which can be considered a proximal marker in euparathyroid
subjects (11,12) was also excreted in increased rate during ECVE in
patients with PBC. This is an additional evidence that the proximal
tubule is the main site of the augmented natriuresis of ECVE in PBC.

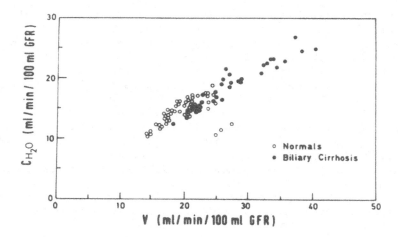

Fig 1.　Relation between C_{H_2O} and V during volume expansion
in normal controls and PBC patients.

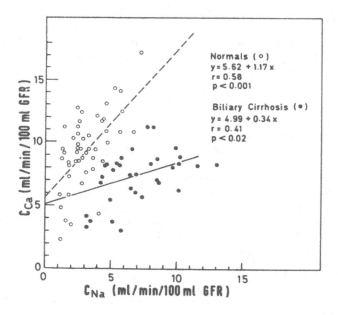

Fig 2.　Effect of ECVE on the relationship between fractional
excretion of sodium and calcium in normal controls
and PBC patients.

In patients with PBC urinary calcium excretion for given rates of sodium excretion was distinctly and significantly subnormal. The phenomenon may be due to diminished intestinal calcium absorption, impaired vitamin D metabolism and secondary hyperparathyroidism (13-16).

The pattern of augmented natriuretic and phosphaturic response to ECVE together with the relative hypocalciuria and the diminished level of 25 hydroxy-vitamin D in PBC suggests enhanced PTH activity in their circulation. In the absence of data on PTH and ionized calcium in PBC this suggestion remains speculative.

Although the above hypothesis seems attractive, other factors must be considered in explaining the rarity of fluid retention in PBC. Among these are the relative sparing of the liver parenchyma in PBC, a disease that is predominantly a biliary obstructive process. Also, protal hypertension which is associated with profound derangment of fluid distribution in Laennec's cirrhosis, is a relatively late phenomenon in PBC (10).

The absence of ascites and edema in our patients is remarkable, particularly in view of conspicuous evidence for portal hypertension (hepatosplenomegaly, oesophageal varies) in 4/5 patients with PBC.

REFERENCES

1. Sherlock, S.: Primary biliary cirrhosis (chronic intrahepatic obstructive jaundice). Gastroenterology, 37:574, 1959.
2. Papper, S.: The role of the kidney in Laennec's cirrhosis of the liver. Med. (Balt.) 37:299, 1958.
3. Schedl, H.P., and Bartter, F.C.: An explanation for experimental correction of the abnormal water diuresis in cirrhosis. J. Clin. Invest. 39:248, 1960.
4. Klingler, E.L., Vasmode, C.A., Vaamonde, L.S., Lancestremere, R.G., Morosi, H.J., Frish, E., and Papper, S.: Renal function changes in cirrhosis of the liver. Arch. Int. Med. 125:1010, 1970.
5. Chaimovitz, C., Szylman, P., Alroy, G., and Better, O.S.: Mechanism of increased renal tubular sodium reabsorption in cirrhosis. Am. J. Med. 52:198, 1972.
6. Better, O.S., and Massry, S.G.: Effect of chronic bile duct obstruction on renal handling of salt and water. J. Clin. Invest. 51:402, 1972.
7. Better, O.S., Tuma, S., Richter-Levin, D., Szylman, P., Geresh, Y., Elbas, S., and Chaimovitz, C.: Intra-renal resetting of glomerulotubular balance in a patient with post obstructive uropathy. Nephron. 9:129, 1972.
8. Better, O.S., Kleeman, C.R., Gonick, F.C., Varrady, P.C., and Maxwell, M.H.: Renal handling of calcium, magnesium and inorganic phosphate in chronic renal failure. Isr. J. Med. Sci. 3:60, 1967.
9. Edelstein, S., Charman, M., Lawson, D.E.M., and Kodicek, E.: Competitive protein-binding assay for 25-hydroxycholecalciferol. Clin. Sci. Molec. Med. 46:231, 1974.
10. Sherlock, S., and Scheuer, P.J.: The presentation and diagnosis of 100 patients with primary biliary cirrhosis. New Eng. J. Med. 289:674, 1973.
11. Wilde, W.S., and Malvin, R.: Graphical placement of transport segments along the nephron from urine concentration pattern developed with stop flow technique. Am. J. Physiol. 195:153, 1958.
12. Massry, S.G., Friedler, R.M., and Coburn, J.W.: Excretion of phosphate and calcium. Arch. Int. Med. 131:828, 1973.
13. Avioli, L.V., and Haddad, J.G.: Vitamin D: Current concepts. Metabolism, 22:507, 1973.
14. Ajdukiewicz, A.B., Agnew, J.E., Byers, P.B., Wills, M.R., and Sherlock, S.: The relief of bone pain in primary biliary cirrhosis with calcium infusions. Gut. 15:788, 1974.
15. Kehayoglou, A.K., Holdsworth, C.D., Agnew, J.E., Whelton, M.J., and Sherlock, S.: Bone disease and calcium absorption in primary biliary cirrhosis with special reference to vitamin D therapy. Lancet 1:715, 1968.

16. Atkinson, M., Nordin, B.E.C., and Sherlock, S.: Malabsorption
     and bone disease in prolonged obstructive jaundice. Quart.
     J. Med. 25:299, 1956.

MINOR INFLUENCE OF PARATHYROID HORMONE ON FRACTIONAL TUBULAR
REABSORPTION OF PHOSPHATE IN CHRONIC RENAL FAILURE

Christensen, M.S., Brøchner-Mortensen, J., Tougaard, L.,
Sørensen, E., and Rødbro, P.
Institute of Pharmacology, University of Aarhus, Aarhus
Departments of Clinical Physiology and Nephrology
Aalborg Hospital (Syd), Aalborg, Denmark

It is well established that a reduction of renal function is
accompanied by both a decrease in fractional tubular reabsorption
of phosphate (fTRP) (1,2) and by secondary hyperparathyroidism (3).
An inverse correlation between the serum concentration of parathyroid hormone (s-PTH) and fTRP is therefore found in chronic renal
failure. However, a correlation does not prove causality, and different opinions have appeared concerning the influence of parathyroid
hormone on tubular handling of phosphate in renal failure.

With the introduction of $1,25(OH)_2$cholecalciferol (1,25-D.H.C.C.)
and 1α-(OH)cholecalciferol (1α-H.C.C.) in clinical medicine it has
become possible to reduce the secondary hyperparathyroidism in
chronic renal failure for sustained periods of time (4). It is
therefore possible to study fTRP in patients with renal failure in
the presence of high concentrations of s-PTH before 1α-H.C.C. treatment and in the presence of much lower or even normal values of
s-PTH after treatment. An increase in fTRP after treatment with
1α-H.C.C. would indicate that parathyroid hormone has a major influence on renal handling of phosphate in renal failure.

PATIENTS

We studied 24 randomly selected patients with a glomerular
filtration rate between 5 and 25 ml/min, known to be relatively
stable. The patients were on a free diet, and continued their
normal medication during the treatment period. None of the patients
received phosphate binders or hormones. After random allocation
12 patients were treated for 11 weeks with an oral daily dose of

1 μg 1α-H.C.C. and 500 mg calcium as calciumlactogluconate. In 3 patients the dose of 1α-H.C.C. was reduced to half because of hypercalcemia. One of the treated patients has been omitted from this study because of unreliable urinary collections.

EXPERIMENTAL PROCEDURE

Before and after 1α-H.C.C. treatment fTRP was measured in the morning after an overnight fast with the patients supine. The glomerular filtration rate (GFR) was determined from the total plasma clearance of ^{51}chromium-EDTA, using a single injection technique without urine sampling (5,6). The renal clearance of phosphate was determined from a five hours urinary collection. Measurements of phosphorus concentrations in urine and serum was done on a Technicon SMA^R 12/60 system. The fractional tubular reabsorption of phosphate was calculated from:

$$fTRP = 1 - \frac{Phosphate\ Clearance}{GFR}$$

The serum concentration of parathyroid hormone (s-PTH) was measured by a sensitive radioimmunoassay on extracts of serum (7), drawn on the days when the fTRP was measured.

RESULTS

Before treatment fTRP was inversely correlated to s-PTH (r = -0.53, p<0.01), and s-PTH was inversely correlated to GFR (r = -0.61, p<0.01). With decreasing renal function fTRP decreased. Because of these closely linked interrelationships it was difficult to evaluate the influence of any one of these factors (PTH and GFR) on fTRP.

Fig. 1 shows the correlation between fTRP and s-PTH before treatment in the patients with GFR values at or below 10 ml/min (left) and in patients with GFR values between 10 and 25 ml/min (right). In patients with the low GFR values no correlation was found between fTRP and s-PTH (r = 0.04, n.s.). This is remarkable because the range of s-PTH in the patients was very broad, from 2 - 30 times upper normal level. The mean fTRP in this group was very low, 0.12. In patients with GFR values between 10 and 25 ml/min there was a significant inverse correlation between fTRP and s-PTH (r = -0.66, p<0.02). The mean fTRP in this group was 0.52.

These observations indicate that s-PTH may have a significant effect on fTRP in patients with GFR values between 10 and 25 ml/min,

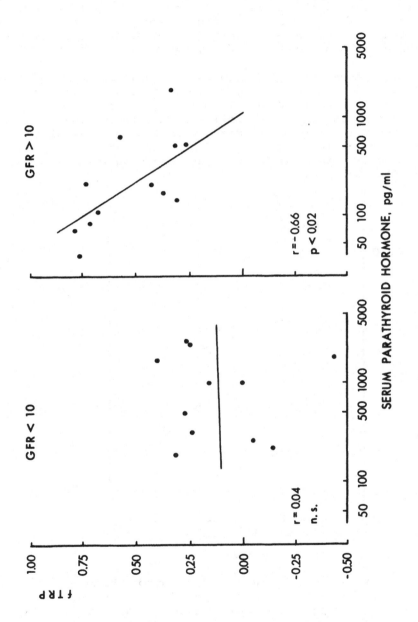

Fig.1 Correlation between fractional tubular reabsorption of phosphate (fTRP) and logarith-
mic values of serum parathyroid hormone in untreated patients with chronic renal failure.
Left: patients with glomerular filtration rate at or below 10 ml/min.
Right: patients with glomerular filtration rate between 10 and 25 ml/min.

whereas the significance of s-PTH for fTRP seems doubtful at very
low renal function (GFR<10 ml/min). If this holds true a decrease
in s-PTH during lα-H.C.C. treatment should cause an increase in
fTRP, demonstrable especially in patients with GFR above 10 ml/min.
In the following figures the values obtained before and after
lα-H.C.C. treatment are given separately for patients with pretreatment GFR values below and above 10 ml/min, respectively.

Fig. 2 shows the decrease in s-PTH on a logarithmic scale
during lα-H.C.C. treatment. S-PTH decreased on average 60%, from
a mean pretreatment value of 840 pg/ml to 335 pg/ml after therapy.
The per cent decrease in s-PTH was similar in the two groups of
patients, although the pretreatment mean s-PTH was twice as high
in the low GFR group as in the high GFR group. After treatment
s-PTH was below upper normal level in 2 patients with low GFR and
in 3 patients with high GFR.

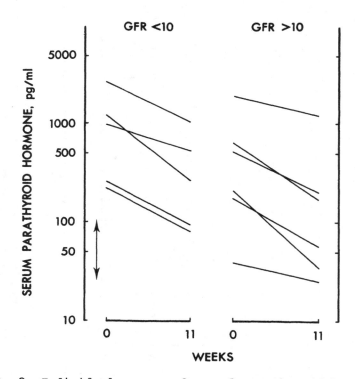

Fig.2 Individual serum values of parathyroid hormone
(logarithmic scale) before and after 11 weeks treatment
with lα-H.C.C. in patients with glomerular filtration
rate below 10 ml/min (left) and above 10 ml/min (right).
Arrows indicate normal range.

Fig. 3 shows the changes in fTRP during 1α–H.C.C. therapy.
There was a significant decrease in fTRP (mean 0.21) slightly
higher in patients with high (0.23) than in patients with low
GFR (0.18).

Fig. 4 shows the changes in GFR during 1α–H.C.C. treatment.
GFR decreased significantly from 11.8 to 8.6 ml/min (27.5%). The
per cent decrease in GFR was almost identical in patients with low
(30%) and in patients with high GFR (26.5%).

Since a reduction in GFR is accompanied by a decrease in
fTRP in spontaneously progressing renal failure, we compared the
mean decrease in fTRP observed during 1α–H.C.C. treatment with
the fall in fTRP occurring in untreated patients with the same
fall in GFR, calculated from the slope of the regression line
between fTRP and GFR found in our patients before treatment.
The observed fall in fTRP corresponded to the expected fall in fTRP.

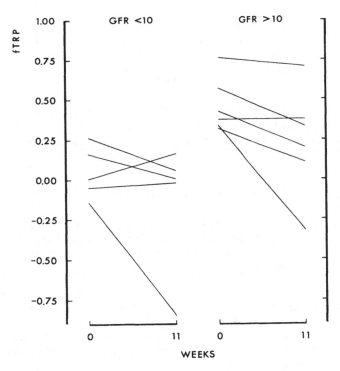

Fig.3 Individual values of fractional tubular reabsorption of phosphate (fTRP) before and after 11 weeks treatment with 1α–H.C.C. in patients with glomerular filtration
rate below 10 ml/min (left) and above 10 ml/min (right).

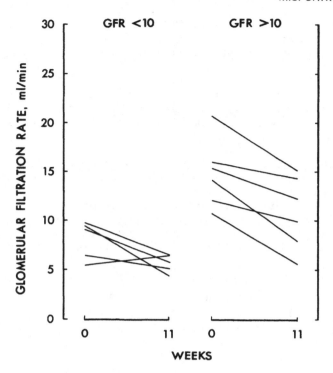

Fig. 4 Individual values of glomerular filtration rate
(GFR) before and after 11 weeks treatment with 1α-H.C.C.
in patients with GFR below 10 ml/min (left) and above
10 ml/min (right).

DISCUSSION

The main result of the present study was that a pronounced
reduction of secondary hyperparathyroidism induced by 1α-H.C.C.
treatment did not increase the fractional tubular reabsorption of
phosphate in renal failure.

The serum concentration of parathyroid hormone decreased on
average to 40% of pretreatment level and was below upper normal
level in 5 patients after treatment, but only in one patient before
treatment. The fractional tubular reabsorption of phosphate and
the glomerular filtration rate both decreased significantly during
1α-H.C.C. treatment.

Our results indicate that parathyroid hormone is of minor importance for the fractional tubular reabsorption of phosphate in chronic renal failure when glomerular filtration rate is below 25 ml/min. This is in accordance with the almost unchanged fractional excretion of phosphate found by Popovtzer et al. (8) in patients with chronic renal failure during normalization of serum calcium and reduction of secondary hyperparathyroidism induced with phosphate binding antacids and oral calcium supplements. Our results are, however, not consistent with the considerable increases of fractional tubular reabsorption of phosphate reported by Slatopolsky et al. (2) after normalization of serum calcium with phosphate binding antacids, oral calcium supplements and very high daily doses of vitamin-D_2 in patients with very low glomerular filtration rates (below 10 ml/min).

Infusions of parathyroid hormone to normal subjects and to patients with moderately impaired renal function has been shown to decrease the fractional tubular reabsorption of phosphate (1,2,9). Contrary to this, no change or a less pronounced decrease in fractional tubular reabsorption of phosphate was caused by parathyroid hormone infusion to patients with advanced renal failure (1,2,9).

It should be mentioned that the decrease in fractional tubular reabsorption of phosphate seen during treatment with 1α-H.C.C. corresponded to the fall that would occur in untreated patients with the same fall in glomerular filtration rate. This supports the hypothesis that renal handling of phosphate in advanced renal failure mainly is determined by other (GFR-related) factors than parathyroid hormone. A connection between renal handling of sodium and phosphate in renal failure has been shown by Coburn et al. (10).

SUMMARY

In <u>untreated</u> patients with chronic renal failure and glomerular filtration rates (GFR) between 10 and 25 ml/min the decrease in fractional tubular reabsorption of phosphate was correlated to the degree of secondary hyperparathyroidism. This correlation was not found in patients with GFR below 10 ml/min.

During treatment with 1α-hydroxycholecalciferol for 11 weeks
a) serum parathyroid hormone concentration decreased in all patients on average 60%, and was normal in 5 patients after treatment
b) fractional tubular reabsorption of phosphate decreased significantly (on average 0.21)
c) glomerular filtration rate decreased significantly (on average 27.5%).

Since the reduction (or normalization) of serum parathyroid hormone concentration did not increase the fractional tubular reabsorption of phosphate, other (GFR-related) factors than parathyroid hormone play the major role for renal handling of phosphate in chronic renal failure when GFR is below 25 ml/min.

REFERENCES

1. Goldman, R., and Bassett, S.H.: Phosphorous excretion in renal failure. J.Clin.Invest. 1623:33, 1954.

2. Slatopolsky, E., Robson, A.M., Elkan, I., and Bricker, N.S.: Control of phosphate excretion in uremic man. J.Clin.Invest. 47:1865, 1968.

3. Bordier, P.J., Marie, P.J., and Arnaud, C.D.: Evolution of renal osteodystrophy: Correlation of bone histomorphometry and serum mineral and immunoreactive parathyroid hormone values before and after treatment with calcium carbonate or 25-hydroxycholecalciferol. Kidney International. Supplementum No 2. S-102, 1975.

4. Tougaard, L., Sørensen, E., Brøchner-Mortensen, J., Christensen, M.S., Rødbro, P., and Sørensen, A.W.S.: Controlled trial of 1α-hydroxycholecalciferol in chronic renal failure. Lancet 1:1044, 1976.

5. Brøchner-Mortensen, J.: A simple routine method for the determination of glomerular filtration rate. Scand.J.clin.Lab.Invest. 30:271, 1972.

6. Brøchner-Mortensen, J., and Rödbro, P.: Selection of routine method for determination of glomerular filtration rate in adult patients. Scand.J.clin.Lab.Invest. 36:35, 1976.

7. Christensen, Merete Sanvig: A sensitive radioimmunoassay of parathyroid hormone using a specific extraction procedure. Scand.J.clin.Lab.Invest. (in press).

8. Popovtzer, M.M., Pinggera, W.F., Hutt, M.P., Robinette, J., Halgrimson, C.G., and Starzl, T.E.: Serum parathyroid hormone levels and renal handling of phosphorus in patients with chronic renal disease. J.Clin.Endocrinol.Metab. 35:213, 1972.

9. Massry, S.G., Coburn, J.W., Lee, D.B.N., Jowsey, J., and Kleeman, C.R.: Skeletal resistance to parathyroid hormone in renal failure. Ann.Intern.Med. 78:357, 1973.

10.   Coburn, J.W., Popovtzer, M.M., Massry, S.G., and Kleeman, C.R.:
      The physiocochemical state and renal handling of divalent ions
      in chronic renal failure. Arch.Intern.Med. 124:302, 1969.

THE MAXIMAL TUBULAR REABSORPTION OF PHOSPHATE IN RELATION TO SERUM PARATHYROID HORMONE

Madsen, S., Ølgaard, K. and Ladefoged, J.

Medical Dept. P, division of nephrology

Rigshospitalet, 2loo Copenhagen Ø, Denmark

The tubular reabsorption of phosphate is affected by multiple factors. It is well established that parathyroid hormone (PTH) causes phosphaturia, by depressing the renal tubular reabsorption of phosphate (1); but the renal function (2), the (intrarenal) calcium concentration (3), the acid-base balance (4), the extracellular volume (5), the circadian rhythm (6), steroids (7), diuretics (8) and vitamin-D (9) have to be taken into account, when the role of the parathyroid hormone in the regulation of the renal handling of phosphate is evaluated.

The maximal tubular reabsorption of phosphate (TmP) is highly correlated to the glomerular filtration rate (GFR) (lo). To reduce or eliminate the contribution of GFR to the variation of TmP, the latter must be expressed in relation to GFR. This TmP/GFR index appears to be the most consistent index of renal phosphate handling (11). This index was used to investigate whether a correlation exists between the renal handling of phosphate and the serum level of immunoreactive PTH (i-PTH) in a group of patients with a wide range of renal function and of i-PTH.

MATERIAL

The material consists of 15 patients (8 females, 7 males) with an age range of 19-58 years (mean 38). Seven patients (4 females, 3 males) had well functioning kidney allografts, with creatinine clearances of 43-65 ml/min (mean 59). Their age range was 22-58 years (mean

35.6). The average time of the present investigation
after the kidney transplantation was 18 months (range
6-6o). The kidney transplanted patients received a
daily prednisone dose of O (one patient)-25 mg (mean
12.9). None of these patients showed clinical or biochemical signs of rejection at the time of the investigation. Eight patients (4 females, 4 males) had varying degrees of chronic progressive renal insufficiency
with creatinine clearances of 27-2 ml/min (mean lo.6).
The age range was 19-58 years (mean 4o.5). No patient
received dialysis treatment. The basic nephrological
diseases were chronic glomerulonephritis in 2, chronic
interstitial nephropathy in 2, polycystic kidney disease
in 2 and congenital nephropathy in 2 patients. The
treatment with oral phosphate-binder (aluminium-amino-
acetate) in these patients was withdrawn 48 hours prior
to the study, and in the entire group any diuretic treatment was withdrawn 24 hours before the study. No patient
received vitamin D treatment.

METHODS
The investigations were carried out at 9 a.m. The seven
kidney transplanted patients, who were normo- or slightly hypophosphatemic (serum phosphate range o.72-1.o4
mmol/l), received an i.v. phosphate infusion in order
to obtain maximal renal phosphate reabsorption. The infusion consisted of a o.1 M solution of phosphate buffered at pH 7.4 delivered at a rate of loo ml/hour with
an infusion pump. After 6o min the seven patients were
hyperphosphatemic (serum phosphate range 1.74-2.47
mmol/l) and during continuous phosphate infusion, a
urine sample was collected in the following l2o min period. (All patients could void on request). Blood samples were collected every 3o min during the urine sampling and analyzed for phosphate. The average serum phosphate in the l2o min period was used in the calculations. In the middle of the investigation-period a blood
sample was collected and analyzed for i-PTH, calcium and
standard bicarbonate.
The eight patients with impaired renal function all had
a considerable degree of phosphate retention (serum
phosphate range 1.62-2.56 mmol/l), so the renal phosphate reabsorption could be regarded as maximal and no
phosphate was administered during the investigation.
GFR was estimated during the study, using the single
injection technique of ^{51}Cr EDTA (12), and similarly the
extracellular volume was calculated as the ^{51}Cr EDTA
distribution space (13). Total phosphate in plasma and
urine was measured as described by Dryer et al. (14),

PATIENT NO	TmP/GFR μMOL/ML	i-PTH NG/ML	TmP μMOL/MIN	GFR ML/MIN	SE-CA MMOL/L	SE-P MMOL/L
1(x)	0.85	2.1	36.9	43.1	2.68	1.74
2(x)	0.77	1.9	50.2	64.9	2.55	1.89
3(x)	0.74	1.9	42.5	57.3	2.48	2.01
4(x)	0.72	2.4	45.3	62.4	2.67	2.11
8	0.70	1.9	5.7	8.1	2.27	2.56
5(x)	0.69	2.8	42.9	61.5	2.41	1.92
9	0.69	1.4	18.3	26.7	2.38	2.47
6(x)	0.58	3.3	34.9	60.1	2.39	2.15
10	0.46	4.1	1.9	6.2	1.95	2.19
11	0.42	3.0	7.7	18.1	2.17	2.05
7(x)	0.38	4.3	24.0	62.1	2.60	2.47
12	0.35	3.5	4.1	11.7	2.08	1.62
13	0.11	9.5	1.1	4.1	2.33	1.81
14	0.08	4.7	0.2	2.3	2.29	1.67
15	0.03	13.0	0.5	7.5	2.49	1.97

Table I TmP/GFR index, i-PTH, TmP, GFR, serum calcium and serum phosphate in 8 uremic and 7 kidney transplanted (x) patients.

all phosphate values being expressed as mmol/l, and the
TmP (µmol/min) in the 12o min period was calculated as
the difference between filtered (GFR x mean serum phosphate) and excreted phosphate (urine phosphate x urine
volume/min). The analysis of PTH in serum was performed
by a radioimmunoassay based on the ability of human PTH
to compete with ^{125}I-labelled bovine PTH for binding to
a guinea-pig antiserum directed against bovine PTH (15).
Normal subjects had a range from 1.1 to 2.5 ng bovine
PTH equivalents/ml.

RESULTS
The values of GFR, TmP, TmP/GFR and i-PTH as determined
in the 15 patients are given in Table I. The GFR values
ranged from 2.3 to 64.9 ml/min (mean 33.1), in the group
of eight patients with chronic nephropathy from 2.3 to
26.7 ml/min (mean lo.6), and in the group of seven kidney transplanted patients from 43.1 to 64.9 ml/min (mean
58.8). The TmP values (mean 44.8 µmol/min) were significantly higher (p < o.ool) in the transplanted patients
than in the patients with chronic nephropathy (mean 4.9
µmol/min) and a linear correlation (r = o.95, p < o.ool)
between GFR and TmP was found in all 15 patients (Fig.
1).

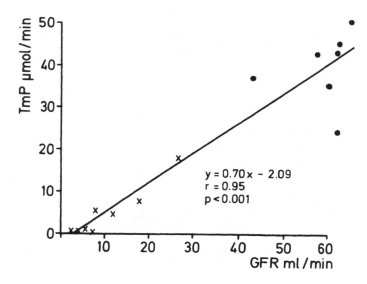

Fig. 1
Correlation between GFR and TmP in 8 uremic (x) and 7
kidney transplanted (●) patients.

To reduce the influence of GFR on TmP, the TmP/GFR index was calculated. This index varied over a wide range
(o.o3-o.85 µmol/ml, mean o.5o), and when related to
i-PTH, which also dispersed over a very wide range (1.4-
13.o ng/ml, mean 4.o) a significant inverse correlation
(r = -o.82, p < o.oo1) was found (Fig. 2). This relation
persisted when the influence of GFR was eliminated by
use of a partial correlation coefficient. Neither i-PTH
nor TmP/GFR showed any significant correlation to the
serum calcium concentration or the extracellular volume.
The serum standard bicarbonate concentration was significantly correlated to the TmP/GFR index (p < o.o5), but
when related to i-PTH, no significance was obtained.
Immunoreactive PTH concentrations were within the same
levels in the two groups of patients (p > o.o5). No correlation could be demonstrated between renal function
and i-PTH concentration (p > o.o5). Serum phosphate concentrations estimated at the same time as i-PTH did not
differ in the two groups, while serum calcium concentrations were higher in the group of transplanted patients
(mean 2.54 mmol/1), than in the group of patients with

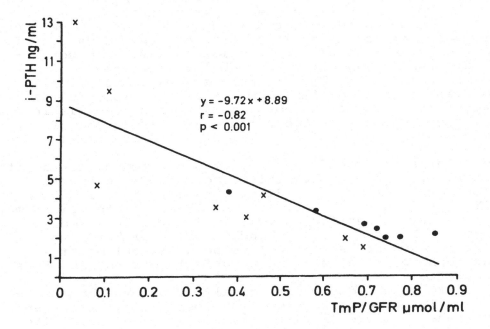

Fig. 2
Correlation between TmP/GFR-index and i-PTH in 8 uremic
(x) and 7 kidney transplanted (●) patients.

chronic nephropathy (mean 2.24 mmol/l) (Table I). A correlation between i-PTH and serum calcium could not be
demonstrated (p > o.l).
Finally, the reproducibility of the estimation of TmP
was calculated. Nine of the 15 patients had the procedure repeated in another 12o min period immediately after the first one. The technique was found to be reproducible, with a coefficient of variation of 14%.

DISCUSSION
In the present investigation the renal handling of phosphate was found to be inverse significantly correlated
to the serum concentration of i-PTH in persons with a
very wide range of TmP, GFR and i-PTH.
The possibility exists that this correlation could be
due to parallel changes in i-PTH and the renal handling
of phosphate without any causal connection. However, of
the mentioned factors known to influence the tubular reabsorption of phosphate, the i-PTH concentration in serum was the only one, which could be highly significantly
correlated to the TmP/GFR index. None of the patients
received vitamin-D, but their serum level of active vitamin-D at the time of the investigation may have affected the results. Only when a sensitive analysis of
1.25dihydroxycholecalciferol in serum has been developed,
this question can be answered. Six of the kidney transplanted patients received steroids (7.5-25 mg predniso-
ne/day), which may alter the tubular reabsorption of
phosphate (16). The TmP in these six patients (mean 39
μmol/min) did not differ from TmP in one transplanted
patient (no. 3) who did not receive prednisone (Table I).
This may suggest that the chronic administration of
prednisone in our patients did not alter the renal phosphate handling.
The material included 3 kidney transplanted patients with
persisting hyperparathyroidism and 6 uremic patients with
secondary hyperparathyroidism. This material, in which
i-PTH levels did not correlate to the renal function, may
explain why a significant correlation was obtained between i-PTH and the renal handling of phosphate, when
other investigators (17, 18) using different materials
(and techniques) have not been able to demonstrate this
correlation.
Thus, although radioimmunological PTH assays should always be interpreted with caution, especially in patients
with renal failure (19, 2o) it can, in accordance with
other investigators (21, 22, 23) be concluded that PTH
has a key role in the regulation of phosphate excretion
in patients with impaired renal function.

SUMMARY

The relation between the renal handling of phosphate and the serum concentration of immunoreactive parathyroid hormone (i-PTH) was investigated in 15 patients with a very wide range of i-PTH, glomerular filtration rate (GFR), maximal tubular reabsorption of phosphate (TmP) and TmP/GFR-ratio. The latter was used as an index of the renal handling of phosphate. Seven patients had well functioning kidney allografts (GFR 43.1-64.9 ml/min), while 8 had varying degrees of chronic nephropathy (GFR 2.3-26.7 ml/min). The TmP, i-PTH, ^{51}Cr EDTA clearance, the extracellular volume and serum concentrations of calcium and standard bicarbonate were estimated. An inverse significant correlation was demonstrated between TmP/GFR and i-PTH ($p < 0.001$), while none of the other investigated factors correlated to the TmP/GFR-index. It is concluded that the parathyroid hormone has a key role in the regulation of the tubular handling of phosphate in patients with impaired renal function.

REFERENCES

1. Hiatt, H.H. & Thompson, D.D.: J. Clin. Invest. 36: 557, 1957.

2. Goldman, R. & Basset, S.H.: J. Clin. Invest. 33: 1623, 1954.

3. Cuche, J.L., Ott, C.E., Marchand, G.R., Diaz-Buxo, J.A. & Knox, F.G.: Am. J. Physiol. 230: 790, 1976.

4. Schiess, W.A., Ayer, J.L., Lotspeich, W.D. & Pitts, R.F.: J. Clin. Invest. 27: 57, 1948.

5. Massry, S.G., Coburn, J.W. & Kleeman, C.R.: J. Clin. Invest. 48: 1237, 1969.

6. Ollayos, R.W. & Winkler, A.W.: J. Clin. Invest. 22: 147, 1943.

7. Nassim, J.R., Saville, P.D. & Mulligan, L.: Clin. Sci. 15: 367, 1956.

8. Eknoyan, G., Suki, W.N. & Martinez-Maldonado, M.: J. Lab. Clin. Med. 76: 257, 1970.

9. Puschett, J.B., Moranz, J. & Kurnick, W.S.: J. Clin. Invest. 51: 373, 1972.

lo. Bijvoet, O.L.M.: Clin. Sci. 37: 23, 1969.

11. Stamp, T.C.B. & Stacey, T.E.: Clin. Sci. 39: 5o5, 197o.

12. Nosslin, B.: Acta Med. Scand., Suppl. 97: 442, 1965.

13. Ladefoged, J.: Europ. J. Clin. Invest. 5: 72, 1975.

14. Dryer, R.L., Tammes, A.R. & Routh, J.I.: J. biol. Chem. 225: 177, 1957.

15. Almqvist, S., Hjern, B. & Wästhed, B.: Acta Endocr. 78: 493, 1975.

16. Roberts, K.E. & Pitts, R.F.: Endocrinology 52: 324, 1953.

17. Gill, G., Palotta, J., Kashgarian, M., Kessner, D. & Epstein, F.H.: Am. J. Med. 46: 93o, 1969.

18. Popovtzer, M.M., Pinggera, W.F., Hutt, M.P., Robinette, J., Halgrimson, C.G. & Starzl, T.E.: J. Clin. Endocr. 35: 213, 1972.

19. Arnaud, C.D.: Kidney Int. 4: 89, 1973.

2o. Reiss, E. & Canterbury, J.M.: Proc. 4th. Int. Congr. Nephrol., Stockholm 2: 164, 1969.

21. Agus, Z.S., Gardner, L.B., Beck, L.H. & Goldberg, M.: Am. J. Physiol. 224: 1143, 1973.

22. Falls, W.F., Carter, N.W., Rector, F.C. & Seldin, D.W.: Clin. Res. 14: 74, 1966.

23. Slatopolsky, E., Robson, A.M., Elkan, I. & Bricker, N.S.: J. Clin. Invest. 47: 1865, 1968.

THE POSTPROXIMAL SITE OF PHOSPHATE REABSORPTION IN PRESENCE AND ABSENCE OF PARATHYROID HORMONE

Greger, R., Lang, F., Marchand, G., Knox, F.G.

Dept. of Physiology & Biophysics, Mayo Foundation

Rochester MN 55901, U.S.A.

From previous studies there is ample evidence that phosphate, in addition to its proximal reabsorption is reabsorbed at some postproximal site (1-3,5,6,8,9,11). In free flow micropuncture studies this reabsorption has at least partially been ascribed to the distal tubule and collecting duct system (1,5). In microinjection studies, on the other hand, no reabsorption of phosphate beyond the loop of Henle could be detected (4,10). These data, however, are methodologically not unequivocal since the phosphate load injected exceeded the amount of phosphate which ought to be expected there under conditions of free flowing tubular fluid. The free flow micropuncture data also are subject to restricted interpretation since it seems likely that nephron heterogeneity in regard to phosphate reabsorption exists between superficial cortical and deeper nephrons.

Therefore, it seemed justified to reinvestigate this question of postproximal phosphate reabsorption (7). The specific refinements of the study reported here included the following. 1. Phosphate determinations in the micropuncture samples were done with a colorimetric determination of higher sensitivity which allowed accurate phosphate measurement even in distal samples in TPTX animals. 2. The microinjection technique was adapted to keep the phosphate load to the injection site well below the expected load to ease the detection even of a small capacity reabsorption mechanism. This was accomplished by: a) blocking the tubular flow proximal to the site of injection, b) microinjection rates as low as 8 nl/min and c) phosphate concentrations in the microinjectate of 2 mmol/l for intact animals and 0.1 mmol/l for TPTX animals. 3. Both micropuncture and microinjection experiments were done in the same intact and TPTX Munich Wistar rats.

The free flow micropunctures in intact rats revealed that
there is a rapid decline in phosphate delivery along the proximal
tubule. Only some 38% of the filtered phosphate load is delivered
to the loop of Henle, here defined arbitrarily as the nephron
segment between the last proximal and the first distal loop
accessible to micropuncture. The distal delivery is still some 37%.
The mean fractional excretion in urine however is only 24%. After
end proximal microinjection in the same animals some 58% of the
injected amount of phosphate is recovered in urine. After distal
microinjection urinary phosphate recovery is complete (101%).
Since no distal reabsorption can be shown,the observed discrepancy
between urinary and distal phosphate delivery is most likely due
to nephron heterogeneity.

Analogous experiments in acutely TPTX-ed rats revealed that
under free flow conditions the decline of phosphate delivery along
the proximal tubule is much steeper than in the intact animals.
Only some 14% of the filtered load of phosphate is delivered to
the loop. There is significant loop reabsorption. The distal delivery of phosphate is only 4%. Fractional urinary excretion of
phosphate averages 1.7%. After end proximal microinjection in the
same animals, only some 5% of the amount of microinjected phosphate
appears in urine. This finding, in accordance with the micropunctures,indicates marked loop reabsorption of phosphate. After
distal microinjection, urinary phosphate recovery is essentially
complete (95%).

The sensitivity of the loop reabsorption of phosphate to PTH
was tested in recollection microperfusion experiments of loop
segments in TPTX-animals in the absence and the presence of exogenous PTH. In the absence of PTH, a marked loop reabsorption of
phosphate can be demonstrated. After i.v. injection of 10 U PTH
this reabsorption decreases significantly and approaches zero.
Thirty minutes after the PTH injection phosphate reabsorption
returns to baseline levels. Therefore,the loop reabsorption of
phosphate is sensitive to PTH.

An attempt was made to localize further the site of phosphate
reabsorption in the loop of TPTX rats by using a modified split
droplet technique. Between 1 and 2 nl of a P32 phosphate and H3
inulin containing fluid were injected into late proximal tubules,
descending limbs, ascending limbs of the loop, and distal convoluted
tubules. After an exposure to the tubular epithelium of up to 100
seconds the fluid was reaspirated and the fractional phosphate recovery measured. The data clearly demonstrated that in proximal
tubules, as in descending limbs of the loop, rapid reabsorption of
phosphate takes place whereas both the ascending limb of the loop
and the distal convoluted tubule appear impermeable to phosphate.

From the above data it can be concluded that: (1) the post proximal site of phosphate reabsorption is localized in the descending limb of the loop of Henle; (2) this reabsorption is sensitive to PTH; and (3) since no phosphate reabsorption beyond the loop could be demonstrated, the discrepancy between urinary and distal phosphate delivery is due to nephron heterogeneity.

Acknowledgment

*This work was supported by travel funds of "Deutsche Forschungs-gemeinschaft".

References

1. Amiel, C., H. Kuntziger, and G. Richet: Micropuncture study of handling of phosphate by proximal and distal nephron in normal and parathyroidectomized rat. Evidence for distal reabsorption. Pflügers Arch. 317:93-109, 1970.
2. Beck, L.H., and M. Goldberg: Effects of acetazolamide and parathyroidectomy on renal transport of sodium, calcium and phosphate. Am. J. Physiol. 224:1136-1142, 1973.
3. Beck, L.H., and M. Goldberg: Mechanism of the blunted phosphaturia in saline-loaded thyroparathyroidectomized dogs. Kidney Int. 6:18-23, 1974.
4. Brunette, M.G., L. Taleb, and S. Carriere: Effect of parathyroid hormone on phosphate reabsorption along the nephron of the rat. Am. J. Physiol. 225:1076-1081, 1973.
5. Chiu, P.J.S., Z.S. Agus, and M. Goldberg: Effect of thyroparathyroidectomy (TPTX) on renal phosphate transport in the rat. Clin. Res. 22:520, 1974 (Abstr.).
6. Knox, F.G., and C. Lechene: Distal site of action of parathyroid hormone on phosphate reabsorption. Am.J.Physiol. 229:1556-1560, 1975.
7. Knox, F.G., E.G. Schneider, L.R. Willis, J.W. Strandhoy, and C.E. Ott: Site and control of phosphate reabsorption by the kidney. Kidney Int. 3:347-353, 1973.
8. Kuntziger, H., C. Amiel, and C. Gaudebout: Phosphate handling by the rat nephron during saline diuresis. Kidney Int. 2:318-323, 1972.
9. Maesaka, J.K., M.F. Levitt, and R.G. Abramson: Effect of saline infusion on phosphate transport in intact and thyroparathyroidectomized rats. Am.J.Physiol. 225:1421-1429, 1973.
10. Staum, B.B., R.J. Hamburger, and M. Goldberg: Tracer microinjection study of renal tubular phosphate reabsorption in the rat. J.Clin.Invest. 51; 2271-2276, 1972.
11. Wen, S.F.: Micropuncture studies of phosphate transport in the proximal tubule of the dog. J.Clin.Invest. 53:143-153, 1974.

SATURATION KINETICS OF PHOSPHATE REABSORPTION IN RATS

F. Lang, R. Greger, G. Marchand and F. Knox

Dept. of Physiology & Biophysics, Mayo Foundation

Rochester MN 55901, U.S.A.

It is a well known fact that increasing plasma concentration
of phosphate is followed by enhancement of phosphate clearance,
a finding which has been ascribed to saturation of phosphate reabsorption. However, although it has been possible to determine a
maximal transport rate for a given experimental situation, further
description of the kinetics has not been possible with the use of
clearance techniques.
In the present paper attempts to define maximal transport rate and
affinity of the reabsorptive transport process in proximal convoluted tubules and loops of Henle will be reported.

Male Munich Wistar rats (n=19) were thyroparathyroidectomized(PX)
and prepared for micropuncture in the usual way. The technique of
continuous in vivo microperfusion was applied to proximal convoluted
tubules (n=96) and loops of Henle (n=104). The perfused segments
were isolated from the remaining nephron by castor oil droplets.
Phosphate concentration in the initial perfusate was varied from
0.1 to 10 mM. Phosphate reabsorption was estimated from the disappearance of ^{32}Phosphate from the luminal fluid. ^{3}H-inulin was
used as a volume marker. Phosphate recovery (R) in the collected
fluid was calculated from the phosphate and Inulin concentrations
in the collected fluid (P,In) and perfusate (Po,Ino): R= (P/In)/
(Po/Ino). In perfusions of proximal convoluted tubules, the perfusate was made up to prevent net water fluxes (110 mM Na^{+}, 70 mM
Mannitol). The perfusion rate was 8 nl/min. The length of perfused
segments was determined with the use of latex casts. In perfusions
of loops of Henle, no mannitol was added to the perfusate (145 mM
Na^{+}), the perfusion rate was varied from 8 to 32 nl/min and the
length of the perfused loops was not accounted for.

In proximal convoluted tubules, the decline of phosphate recovery in the collected fluid as a function of the length of perfused segments was linear with high phosphate concentrations in the perfusate and approached an exponential slope with low concentrations. Therefore, linear regressions were calculated from the experiments with high concentrations in the perfusate, and regressions based on an integrated Michaelis-Menten kinetic were calculated from the data points with low concentrations. From the slopes of the respective regressions, the luminal concentrations of phosphate (C) and the perfusion rate, the reabsorptive transport rate (I) could be calculated for each experiment. If transport rate is in linear proportion to the concentration of a hypothetical substrate-carrier complex and if the concentration of this complex is in linear proportion to the product of the concentration of free carrier and free substrate, Michaelis-Menten kinetics can be applied for the description of transport: $I = C \ I_{max}/(C + K_M)$, where I_{max} is the maximal transport rate and K_M the concentration at half saturation. Plotting $1/I$ versus $1/C$, I versus I/C, and C/I versus C should result in a linear pattern of the data points. Indeed no systematic deviation from linearity was apparent in any of the plots. Obviously, minor deviations from linearity might have been obscured by the scatter of the data. Analysis of the linear regressions allowed estimates of I_{max} and K_M from the slopes and intercepts. I_{max} was, as derived from the respective plots 15.1, 13.3 and 14.3 pmol/min mm, K_M was 1.2, 0.8 and 1.1 mM. The regression coefficients of the linear regressions were .96, .77, and .92, respectively. Since various segments from the entire length of the proximal tubule (excluding the first 0.5 - 1 mm and the portion beyond the reach of micropuncture) were perfused, the data should be understood as an average of early and late segments and do not address inhomogeneity of the proximal tubule. Comparison with free flow data reveals that phosphate reabsorption is more avid in the first mm of the proximal tubule than in the segments microperfused in this study.

In loops of Henle, transport rate was calculated from the perfusion rate, phosphate concentration in the initial perfusate, and recovery of phosphate in the collected fluid. As with the data from proximal tubules, $1/I$ was plotted versus $1/C$, I versus I/C and C/I versus C. As derived from the respective plots, I_{max} was 16.9, 17.5 and 18.5 pmol/min and K_M was 0.2, 0.2, and 0.3 mM. The regression coefficients were .93, .79, and .99, respectively. Again, no systematic deviation from linearity was apparent in any of the plots. The data clearly show that the affinity of phosphate reabsorption is much higher in loops of Henle than proximal convoluted tubules. Since, during maximal reabsorption, the loop of Henle reabsorbs only slightly more phosphate than 1 mm of proximal tubule, the maximal transport rate in the loops appears relatively low. At luminal concentrations of $\geq$ 2 mM, phosphate reabsorption was 16.3, 17.7, and 16.1 pmol/min with luminal flow rates of 8,20, and 32 nl/min, respectively. Therefore, luminal flow rate appears to be no determinant of maximal transport rate in the loop of Henle. The high affinity of the transport process especially in the loop of Henle allows phosphate reabsorption to be almost complete and excretion to be minimal even when the reabsorptive process operates close to saturation. The high affinity and limited transport capacity allow therefore efficient regulation of plasma concentration even in absence of parathyroid hormone (PTH).

The effect of PTH was tested by injection of synthetic PTH during the microperfusion experiments. No significant effect of PTH could be demonstrated in proximal convoluted tubules. This might be related to the blockage of tubule flow. In loops of Henle, PTH was effective despite the isolation of the perfused segments from the tubule flow. The effect, however, appeared to be smaller than would be expected from free flow data. The effect of PTH was smaller at low than at high luminal concentrations. Therefore, PTH appears to exert its regulatory effect by reducing the maximal transport rate. A similar conclusion can be derived from clearance data, where the magnitude of the effect of PTH on phosphate reabsorption was similar at endogenous and increased plasma concentrations.

Acute systemic phosphate infusion had no appreciable effect on phosphate reabsorption in microperfused segments of the proximal tubule. In additional micropuncture (n=2) and clearance experiments, systemic phosphate infusion failed to increase net phosphate reabsorption. In contrast with prolonged exposure (2h) to increased plasma concentrations (> 4 mM) a significant decline of phosphate reabsorption could be observed in PX animals both in absence and presence of exogenous PTH. The failure of systemic phosphate infusion to result in significant enhancement of phosphate reabsorption is at least partially due to the high affinity and limited transport capacity of phosphate reabsorption as apparent from the microperfusion experiments.

This study has been supported by a travel grant from the Deutsche Forschungsgemeinschaft.

HYPOCALCIURIC EFFECT OF LITHIUM IN MAN

P.D. Miller, M.D., S.L. Dubovsky, M.D., R.W. Schrier,
M.D., K.M. McDonald, M.D., and C. Arnaud, M.D.
Renal Div., Dept. of Med. and Dept. of Psychiatry, Univ.
of Colo. Med. Ctr., and Endocr. Res. Lab., Mayo Clinic
Denver, Colorado and Rochester, Minnesota

Lithium has been shown to inhibit the adenylate cyclase,
cyclic-AMP responses to arginine vasopressin in both in vivo (1-3)
as well as in vitro assay systems (3-5). Alternatively, it has
been shown that lithium may potentiate the cyclic AMP responses to
other polypeptide hormones (6-7) although these effects have not
been consistent (8). Additionally, lithium has been reported to
have divergent effects on urinary calcium excretion in experimental
animals (7-10) and man (11). Consequently, we studied the effects
of chronic lithium administration on the renal handling of calcium
and the renal response to the administration of parathyroid hormone.
Though we demonstrated neither a potentiating nor inhibiting effect
of lithium on the renal response to parathyroid hormone, we did
observe a significant reduction in basal twenty-four hour urinary
calcium excretion during lithium therapy.

METHODS

Seven patients who were previously diagnosed as having a manic
depressive disorder and were to receive lithium therapy were ad-
mitted to the Clinical Research Center. Informed consent was
obtained. There were five men (ages: 21 to 53) and two women
(ages: 46 and 51). Each subject was placed on a constant normal
diet of sodium (120-194 mEq/day), potassium (75-95 mEq/day), calcium (575-1300 mg/day) and phosphorus (760-1740 mg/day) for 3 days
prior to the initiation of any studies. None had received any
lithium carbonate previously and had had all other medications discontinued four weeks prior to their admission. Except for P.D. who
was found to have mild primary hypothyroidism during her control
study and J.B. who had a normal free T_4 but a high TSH level before

lithium and a low free T$_4$ and higher TSH after lithium despite
being clinically euthyroid, none had any known prior significant
chronic medical illnesses. Patient P.D. was subsequently studied
on lithium while euthyroid on 200 µg of synthyroid per day. Subject J.Ca. was studied on three occasions: before lithium administration, during lithium administration, and again six weeks after
lithium administration had been discontinued. After control, pre-
lithium studies had been completed, each subject was given lithium
carbonate, 900-1800 mg/day and were discharged to the Colorado State
Hospital where frequent plasma lithium levels were monitored and
dietary constituents approximating the diets on the Clinical Research Center were continued. During a three to four week period,
the plasma lithium was maintained at between 0.5-1.50 mEq/L, and
the subjects were then all readmitted to the Clinical Research
Center of the University of Colorado Medical Center for repeat
studies on lithium. Both before and during lithium administration,
the subjects were evaluated psychiatrically by one of us (S.D.)
and the level of activity of the subjects was not different during
the control or experimental periods.

Both before and during lithium administration, subjects underwent the following studies after 3 days on their constant diets:

Days 1-3: At 7:00 A.M. peripheral venous blood was drawn
without tourniquet application for the measurement of total protein,
hematocrit, total and ionized calcium, magnesium, phosphorus,
creatinine, parathyroid hormone, lithium, sodium, potassium,
chloride, and bicarbonate. Plasma total and free thyroxin and
thyroid stimulating hormone were also measured on the first day.
Twenty-four hour urine collections were evaluated for creatinine,
calcium, phosphorus, magnesium, sodium, and cyclic-AMP.

On the fourth day after baseline blood was drawn at 7:00 A.M.,
six of the seven subjects voided at 8:00 A.M. and then received an
intravenous infusion of 1000 ml of 5% dextrose in water (D^{5}W) at a
constant rate of 1.0 ml/min from 8:00 A.M. to 4:00 P.M. Infusions
could not be performed on one subject (J.B.) because of technical
difficulties with intravenous catheters. Hourly urine and bloods
were collected and analyzed for previously mentioned chemistries.
The subjects remained supine throughout the 8 hour study except to
void and ate all meals during this time. Blood was drawn by the
use of a second intravenous catheter kept patent between blood
drawings by a heparized saline solution. On the fifth day of the
study, the exact same D^{5}W procedure as performed on day 4 was repeated with the exception that on this fifth day 10 units/kg of
parathyroid hormone (Lilly) was added to the D^{5}W solution.

Total calcium (normal: 9.0-10.6 mg%), magnesium (normal:
1.8-2.3 mg%), and phosphorus (normal: 2.5-4.5 mg%) were measured

by atomic absorption spectrophotometry while ionized calcium (normal: 4.1-4.8 mg%) was measured using the orion flow-through elec-
trode ionalyzer. In vitro, lithium concentrations ranging between
0-90 mg% were shown not to alter the atomic absorption determination
of calcium. Creatinine was measured by the modification of the
Jaffe reaction while the sodium was determined by flame photometry.
Parathormone (normal: 9-40 mEq/L) was measured by one of us (C.A.)
using an antibody (GP-1) which detects predominately the carboxy
terminal portion of the parathormone molecule. Urinary cyclic-AMP
was determined by a modification of the competitive protein binding assay of Gilman (12). Serum lithium was measured by autoanalyzer. Total and free thyroxine (normals: 4.7-10.7 μg% and .45-
1.1 μg%, respectively) were measured by competitive protein binding while the thyroid stimulation hormone (normal: 1.0-11.0 mμ/
ml) level was measured by radioimmunoassay.

RESULTS

The individual and mean results of the first three control
and experimental days are shown in Table I. There was a significant decrease in the mean 24 hour urinary calcium excretion in the
seven subjects from 210 ± 52 SEM mg/24 hours to 93 ± 21 mg/24
hours (p<.025). Figure 1 shows these results graphically. Each
subject except for W.B. had a decrease in calcium excretion on
lithium. No change in urinary calcium excretion was observed in
W.B. whose control calcium excretions were very low. There was no
obvious explanation for this low calcium excretion in this subject
whose serum calcium, phosphorus, magnesium, alkaline phosphatase
and PTH levels were normal as were his bone x-rays and creatinine
clearance. He was on no medication which could alter calcium
excretion. Two subjects (J.Ca. and S.V.) had persistent hypercalciuria before lithium and became normocalciuric during lithium
treatment. The effect of lithium to decrease urinary calcium
excretion was abolished in patient J.Ca. when he again became persistently hypercalciuric four weeks after discontinuation of his
lithium. The reduction in urinary calcium excretion was seen despite no significant decrease in urinary sodium, phosphorus or magnesium excretion (Table I) or creatinine clearance (Table I). Although there was no significant change in the mean urinary cyclic-
AMP excretion in the seven subjects, urinary cyclic-AMP did fall
substantially in two subjects (K.R. and W.B.) and increased slightly in one other (J.B.) (Table II). None of these patients, however,
were the hypercalciuric subjects. Although there was no change in
the total serum calcium, there was a significant increase in the
mean ionized serum calcium concentration during lithium therapy
(4.59 ± .10 to 4.88 ± .11, p<.05) (Table II). The rise in ionized
calcium, however, only slightly exceeded the upper limit for the
normal range in our laboratory. There was no significant change

TABLE I

PATIENT	DAY	WEIGHT KG		$U_{Na}V$ MEQ/DAY		$U_{Ca}V$ MG/DAY		U_PV MG/DAY		$U_{Ma}V$ MG/DAY		C_RCL ML/MIN	
		PRE-Li	Li	PRE-Li	Li	PRE-Li	Li	PRE-Li	Li	PRE-Li	Li	PRE-Li	Li
J.Ca.	1	160.2	165.5	177	196	352	128	1309	1283	169	141	154	120
	2	163.5	165.6	137	153	342	115	1240	1342	156	153	129	135
	3	161.0	164.7	181	123	296	74	1408	1430	152	172	165	159
	X̄	161.5	165.2	165	157	330	106	1319	1352	159	155	149	138
K.R.	1	158.7	159.7	68	95	260	143	1101	794	141	154	90	87
	2	161	160.7	129	184	254	198	1222	1150	126	179	96	96
	3	160	159.2	106	186	219	150	1131	1285	155	178	98	108
	X̄	159.9	159.8	101	155	244	163	1151	1076	141	170	95	97
J.B.	1	134	136	71	100	88	17	712	622	40	67	47	72
	2	132	134	45	90	40	13	647	642	30	49	36	60
	3	134	134	120	65	72	8	930	930	42	34	45	47
	X̄	133	134	77	85	67	13	763	763	37	50	43	59
W.B.	1	175.5	174	111	145	15	18	1136	751	106	116	135	139
	2	175.7	175.7	116	142	19	16	943	1069	108	159	153	146
	3	175.2	173.2	112	118	14	23	609	841	91	134	115	147
	X̄	175.3	174.3	113	135	16	19	896	887	102	136	134	144
J.C.	1	141.5	145	114	181	167	165	1172	1255	151	173	140	110
	2	141.5	145	150	118	275	125	1486	1205	202	146	111	99
	3	141.5	144	81	52	127	58	957	660	92	60	99	65
	X̄	141.5	145	115	117	190	116	1205	840	148	126	117	92

TABLE I (continued)

PATIENT	DAY	WEIGHT KG		$U_{Na}V$ MEQ/DAY		$U_{Ca}V$ MG/DAY		U_PV MG/DAY		$U_{Ma}V$ MG/DAY		C_RCL ML/MIN	
		PRE-Li	Li	PRE-Li	Li	PRE-Li	Li	PRE-Li	Li	PRE-Li	Li	PRE-Li	Li
P.D.	1	144.5	136.0	91	59	207	108	731	1114	101	115	94	116
	2	145.0	133.5	99	54	195	128	760	1183	85	132	81	107
	3	145.0	133.2	142	53	243	115	962	956	92	115	87	91
	X̄	144.8	134.2	111	55	215	117	816	1084	93	121	87	105
S.V.	1	159.2	157.2	173	142	395	144	1219	1236	146	128	129	94
	2	155.0	157.0	134	122	402	58	1482	1558	148	68	111	102
	3	155.0	157.0	134	70	422	149	1381	1019	132	122	106	80
	X̄	156.4	157.0	147	111	406	117	1360	1271	152	106	115	92
MEAN		153	153	118	116	210	93	1073	1017	117	123	106	104
SE		5.4	5.9	11	14	52	21	92	97	16	15	13	11
P		NS		NS		<.025		NS		NS		NS	

TABLE II

PATIENT	DAY	URINE C-AMP μM/G CREATININE		SERUM CALCIUM TOTAL MG%		SERUM CALCIUM IONIZED MG%		PTH MEQ/L	
		PRE-Li	Li	PRE-Li	Li	PRE-Li	Li	PRE-Li	Li
J.Ca.	1	4.22	5.72	10.2	11.0	-	4.80	19	20
	2	4.29	3.74	9.2	10.5	-	4.56		
	3	3.56	3.64	10.0	10.7	-			
	$\overline{X}$	4.02	4.36	9.8	10.7	-			
K.R.	1	6.53	3.99	9.5	9.4	4.08	4.64	17	26
	2	7.34	4.66	9.8	9.2	4.56	4.64		
	3	9.39	3.80	9.0	9.5	4.68	4.84		
	$\overline{X}$	7.75	4.15	9.43	9.36	4.44	4.70		
J.B.	1	3.48	6.56	9.7	9.5	4.28	4.48	27	35
	2	3.54	7.11	9.8	9.8	4.52	4.76		
	3	5.01	6.85	9.3	9.5	4.48	4.72		
	$\overline{X}$	4.01	6.84	9.6	9.6	4.42	4.65		
W.B.	1	6.13	3.83	9.3	9.3	4.64	4.60	20	21
	2	6.04	3.39	9.3	9.5	4.84	4.60		
	3	6.19	3.67	9.3	9.4	4.68	4.52		
	$\overline{X}$	6.12	3.63	9.3	9.4	4.72	4.57		
J.C.	1	3.88	6.38	9.9	9.9	4.60	4.96	29	34
	2	5.32	3.04	9.7	9.3	4.53	5.16		
	3	4.61	3.81	9.5	9.3	4.44	5.28		
	$\overline{X}$	4.60	4.41	9.7	9.5	4.52	5.13		
P.D.	1	5.23	6.03	9.3	9.5	4.20	5.04	25	29
	2	5.07	5.62	10.4	9.5	4.40	4.76		
	3	5.06	5.41	10.0	8.3	4.72	5.16		
	$\overline{X}$	5.12	5.68	9.9	9.1	4.44	4.98		
S.V.	1	3.43	4.24	10.2	9.2	5.04	4.96	30	26
	2	3.29	4.24	9.8	10.0	4.76	5.36		
	3	3.35	4.24	10.3	9.6	5.32	5.48		
	$\overline{X}$	3.36	4.24	10.1	9.6	5.04	5.26		
MEAN		4.99	4.75	9.69	9.60	4.59	4.88	24	28
SE		.57	.43	.10	.19	.10	.11	2	2
P		NS		NS		<.05		NS	

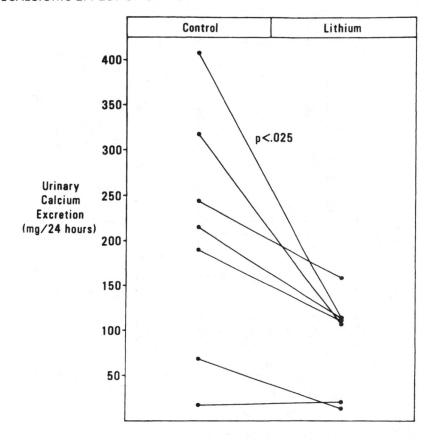

FIGURE 1. Effect of Lithium on Urinary Calcium Excretion in Patients with Affective Psychiatric Disorders

in the mean parathyroid hormone level, although the PTH level did rise in six of seven subjects. In no subject, however, did the PTH exceed the upper normal limit (Table II).

The results of the infusions of 5% dextrose in water without and with the addition of exogenous parathyroid hormone are shown in Table III and Figure 2. The data for each patient in Table III represent the mean clearance data of eight one hour urine and blood collections during the infusions. Proof that the exogenous para-thormone was metabolically active is shown by the significant in-creases in the tubular reabsorption of ionized calcium (TRCa++) and urinary cyclic-AMP excretions and the decrease in the tubular re-

TABLE III

	TUBULAR REABSORPTION TOTAL CALCIUM (%)				TUBULAR REABSORPTION IONIZED CALCIUM (%)				TUBULAR REABSORPTION PHOSPHORUS (%)				URINE CYCLIC AMP (μM/G GREAT)			
	PRE-Li		Li		PRE-Li		Li		PRE-Li		Li		PRE-Li		Li	
PT.	D^5W	PTH	D^5W	PTH	D^5W	PTH	D^5W	PTH	D^5W	PTH	D^5W	PTH	D^5W	PTH	D^5W	PTH
J.Ca.	98.6	99.2	99.8	99.7					87.7	78.7	84.5	70.0	3.52	8.87	3.65	13.12
K.R.	97.5	98.3	98.1	99.3	94.9	96.4	97.2	98.6	81.4	66.5	79.7	59.4	8.13	25.3	3.95	17.4
W.B.	99.9	99.8	99.8	99.9	99.8	99.7	99.7	99.9	89.4	75.9	87.9	72.4	5.37	15.6	3.19	12.9
J.C.	97.8	98.7	99.1	99.9	96.5	97.3	98.3	99.9	82.5	68.1	81.5	73.6	4.85	10.5	3.49	10.3
P.D.	97.1	98.4	98.8	99.5	96.7	97.2	97.2	99.2	76.2	63.5	81.8	66.1	7.13	15.9	5.34	13.83
S.V.	97.8	96.1	98.9	99.2	95.2	96.1	97.7	98.3	72.9	67.4	84.4	66.3	4.47	19.04	3.11	16.98
MEAN	98.1	98.4	99.2	99.6	96.6	97.3	98.0	99.2	81.7	70.0	83.3	67.9	5.58	15.89	3.78	14.1
SE	.41	.51	.28	.13	.86	.63	.47	.33	2.61	2.41	1.19	2.12	.70	2.42	.33	1.10
P		NS		NS		<.05		<.025		<.001		<.001		<.005		<.001
MEAN CHANGE		+.255		+.540		+.690		+1.16		-11.7		-15.3		+10.30		+10.30
SE		+.465		.197		+.258		+3.25		- 1.5		- 1.7		1.94		1.14
P			NS				NS				NS				NS	

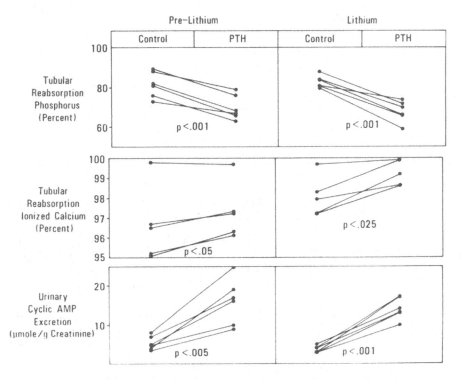

FIGURE 2.   Effect of Parathyroid Hormone (PTH) on the Tubular Re-
absorption of Phosphorus and Ionized Calcium and Urinary Cyclic-
AMP Excretion Before and During Lithium Therapy in Patients with
Affective Psychiatric Disorders

absorption of phosphorus.   However, there were no significant differences in these effects of PTH during the lithium treatment.
There were also no differences in the creatinine clearances during
the infusions.   It should be noted that despite a significant effect
of exogenous parathyroid hormone to increase the tubular reabsorption of ionized calcium, no such effect could be demonstrated for
the total serum calcium.   Although the change brought about by the
parathyroid hormone was in the positive direction for the biological effect of the hormone on total renal calcium reabsorption, this
did not reach statistical significance.   Since the ionized calcium
is a better representation of the filtered calcium load than is
the total calcium and many of the control tubular reabsorptions of
total calcium were already greater than 99%, any increase in the
TRCa++ induced by PTH is more difficult to demonstrate.   The ionized
calcium data are a more accurate index of the metabolic activity of

TABLE IV

PATIENT	DAY	TOTAL T_4 PRE-Li	Li	FREE T_4 PRE-Li	Li	TSH LEVELS PRE-Li	Li
J.Ca.	1	7.8	8.4	.70	.60	4.0	2.0
K.R.	1	6.7	4.5	.87	.50	1.0	1.0
J.B.	1	1.1	1.0	.40	.15	50	75
W.B.	1	5.8	6.4	.50	.53	7.0	4.5
J.C.	1	5.6	6.5	.55	.47	3.5	4.4
P.D.	1	1.8	8.7	.20	.80	50	1.2
S.V.	1	6.6	5.8	.50	.53	2.3	4.2
MEAN		4.95	6.01	.57	.54	19.2	14.9
SE		.95	.98	.08	.21	9.7	12.0
P		NS		NS		NS	

PTH on renal calcium transport.

Table IV shows the results of the thyroid function tests in our subjects. Both J.B. and P.D. had abnormal values prior to lithium therapy. J.B. had a normal free thyroxine (T$_4$) but an elevated TSH level. She developed free T$_4$ values into the hypothyroid range and higher TSH levels on lithium. P.D. was found to be chemically hypothyroid prior to the initiation of lithium. Both subjects were clinically euthyroid. P.D. was placed on exogenous thyroid (synthroid 200 µg per day) for eight weeks prior to the repeat studies on lithium at which time she was chemically euthyroid as well. When the total group of patients were examined, there were no significant changes in the total or free thyroxine or TSH levels (Table IV).

DISCUSSION

The most important observation made in this study is the reduction in urinary calcium excretion during lithium administration. This decrease was not associated with any decrease in creatinine clearance or fall in serum calcium. In fact, there was a significant increase in the ionized serum calcium concentration during lithium administration. Hence, the reduction in urinary calcium excretion occurred despite a slight increase in a major portion of the ultrafilterable calcium. In addition, parathormone levels did not change significantly during lithium administration. Therefore, we cannot attribute the increased renal calcium reabsorption to any increased PTH levels. There was neither potentiation of the renal cell response to exogenous parathyroid hormone, nor any blunting of the biological effect of PTH by lithium. Hence, we could not confirm previous reports of a blunting (8) or enhancing effect (7) of lithium administration on the action of PTH. Although we could not demonstrate any alteration in the effect of acutely administered parathormone, we cannot rule out a chronic potentiation of the effect of PTH. However, our daily 24 hour urinary cyclic-AMP excretions were not higher during lithium administration and no enhanced phosphorus clearance could be demonstrated despite hypocalciuria. Thus, it seems unlikely that a chronic enhancement of the effect of PTH was occurring. Since only one ion whose transport might be altered by PTH was affected and not other ions, the alteration in calcium excretion was probably not mediated by an isolated, selective renal tubular effect of PTH. Such an independent action of PTH on the kidney has never been demonstrated.

It is unlikely that lithium depressed the gastrointestinal absorption of calcium. Previous reports have shown that less than 1% of lithium carbonate leaves the human body in feces (14). Additionally, one would not expect to see an increase in the ionized serum calcium if decreased gastrointestinal absorption had taken place.

The fact that the parathyroid hormone levels were not suppressed despite a significant increase in ionized serum calcium deserves comment. This observation could suggest that lithium in some way either stimulated PTH release, decreased PTH metabolic clearance, or interfered with the negative feedback of calcium on PTH secretion. The first proposal is not unreasonable in light of observations showing that magnesium, a closely related cation, may be necessary for optimum PTH release (15-17). The last proposal is more difficult to rationalize. However, it is now becoming recognized that factors other than calcium may regulate parathyroid hormone secretion (18-20). Catecholamines may be one of these non-calcium factors (20). Thus, the reported interaction of lithium with epinephrine (21) might in some way be related to the extra-calcium parathyroid hormone secretion pathways. It might more simply be that our measured parathyroid hormone levels did not decrease because although the ionized serum calcium did increase significantly they barely exceeded the upper normal range and remained normal in several subjects. Previous studies have either shown no change in total (9-10,22) or ionized (22) serum calcium with chronic lithium administration although one acute experiment did report a rise in total serum calcium concentration (23).

The hypocalciuric effect occurred regardless of the initial starting level of urinary calcium excretion with one exception (W.B.) whose starting urinary Ca++ excretion was very low. In the two subjects with persistent hypercalciuria, the urinary calcium excretion became persistently normocalciuric. Subject J.C. became persistently hypercalciuric again four weeks after lithium was discontinued. In none of our subjects could this hypocalciuric effect be attributed to changes in diet or degree of activity. In addition, the mean thyroid levels for the group did not change. Thus, we cannot attribute the decrease in calcium excretion to the development of hypothyroidism. In fact, P.D. had a consistent decrease in urinary calcium excretion despite going from a chemical hypo-thyroid state to a euthyroid state.

Thus, without any direct evidence for an increase in PTH levels or PTH effect, or indirect evidence for any calcium malabsorption, we observed a hypocalciuric effect despite an increase in the filtered calcium load. This evidence suggest that lithium exerts a direct tubular effect to promote calcium transport. Although we can suggest that this hypocalciuric effect is a direct tubular effect, we cannot state for certainty what the direct mechanism is.

Since we did not observe any change in urinary sodium excretion while a reduction in urinary calcium excretion was seen, a dissassociation between the excretion of sodium and calcium occurred. Normally a linear relationship exists between the clearances of sodium and that of calcium (24-25). The disassociation mimics that induced by thiazides or parathyroid hormone (26-29). Since we did not demonstrate any PTH alterations, the possibility exists that there may be a link between the mechanism whereby lithium reduces urinary calcium excretion and the hypocalciuric effect of thiazides. It is known that lithium administration initially induces a natriuresis and negative sodium balance that is transient and lasts for only 2-3 days. Subjects then return to sodium balance, but at a level of reduced total body sodium (11,14). Such a sequence is reminescent of the effect of thiazides on sodium metabolism, which also results in a reduced urinary calcium excretion. Thus, it is possible that the hypocalciuric effect of lithium is mediated by a slight drop in extracellular fluid volume and negative sodium balance. If so, the effect should be capable of being abolished by sodium replacement and maintenance of sodium balance. Our patients were discharged from the research center to the state mental hospital immediately after initiating lithium therapy. Hence, early sodium repletion studies could not be done. However, the fact that there were no significant differences in body weight, hematocrit, or total protein during lithium administration any substantial reduction in extracellular fluid volume to explain the hypocalciuric effect was probably not present.

In conclusion, lithium has been shown in this study to reduce urinary calcium excretion through a mechanism which appears independent of parathyroid hormone metabolism or effect, sodium excretion, or glomerular filtration rate. Thus, lithium deserves further study into this urinary calcium lowering effect and trials to examine its potential efficacy in hypercalciuric disorders.

REFERENCES

1. Forrest, J.N., Cohen, A.D., Torretti, J., Himmelitoat, J.M., and Epstein, F.H.: On the mechanism of lithium-induced diabetes insipidus in man and the rat. J. Clin. Invest. 53:1115, 1974.

2. Martinez-Maldonado, M., Stuaroulari-Tsapara, A., Tsaparas, N., Suki, W.N., and Eknoyan, G.: Renal effects of lithium administration in rats. Alterations in water and electrolyte metabolism and the response to vasopressin and cyclic-adenosine monophosphate during prolonged administration. J. Lab. Clin. Med. 86:445, 1975.

3. Singer, I., Rottenberg, D., Puschett, J.B.: Lithium-induced

nephrogenic diabetes insipidus.   In vivo and in vitro studies.
J. Clin. Invest. 51:1081, 1972.

4. Singer, I. and Franko, E.A.:   Lithium-induced ADH resistance
    in toad urinary bladders.   Kid. Internat. 3:151, 1973.

5. Dousa, T.P.:   Interaction of lithium with vasopressin-sensi-
    tive cyclic AMP system of human renal medulla.   Endocrinology
    95:1359, 1974.

6. Olesen, O.V., Jensen, J., and Thomsen, K.:   Effect of lithium
    on glucagon-stimulated cyclic AMP excretion in rats.   Acta
    Pharmacol. et Toxico. J. 35:403, 1974.

7. Olesen, O.V. and Thomsen, K.:   Effect of prolonged lithium in-
    gestion on glucagon and parathyroid hormone responses in rats.
    Acta Pharmacol. et Toxicol. 34:225, 1974.

8. Dousa, T. and Hechter, O.:   Lithium and brain adenyl cyclase.
    Lancet 1:834, 1970.

9. Gotfredsen, C.F. and Rafaelsen, O.J.:   Effect of lithium and
    other psychopharmaca on rat electrolyte metabolism.   Int. Phar-
    macopsychiat. 5:242, 1970.

10. Birch, N.J. and Jenner, F.A.:   The distribution of lithium and
    its effect on the distribution and excretion of other ions in
    the rat.   Br. J. Pharmac. 47:586, 1973.

11. Tupin, J.P., Schlagenhauf, G.K., and Creson, D.L.:   Lithium
    effects on electrolyte excretion.   Am. J. Psychiat. 125:536,
    1968.

12. Gilman, A.G.:   Protein binding assay for cyclic nucleotides.
    Adv. Cyclic Nucleotide Res. 2:9, 1972.

13. Richardson, J.M., Wolfson, J.A., and Kurtzman, N.A.:   Lithium
    administration and phosphate excretion.   Clin. Res. 541A, 1975.

14. Hullin, R.P., Swinscoe, J.C., McDonald, R., and Dransfield,
    G.A.:   Metabolic balance studies on the effect of lithium
    salts in manic-depressive psychosis.   Brit. J. Psychiat. 114:
    1561, 1968.

15. Arnst, C.S., Mohs, J.M., Kaplan, S.L., and Burns, T.W.:   Evi-
    dence for parathyroid failure in magnesium deficiency.   Science
    177:606, 1972.

16. Muldowney, F.P., McKenna, T.J., Kyle, L.H., Fraeney, R., and

Swan, M.: Parathormone-like effect of magnesium replenishment in steatorrhea. N. Engl. J. Med. 282:61, 1970.

17. Suh, S.M., Tashjian, A.H., Matsuo, N., Parkinson, D.K., and Fraser, D.: Pathogenesis of hypocalcemia in primary hypomagnesemia: normal end-organ responsiveness to parathyroid hormone, impaired parathyroid gland function. J. Clin. Invest. 52:153, 1973.

18. Chertow, B.S., Baylink, D.J., Wergedal, J.E., Su, M.H.H., and Norman, A.W.: Decrease in serum immunoreactive parathyroid hormone in rats and in parathyroid hormone secretion in vitro by 1,25 dihydroxycholecalciferol. J. Clin. Invest. 56:668, 1975.

19. Mayer, G.P., Habener, J.F., and Potts, J.T., Jr.: Parathyroid secretion in vivo. Demonstration of a calcium independent nonsuppressible component of secretion. J. Clin. Invest. 57:678, 1976.

20. Fischer, J.A., Blum, J.W., and Binswanger, U.: Acute parathyroid response to epinephrine in vivo. J. Clin. Invest. 52: 2434, 1973.

21. Singer, I. and Rotenberg, D.: Mechanisms of lithium action. N. Engl. J. Med. 289:254, 1973.

22. Frizel, D., Coppen, A., and Marks, V.: Plasma magnesium and calcium in depression. Brit. J. Psychiat. 115:1375, 1969.

23. Mellerup, E.T., Plenge, P., Ziegler, R., and Rafaelsen, O.J.: Lithium effects on calcium metabolism in rats. Int. Pharmacopsychiat. 5:258, 1970.

24. Walser, M.: Calcium clearance as a function of sodium clearance in the dog. Am. J. Physiol. 200:1099, 1961.

25. Massry, S.G., Coburn, J.W., Chapman, L.W., and Kleeman, C.R.: Effect of Na Cl infusion on urinary Ca++ and Mg++ during reduction in their filtered loads. Am. J. Physiol. 213:1218, 1967.

26. Brickman, A.S., Massry, S.G., and Coburn, J.W.: Changes in serum and urinary calcium during treatment with hydrochlorothiazide. J. Clin. Invest. 51:945, 1972.

27. Costanzo, L.S. and Weiner, I.M.: On the hypocalciuric action of chlorothiazide. J. Clin. Invest. 54:625, 1974.

28. Widrow, S.H., and Levinsky, N.G.: The effect of parathyroid extract on renal tubular calcium reabsorption in the dog. J. Clin. Invest. 41: 2151, 1962.

29. Agus, Z.S., Gardner, L.B., and Goldberg, M.: Effects of parathyroid hormone on renal tubular reabsorption of calcium, sodium, and phosphate. Am. J. Physiol. 224: 1143, 1973.

THE RENAL HANDLING OF PHOSPHATE BY RENAL TRANSPLANT PATIENTS:
CORRELATION WITH SERUM PARATHYROID HORMONE (S$_{PTH}$),
CYCLIC 3',5'-ADENOSINE MONOPHOSPHATE (cAMP) URINARY
EXCRETION, AND ALLOGRAFT FUNCTION

H.N. Ward, R.C. Pabico, B.A. McKenna, and R.B. Freeman

Nephrology Unit, Department of Medicine
University of Rochester Medical Center
Rochester, New York

Hypophosphatemia and hyperphosphaturia have been observed in renal transplant patients (1). Numerous factors can affect urinary phosphate excretion in the post-transplant state, but PTH is probably the most important. The persistence of an elevated S$_{PTH}$ level in the post-transplant period, despite good allograft function, suggests that phosphaturia may be directly related to the hyperparathyroid state. Since PTH-induced phosphaturia is mediated by cAMP (2), there should be a correlation between S$_{PTH}$ and urinary cAMP excretion (U$_{cAMP}$). Our study was initiated with the following objectives:

a. To correlate the level of allograft function (determined by endogenous creatinine clearance, C$_{creat}$) and S$_{PTH}$ concentration.
b. To define the relationship between S$_{PTH}$ level and U$_{cAMP}$.
c. To correlate phosphate handling by the allograft with S$_{PTH}$ and U$_{cAMP}$ excretion.

PATIENTS AND METHODS
Patients
Forty renal allograft recipients (25 men and 15 women) with a mean age of 34 years and a mean duration post-renal transplantation of 23 months were investigated. These patients were anatomically or physiologically anephric prior to transplantation. All patients were receiving standard immunosuppressive treatment. Twenty-seven patients were on diuretics and/or propranolol for sustained arterial hypertension. None of the patients were receiving phosphate-binding antacids, calcium, vitamin D, or phosphate supplements. The urine

was sterile at the time of the study. These patients were divided into 2 groups:

Group I consisted of 18 patients with $C_{creat} \geq 70ml/min/1.73m^2$
Group II consisted of 22 patients with $C_{creat} < 70ml/min/1.73m^2$

In a previous study we showed that the remaining kidney of uninephrectomized donors could achieve a C_{creat} of at least 70 ml/min/1.73m^2 (3). Hence, this value is used as a dividing level of function.

Controls

Eight healthy uninephrectomized donors (6 men and 2 women) served as controls.

Analytical Methods

Urine specimens were collected for 24 hours; venous blood samples were obtained before breakfast on the morning when urine collections ended. Serum and urine creatinine, and inorganic phosphate were determined by the methods adapted for the Technicon Auto-Analyzer. Plasma and urinary calcium were determined by atomic absorption spectroscopy. S_{PTH} was measured by radioimmunoassay*. U_{cAMP} was measured by the cAMP RIA kit of Schwarz/Mann and expressed in nM/min/100 ml C_{creat}. C_{creat}, C_{PO_4}, and tubular reabsorption of phosphate (% TRP)) were calculated by the standard formulas. The tubular threshold of phosphate (Tm_{PO_4}/C_{creat}) was calculated from Bijvoet nomogram (4). The statistical analysis was performed using student's t test.

RESULTS

Table I summarizes the results in the 3 groups studied.

C_{creat} and S_{PTH}

The mean C_{creat} in Group I and in the control group were not significantly different, statistically. However, the mean S_{PTH} in Group I patients was significantly higher compared to the control group. Patients in Group II had a lower mean C_{creat} and a higher mean S_{PTH} compared to patients in Group I.

Calcium and Phosphate

The mean serum calcium values for the 3 groups were not statistically different; nor was the mean S_{PO_4} concentration. However, 6 Group I and 5 Group II patients were hypophosphatemic ($S_{PO_4} < 2.5$ mg/100 ml). The mean Tm_{PO_4}/C_{creat} in the 3 groups were not statistically different. The % TRP in the control group, and in Group I patients, were virtually identical. Patients in Group II had a significantly lower mean % TRP, compared with mean % TRP in Group I patients.

*Done in Dr. Claude Arnaud's Laboratory, Rochester, Minnesota USA

U_{CAMP} Excretion

The mean U_{CAMP} excretion in the control group was not statistically different from that in Group I. However, the mean U_{CAMP} excretion in Group II, was significantly higher than that in the control group and Group I.

Correlation between C_{creat}, S_{PTH}, and U_{CAMP}

Figure I illustrates the relationship between C_{creat} and S_{PTH} in the transplanted patients. The shaded area and the area between the interrupted lines represent the range of values obtained in the control group. There is a significant inverse relationship between C_{creat} and S_{PTH}.

Figure 2 shows a significant negative linear relationship between C_{creat} and U_{CAMP} in the transplanted population ($r = -0.32$, $p < 0.05$).

Correlation between S_{PTH} and U_{CAMP}:

Figure 3 illustrates a significant positive linear relationship between S_{PTH} and U_{CAMP} in the transplant population ($r = 0.32$,

Table I: Mean ($\pm$ SEM) C_{creat}, S_{PTH}, $S_{Ca^{++}}$, S_{PO_4}, Tm_{PO_4}/C_{creat}, %TRP, and U_{CAMP} in the Control Group and Transplanted Patients

	Control n = 8		Group I n = 18		Group II n = 22
C_{creat} ml/min/1.73m^2	89.5 $\pm$ 7.9	p = NS	94.5 $\pm$ 4.6	p = < 0.0001	41.4 $\pm$ 3.3
S_{PTH} µlEq/ml	26.6 $\pm$ 2.6	p = < 0.01	65.8 $\pm$ 8.9	p = < 0.002	148.6 $\pm$ 20.6
$S_{Ca^{++}}$ mg/dl	9.73 $\pm$ 0.12	p = NS	10.02 $\pm$ 0.09	p = NS	9.82 $\pm$ 0.14
$S_{PO_4^=}$ mg/dl	2.9 $\pm$ 0.13	p = NS	2.75 $\pm$ 1.6	p = NS	3.04 $\pm$ 0.20
$Tm_{PO_4^=}/C_{creat}$ mg/ml	2.22 $\pm$ 0.098	p = NS	2.22 $\pm$ 0.22	p = NS	1.85 $\pm$ 0.18
% TRP	76.8 $\pm$ 1.4	p = NS	76.1 $\pm$ 2.51	p = < 0.001	59.0 $\pm$ 3.53
U_{CAMP} nM/min/100 ml C_{creat}	3.03 $\pm$ 0.17	p = NS	3.59 $\pm$ 0.24	p = < 0.005	5.89 $\pm$ 0.32

p < 0.05). The shaded area represents the range of values obtained in the control group. The closed and open circles represent the patients in Group I and II, respectively.

Correlation between allograft phosphate handling, S_{PTH}, and U_{cAMP} (Figure 4)

There is a linear correlation between S_{PTH} and % TRP in the transplanted population (r = -0.41, p < 0.01). No such relationship exists between S_{PTH} and Tm_{PO_4}/C_{creat}. The Tm_{PO_4}/C_{creat} and % TRP in the transplanted patients are inversely related to U_{cAMP} excretion (r= -0.46, p < 0.005 and r = -0.64, p < 0.0001, respectively).

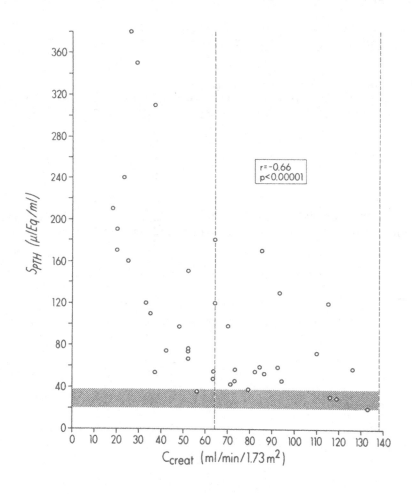

Figure 1: Relationship between S_{PTH} and C_{creat}

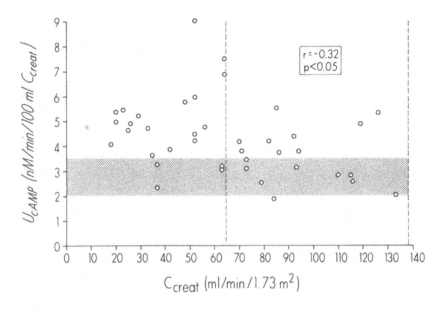

Figure 2: Relationship between U_{cAMP} and C_{creat}.

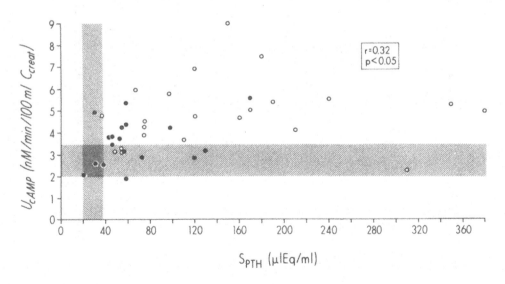

Figure 3: Relationship Between U_{cAMP} and S_{PTH}.

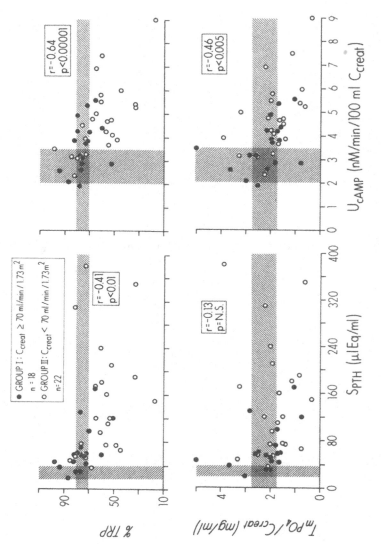

Figure 4: Relationship Between Allograft Phosphate Handling, S_{PTH}, and U_{cAMP}.

DISCUSSION

Following successful renal allotransplantation, hyperparathyroidism of renal failure apparently improves and parathyroid function becomes normal. What is not clearly defined is when this change occurs (5,6). Our results demonstrate an inverse relation between the level of allograft function and circulating PTH. The elevated S_{PTH} may exert biologic effects on the allograft, but this has not yet been clarified. Studies have shown that there are at least 3 distinct immunoreactive species of PTH in human hyperparathyroid serum with different physiologic properties (5). The biologic heterogeneity of S_{PTH} in the transplant patients has not yet been defined. Furthermore, the persistently elevated S_{PTH} may make the receptor sites in the renal cortex less responsive.

Since the original work of Chase and Aurbach (6), confirmation of the cAMP-mediated phosphaturic action of PTH has been provided by Agus, et al (2), and Goldberg, et al (7). Broadus, et al (8) showed that PTH administration increased U_{cAMP} excretion in man and the source of the PTH-induced increase in U_{cAMP} is the kidney itself (nephrogenous cAMP) and not an increased renal clearance of cAMP from the blood. Clinically, the increased U_{cAMP} has been correlated with the elevated S_{PTH} of primary hyperparathyroidism and was useful in distinguishing this entity from other hypercalcemic states (9). In our study, we used the urinary excretion of cAMP as a marker to assess the effects of S_{PTH} on allograft phosphate handling.

At the time of the study, the transplanted patients receiving diuretic therapy were in stable edema-free state. With the exception of Triflocin, the phosphaturic/anti-phosphaturic property of a diuretic agent depends on the fluid balance of the individual (10). The contribution by the diuretics to the phosphaturia encountered in some of our patients is probably minor or non-existent. Propranolol has no known effect on phosphate handling by the kidney, nor on urinary cyclic nucleotide kinetics. Glucocorticosteroids are known to be phosphaturic agents (11), and their relative contribution to the phosphaturia post-renal transplantation cannot be determined accurately. Steroids have a permissive effect on cAMP-mediated processes probably via a decreased phosphodiesterase activity (12); however, they do not cause an increase in U_{cAMP} excretion. None of the transplanted patients had evidence of tubular dysfunction. Acquired tubular disorders, therefore, cannot be incriminated as a cause of phosphaturia in our patients.

As the C_{creat} declines, the absolute amount of U_{cAMP}, expressed in nMoles per day, diminishes. In the presence of depressed renal function and decreased filtered load of cAMP, the finding of a higher fractional U_{cAMP} excretion suggests increased secretion by the remaining tubules under the influence of S_{PTH} (and/or other factors).

Figure 3 shows that S_{PTH} correlated significantly with the rate of U_{cAMP} excretion in the transplantation population ($r = 0.32$, $p < 0.05$) attesting to significant biological activity with an appropriate U_{cAMP} response.

As shown in Figure 4, and in agreement with Slatopolsky's data, transplant patients showed a significant negative linear relationship between S_{PTH} and % TRP. This was most evident in Group I, but not in Group II patients. Two possibilities can explain the results in the pattern of U_{cAMP}: 1. the presence of other factors causing phosphaturia (thyrocalcitonin, lack of Vitamin D metabolites, glucocorticosteroids); 2. Refractory state to S_{PTH} action of tubular receptors as a result of the persistent high level of S_{PTH}. The absence of a negative relationship between S_{PTH} and Tm_{PO_4}/C_{creat} in the transplanted patients could be related to the use of a nomogram for patients with two kidneys and not one kidney. It is interesting to note that the mean Tm_{PO_4}/C_{creat} of the uninephrectomized controls is lower than values for normal published by Bijvoet (4). The Tm_{PO_4}/C_{creat} and the % TRP were inversely related to U_{cAMP} in the transplanted population, particularly in Group II patients. The variation in PTH-cAMP-allograft phosphate handling interrelations in Groups I and II indicates that other important mechanisms may be involved, either an alteration in cortical renal tubular epithelial cell cAMP responsiveness to S_{PTH} or modulation of cAMP-mediated phosphaturia.

In conclusion, diminished renal allograft function stimulates PTH secretion by already defined mechanism(s). The biologically active S_{PTH} triggers an increased synthesis and excretion of cAMP by the renal allograft allowing for an increase in fractional phosphate excretion.

ACKNOWLEDGMENTS

The authors wish to thank Mr. Craig Dickstein for performing the statistical analyses, Mrs. Barbara Byer and Mrs. Jenny Yarger for their invaluable assistance in obtaining the required specimens from the transplanted patients, and Mrs. Christine Clarke for her secretarial excellence.

References

1. Gyory, A.Z., Stewart, J.H., George, C.R.P., Tiller, D.J., and Edwards, K.D.G.: Renal tubular acidosis, acidosis due to hyperkalemia, hypercalcemia, disordered citrate metabolism and other tubular dysfunctions following human renal transplantation. Quart. J. Med. 38:231, 1969.
2. Agus, S.G., Puschett, J.B., Senesky, D., and Goldberg, M.: Mode of action of parathyroid hormone on cyclic adenosine 3', 5'-monophosphate on renal tubular phosphate reabsorption in the dog. J. Clin. Invest. 50:617, 1971.
3. Pabico, R.C., McKenna, B.A., Freeman, R.B.: Renal function before and after unilateral nephrectomy in renal donors. Kid. Intern. 8:166, 1975.
4. Walton, R.J., and Bijvoet, E.L.M.: Nomogram for derivation of renal threshold phosphate concentration. Lancet 2:309, 1975.
5. Canterbury, J.M., and Reiss, E.: Multiple immunoreactive molecular forms of parathyroid hormone in human serum. Proc. Soc. Exp. Biol. Med. 140:1393, 1972.
6. Chase, L.R., Aurbach, G.D.: Parathyroid function and the renal excretion of 3',5'-adenylic acid. Proc. Nat. Acad. Sci. 58: 518, 1967.
7. Goldberg, M., Agus, Z.S., Puschett, J.B., and Senesky, D.: Mode of phosphaturic action of parathyroid hormone: micropuncture studies, in Calcium, Parathyroid Hormone and the Calcitonins. Ed. Talmage, R.V., and Munson, P.L. p. 273 Amsterdam: Excerpta Medica. 1972.
8. Broadus, A.E., Hardman, J.G., Kaminsky, N.I., Ball, J.H., Sutherland, E.W., Liddle, G.W.: Extracellular cyclic nucleotides. Ann. N.Y. Acad. Sci. 50:50, 1971.
9. Murad, F., Pak, C.Y.C.: Urinary excretion of adenosine 3',5'-monophosphate and guanosine 3',5'-monophosphate. N. Engl. J. Med. 286:1382, 1972.
10. Steele, T.H.: Dual effect of potent diuretics on renal handling of phosphate in man. Metabolism 20: 749, 1971.
11. Camanni, F., Losana, O., Massara, F., Molinatti, G.M.: Increased renal phosphate   excretion in cushing's syndrome. Acta Endocrinologica 56:85, 1967.
12. Thompson, E.B., and Lippman, M.E.: Mechanism of action of glucocorticoids. Metabolism 23:159, 1974.

INDEPENDENCE OF PHOSPHATE HOMEOSTASIS FROM

PARATHYROID FUNCTION IN THE PHOSPHATE-DEPLETED RAT

Thomas H. Steele

Dept. of Medicine, University of Wisconsin

Madison, Wisconsin   USA

Parathyroid hormone (PTH) performs many functions important to the optimum maintenance of phosphate homeostasis. One of these is to maintain the plasma inorganic phosphate (P_i) concentration at a relatively constant level in order to avoid episodic fluctuations in plasma P_i which could accompany variations in the dietary phosphorus intake. PTH can prevent hyperphosphatemia by eliciting a phosphaturic response, secondary to its inhibition of the renal tubular reabsorption of P_i.

Recent observations have established the existence of an additional PTH-independent system for the regulation of renal P_i reabsorption in the rat (1,2). In studies performed in our laboratory, the infusion of phosphate in thyroparathyroidectomized (TPTX) rats maintained on a phosphorus-deficient diet elicited rates of tubular P_i reabsorption greatly in excess of those observed in other TPTX rats maintained on a normal phosphorus intake (2). A particularly striking observation was that TPTX phosphorus-deficient rats could maintain a phosphate-free urine, with fractional P_i excretions (FE_{P_i}) less than 1 percent, even when the plasma P_i exceeded 20 mg/100 ml (2). Similarly avid P_i conservation was observed in phosphorus-depleted vitamin D-deficient TPTX rats (3).

Such a putative system, by promoting P_i retention in the phosphorus-depleted animal during the administration of phosphate, could perform an important homeostatic function by promoting P_i retention during the repletion

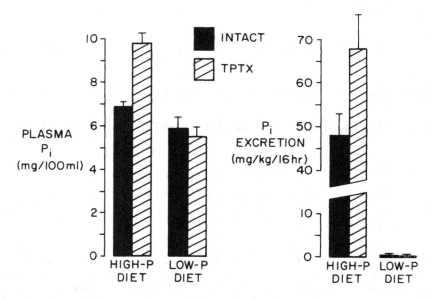

<u>Figure 1</u>: Plasma P_i and P_i excretion after a 16-hour
fast. Significant hyperphosphatemia occurred in TPTX
rats stabilized on the high-phosphorus diet. Note the
vanishingly small P_i excretion in both the intact and
TPTX rats stabilized on the low-phosphorus diet. Values
are mean and SEM.

of body phosphorus stores. On the other hand, the clinical utility of this system for the correction of phosphorus depletion would be limited severely if PTH secretion occurred and permitted significant urinary P_i wastage during the repletion process. The ingestion of
relatively small amounts of phosphate can elicit an increase in serum PTH levels in normal man (4), and it
seems likely that PTH release also would occur during
phosphate administration to rats. The present studies
were undertaken to explore the effect of the parathyroids
upon the renal response during correction of phosphorus
depletion.

We compared baseline P_i excretion in mature hydropenic fasted rats which had been stabilized for one month
on a diet containing either 1% calcium and 0.07% phosphorus, ("low-phosphorus") or 1.6% calcium and 1% phosphorus ("high-phosphorus"). Animals were studied either
with intact parathyroid glands or 48 hours after TPTX,

and were fasted during the 16-hour urine collections depicted in Figure 1. During fasting, the plasma P_i increased an average of 1.3 $\pm$ 0.5 mg/100 ml (mean $\pm$ SEM) in the low-phosphorus intact rats, and decreased by 0.7 $\pm$ 0.2 mg/100 ml in the high-phosphorus group. Thus, in the presence of the parathyroids, after 16 hours of fasting, plasma P_i differed by only 1.1 mg/100 ml in hydropenic intact high and low dietary phosphorus animals (Figure 1).

Among the rats stabilized on the low-phosphorus diet, P_i excretion was very low in both the intact and TPTX animals. P_i excretion was more than 100 times greater in both groups stabilized on the high-phosphorus diet (Figure 1). Of these high-phosphorus rats, significant hyperphosphatemia occurred in the TPTX animals. In contrast, rats stabilized on the low phosphorus diet had similar plasma P_i values irrespective of the presence or absence of the parathyroids.

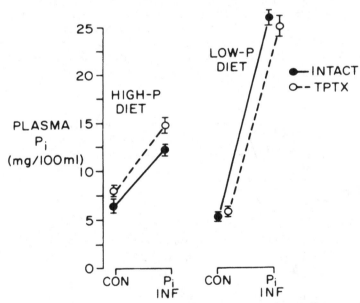

Figure 2: Response of plasma P_i to phosphate infusion, 2.3 mmol/kg/hour, in NaCl-loaded rats. Significantly greater hyperphosphatemia was elicited by the same amount of phosphate in animals stabilized on the low-phosphorus intake, irrespective of the presence or absence of the parathyroids. Values are mean and SEM.

During phosphate loading, phosphaturia might be elicited through at least two mechanisms. First, an increase in PTH secretion could result in the inhibition of the tubular reabsorption of P_i (4). Second, extracellular volume expansion accompanying phosphate loading could inhibit P_i reabsorption through mechanisms independent of PTH (5,6). In order to explore these possibilities, fasted adult rats stabilized on the low and high-phosphorus diets underwent clearance studies, either in the intact state or 48-72 hours after TPTX. Sixty minutes prior to and during control clearance periods, each animal received an NaCl infusion delivering 9 mmol/kg/hour. They then received neutral sodium phosphate at 2.3 mmol/kg/hour for 40 minutes, after which specimens were collected for additional clearance periods. In addition, each animal received calcium at 7 mg/kg/hour.

In the <u>high dietary phosphorus</u> animals, control plasma P_i after NaCl loading averaged 6.3 ± 0.4 mg/100 ml in intact and 7.3 ± 0.5 mg/100 ml in TPTX rats (Figure 2). Absolute and fractional P_i excretions did not differ significantly between the intact and TPTX animals (Figure 3). Following P_i infusion, plasma P_i increased to 11.8 ± 0.5 mg/100 ml in the intact and 14.7 ± 1.1 mg/100 ml in the TPTX high phosphorus animals (Figure 2). Both the

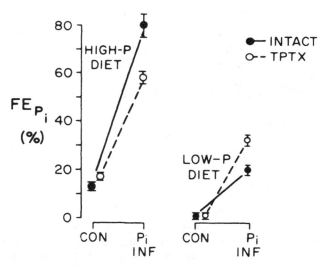

<u>Figure 3</u>: Fractional P_i excretion (FE_{P_i}) in the experiments depicted in Figure 2. FE_{P_i} was depressed significantly in both groups of low-phosphorus animals (right).

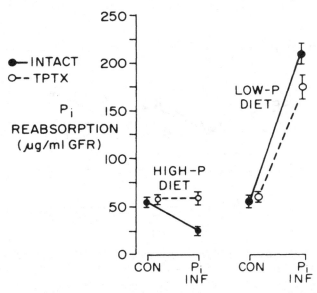

Figure 4: P_i reabsorption was depressed by phosphate infusion in the intact high dietary phosphorus group, but unaffected after TPTX (left). P_i reabsorption increased during phosphate infusion in both groups of low-phosphorus rats (right).

absolute and fractional P_i excretions increased significantly more in the intact than in the TPTX rats during phosphate infusion (Figure 3). P_i reabsorption decreased significantly in the intact group after phosphate infusion, but remained constant in the TPTX animals (Figure 4). Fractional sodium excretion exceeded 7% throughout in both high-phosphorus groups (Figure 5).

In contrast, rats stabilized on the <u>low dietary phosphorus</u> intake exhibited few differences between the intact and TPTX state. In the low-phosphorus animals, baseline plasma P_i values were similar in the intact and TPTX groups (Figure 2). Despite massive volume expansion, with fractional sodium excretions in excess of 9% (Figure 5), FEp_i values remained less than 1% during the control periods (Figure 3). Following P_i loading, plasma P_i values increased to 26 $\pm$ 1.1 mg/100 ml and 25.3 $\pm$ 2.2 mg/100 ml in the intact and TPTX low-phosphorus animals, respectively (Figure 2). Despite this degree of hyperphosphatemia, mean FEp_i values climbed to only

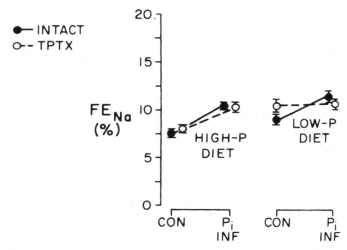

Figure 5: Fractional sodium excretion (FE_{Na}) in experiments summarized in Figures 2-4. The high FE_{Na} values reflect the infusion of the same amounts of NaCl (9 mmol/kg/hour) and sodium phosphate (2.3 mmol/kg/hour) in all 4 groups.

21.1% and 32.0%, respectively, which were significantly less than the analogous levels in the high-phosphorus rats following phosphate infusion (Figure 3). Instead of decreasing or remaining constant, P_i reabsorption increased substantially in both low-phosphorus groups (Figure 4).

One laboratory recently has reported that hypercapnia may elicit a phosphaturic response by decreasing P_i reabsorption (7). In the present studies, no correlation could be made between pCO_2 and P_i excretion or reabsorption. Spontaneous changes in pCO_2 did not occur in any consistent relationship to alterations in P_i transport. Likewise, changes in urine pH (8) and in tubular fluid pH (9,10) have been related to changes in P_i reabsorption. In the present studies, no relationships between urine pH and P_i transport were evident.

On the other hand, bicarbonate loading <u>does</u> appear to depress P_i reabsorption (11). When TPTX rats were loaded with $NaHCO_3$, 9 mmol/kg/hour, P_i reabsorption during phosphate infusion was depressed (Figure 6), as compared to animals loaded with equivalent amounts of NaCl. Nevertheless, P_i reabsorption after bicarbonate

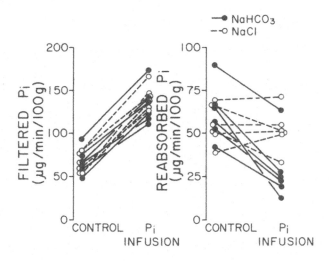

Figure 6: Effect of NaHCO3 loading on Pi reabsorption
in rats studied 48-72 hours after TPTX. Animals received
NaCl or NaHCO3, 9 mmol/kg/hour. The inhibitory effect
of NaHCO3 on Pi reabsorption became evident only after
phosphate infusion, in rats stabilized on the high-phosphorus diet.

loading remained greater in TPTX rats stabilized on the
low-phosphorus diet than in similarly NaHCO3-loaded
animals stabilized on the high-phosphorus diet.

In summary, the presence of the parathyroid glands
in phosphorus-depleted rats does not interfere with Pi
conservation during rapid phosphorus repletion - even in
the presence of substantial NaCl volume expansion.
Rather, the antecedent dietary phosphorus intake appears
to be a more important determinant of phosphorus conservation, independently of the parathyroids and of the
degree of extracellular volume expansion. The parathyroids influence Pi reabsorption importantly in normal
rats, but have little effect upon Pi transport in phosphorus-depleted animals. This could arise as a consequence of either defective PTH secretion or a diminished
phosphaturic response to PTH following phosphorus deprivation. Recent results in our laboratory have indicated
that the phosphaturic response to PTH is almost eliminated in acutely TPTX phosphorus-depleted rats, as compared to appropriate controls, despite the preservation
of a normal urinary cyclic AMP response to PTH. In

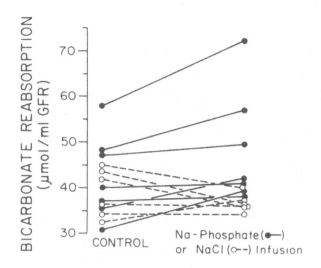

Figure 7: Bicarbonate reabsorption in TPTX rats during phosphate infusion. Animals were loaded with sufficient NaHCO$_3$ to maintain plasma bicarbonate at 47-58 mmol/l throughout. Although bicarbonate inhibited P$_i$ reabsorption during hyperphosphatemia (Figure 6), phosphate did not interfere with bicarbonate reabsorption.

addition, the phosphaturic response to dibutyryl cyclic AMP infusion in phosphorus-deprived animals is strikingly diminished. Therefore, a defect in the renal response to either PTH itself or a PTH-induced "second messenger", as well as decreased PTH secretion, could account for a diminished influence of the parathyroids on phosphate homeostasis during phosphorus depletion.

REFERENCES

1. Tröhler, U., Bonjour, J.-P., and Fleisch, H.:
    Inorganic phosphate homeostasis. Renal adaptation
    to the dietary intake in intact and thyroparathy-
    roidectomized rats. J. Clin. Invest. 57:264, 1976.

2. Steele, T.H., and DeLuca, H.F.: Influence of the
    dietary phosphorus on renal phosphate reabsorption
    in the parathyroidectomized rat. J. Clin. Invest.
    57:867, 1976.

3. Steele, T.H., Engle, J.E., Tanaka, Y., Lorenc, R.S.,
    Dudgeon, K.L., and DeLuca, H.F.: Phosphatemic
    action of 1,25-dihydroxyvitamin D_3. Am. J. Physiol.
    229:489, 1975.

4. Reiss, E., Canterbury, J.M., Bercovitz, M.A., and
    Kaplan, E.L.: The role of phosphate in the secre-
    tion of parathyroid hormone in man. J. Clin. Invest.
    49:2146, 1970.

5. Massry, S.G., Coburn, J.W., and Kleeman, C.R.:
    The influence of extracellular volume expansion on
    renal phosphate reabsorption in the dog. J. Clin.
    Invest. 48:1237, 1969.

6. Suki, W.N., Martinez-Maldonado, M., Rouse, D., and
    Terry, A.: Effect of expansion of extracellular
    fluid volume on renal phosphate handling. J. Clin.
    Invest. 48:1888, 1969.

7. Webb, R.K., Woodhall, P.B., Tisher, C.C., Neelon,
    F.A., and Robinson, R.R.: Mechanism of phosphaturia
    during acute hypercapnia. Clin. Res. 24:415A
    (Abstract), 1976.

8. Fulop, M., and Brazeau, P.: The phosphaturic
    effect of sodium bicarbonate and acetazolamide in
    dogs. J. Clin. Invest. 47:983, 1968.

9. Bank, N., Aynedjian, H.S., and Weinstein, S.W.:
    A microperfusion study of phosphate reabsorption
    by the rat proximal renal tubule. Effect of para-
    thyroid hormone. J. Clin. Invest. 54:1040, 1974.

10. Baumann, K., Rumrich, G., Papavassiliou, F.,
     and Klöss, S.: pH dependence of phosphate reab-
     sorption in the proximal tubule of rat kidney.
     Pflügers Arch. Ges. Physiol. 360:183, 1975.

11. Mercado, A., Slatopolsky, E., and Klahr, S.: On
     the mechanisms responsible for the phosphaturia
     of bicarbonate administration. J. Clin. Invest.
     56:1386, 1975.

Regulation of Vitamin D Metabolism:

Role of Phosphate

REGULATION OF VITAMIN D METABOLISM IN THE KIDNEY

Hector F. DeLuca

Department of Biochemistry, University of Wisconsin-

Madison, Madison, Wisconsin 53706 USA

HISTORICAL CONSIDERATIONS

With the discovery that the kidney is the sole site of biosynthesis of what is believed to be the metabolically active form
of vitamin D, namely 1,25-dihydroxyvitamin D_3 (1,25-$(OH)_2D_3$), came
the idea that this substance can be regarded as a hormone with its
targets as intestine and bone (1-3). This led to the initial idea
by Boyle et al. in 1971 (3, 4) that the biosynthesis of this
active form of vitamin D might be feed-back regulated by the need
for calcium and phosphorus. Because it was not possible, and is
still not possible, to measure directly the hydroxylases in mammalian renal tissue (5), Boyle et al. (3) chose the approach of
injecting the precursor ^{3}H-25-hydroxyvitamin D_3 (25-OH-D_3) into
rats and determining the in vivo conversion of the 25-OH-D_3 to the
more polar metabolites as a method of measuring the ability of the
animals to hydroxylate and accumulate the active form of vitamin D.
Using this approach, these investigators were able to show that
regardless of the dietary level of calcium and phosphorus, vitamin
D-deficient rats accumulate large amounts of a single polar metabolite which was identified as 1,25-$(OH)_2D_3$. Thus vitamin D-deficient
animals showed no tendency to regulate their production or accumulation of the 1,25-$(OH)_2D_3$ as a function of calcium and phosphorus,
an important fact which later proved to be a key issue in the
regulation of the vitamin D hydroxylases located in the kidney. On
the other hand, rats maintained on 25 ng of vitamin D daily, showed
a remarkable ability to regulate the synthesis and accumulation of
their radioactive 1,25-$(OH)_2D_3$: low calcium animals showing a very
large accumulation in a defined period of time, while those on a
high calcium diet showing virtually no accumulation of this metabolite. Boyle also noted that as the accumulation of the 1,25-

$(OH)_2D_3$ was suppressed, another polar metabolite appeared in the profile which was later identified as 24,25-dihydroxyvitamin D_3 (24,25-$(OH)_2D_3$) (6). It, therefore, became evident that dietary calcium and hence serum calcium concentration plays an important regulatory role on the vitamin D renal hydroxylases. Because this was not a direct enzymatic measurement, further work in our laboratory by Omdahl et al. in 1972 using in vitro measurements (7) illustrated that chicks given a source of vitamin D and low calcium diets have high renal 25-OH-D_3-1-hydroxylase activity whereas those given vitamin D and high calcium diets showed minimal amounts of this activity and instead the kidney preparations in vitro produced predominantly the 24,25-$(OH)_2D_3$. The results of Omdahl, which are rarely quoted, were confirmed some three years later (8) and illustrate clearly that dietary calcium and hence serum calcium concentration regulates the accumulation of 1,25-$(OH)_2D_3$ by regulating the level of renal 25-OH-D_3-1-hydroxylase activity in the kidney. To gain further insight into how calcium might regulate biosynthesis of 1,25-$(OH)_2D_3$, it appeared that involvement of the parathyroid glands might be possible (9). Again, because of the simplicity with which thyroparathyroidectomy can be executed in rats, it was necessary to carry out the initial investigation in this species. Garabedian et al. (9), therefore, thyroparathyroidectomized vitamin D-deficient rats maintained on a small amount of 1,25-$(OH)_2D_3$ and a low calcium diet. These animals accumulate mainly ^3H-1,25-$(OH)_2D_3$ from ^3H-25-OH-D_3 in their tissues prior to thyroparathyroidectomy. Following this surgery, their ability to produce the 1,25-$(OH)_2D_3$ and thus accumulation in the blood is suppressed until at 48 hours they can no longer synthesize this metabolite and instead they produce 24,25-$(OH)_2D_3$. This change occurred in the face of extreme hypocalcemia and could be reversed by the administration of parathyroid hormone, restoring the ability to produce 1,25-$(OH)_2D_3$. Fraser and Kodicek (10) were able to demonstrate in intact chickens that parathyroid hormone injections stimulate 25-OH-D_3-1-hydroxylase as measured in vitro, a result which we have also obtained in thyroparathyroidectomized chicks. Thus it appears that low serum calcium levels stimulate the parathyroid glands to secrete parathyroid hormone which in turn has, as one of its roles, stimulation of 25-OH-D_3-1-hydroxylase activity in the kidney, illustrating the importance of the parathyroid hormone in the regulation of 25-OH-D_3-1-hydroxylase. The third and important regulatory discovery was the work of Tanaka et al. (11, 12), which demonstrated that phosphate-depleted animals accumulate large amounts of 1,25-$(OH)_2D_3$ in their blood and tissues even in the thyroparathyroidectomized state. Hyperphosphatemia, on the other hand, suppressed accumulation of this metabolite and instead stimulated the accumulation of the 24,25-$(OH)_2D_3$. It, therefore, became apparent that the major controlling factors known for the vitamin D hydroxylases in the kidney are: 1) vitamin D, 2) calcium and the parathyroid hormone, and 3) serum inorganic phosphorus concentration. Since these original discoveries, these basic regulatory phenomenon have been

confirmed in several laboratories. This presentation will attempt
to bring together some of the more recent results relating to these
regulatory phenomenon and their physiologic meaning.

THE ROLE OF 1,25-(OH)$_2$D$_3$

The discovery by Boyle et al. (3, 4) that vitamin D-deficient
rats accumulate ^{3}H-1,25-(OH)$_2$D$_3$ from ^{3}H-25-OH-D$_3$ regardless of
dietary levels of calcium and phosporus led to further examination
of this important question. It soon became evident that in some
manner vitamin D permitted the hydroxylases of the kidney to
become sensitive to regulation by such factors as serum calcium,
parathyroid hormone and serum phosphorus concentration (13). A
further examination of this question led to the discovery that of
the vitamin D metabolites, 1,25-(OH)$_2$D$_3$ appeared to be specific in
permitting this regulation. Thus the administration of 1,25-
(OH)$_2$D$_3$ to vitamin D-deficient rats permitted the accumulation of
24,25-(OH)$_2$D$_3$ in the blood and tissues (13). Additional experiments have shown that administration of a single dose of 1,25-
(OH)$_2$D$_3$ to a rachitic chick brings about a suppression of the 25-
OH-D$_3$-1-hydroxylase and a stimulation of the 25-OH-D$_3$-24-hydroxylase
as measured in vitro (14). It, therefore, appears that the 1,25-
(OH)$_2$D$_3$, among its other functions, is responsible for the induction of the 25-OH-D$_3$-24-hydroxylase whose role is not fully understood. It is of some interest that the 1,25-(OH)$_2$D$_3$ suppresses the
25-OH-D$_3$-1-hydroxylase, but whether this is a direct effect of the
1,25-(OH)$_2$D$_3$ or mediated by the appearance of the 24-hydroxylase or
by the changes in calcium and phosphorus flux across the renal
cells remains to be determined. The specificity of the 1,25-
(OH)$_2$D$_3$ in this system has been tested with the result that of the
vitamin D metabolites, the 1,25-(OH)$_2$D$_3$ is the specific one causing
these changes (13, 14). The mechanism whereby 1,25-(OH)$_2$D$_3$ induces
these changes in the renal hydroxylases remains to be established.
We have not yet been successful in solubilizing the 25-OH-D$_3$-24-
hydroxylase and hence are unable to determine whether this is a
direct induction of a component of this enzyme system or not.
However, 1,25-(OH)$_2$D$_3$ does increase nuclear RNA synthesis in kidney
very soon after injection. It may well be that RNA synthesis may
in part represent the RNA which codes for some components of the
renal 24-hydroxylase. It, therefore, may be that following the
appearance of the messenger RNA from this induction the regulation
phenomenon can become sensitive to calcium, parathyroid hormone and
inorganic phosphorus concentration.

THE ROLE OF CALCIUM AND OF PARATHYROID HORMONE

The work of Boyle et al. (3, 4) demonstrated that there is a
relationship between serum calcium concentration and the accumula-

tion of either $1,25-(OH)_2D_3$ or $24,25-(OH)_2D_3$ in the blood and tissues of rats on a variety of diets provided the animals have received a vitamin D supplement. Garabedian et al. demonstrated that, under the conditions of hypocalcemic challenge, the parathyroid glands play an important role in sensing the hypocalcemia and the parathyroid hormone plays some role in stimulating production of $1,25-(OH)_2D_3$ and suppressing production of $24,25-(OH)_2D_3$. Fraser and Kodicek[3] have provided evidence that parathyroid hormone injections stimulate the $25-OH-D_3$-1-hydroxylase activity as measured in vitro, an effect which was confirmed in our laboratory. Thus the role of the parathyroid hormone and of hypocalcemia through the parathyroid hormone is to stimulate the $25-OH-D_3$-1-hydroxylase, an observation which was confirmed some time later[3] by Henry et al. (8). However, the relationship between the parathyroid hormone and the $25-OH-D_3$-24-hydroxylase activity was not described. When we demonstrated[3] that it was possible to induce the appearance of the 24-hydroxylase by means of nonradioactive $1,25-(OH)_2D_3$ (see the

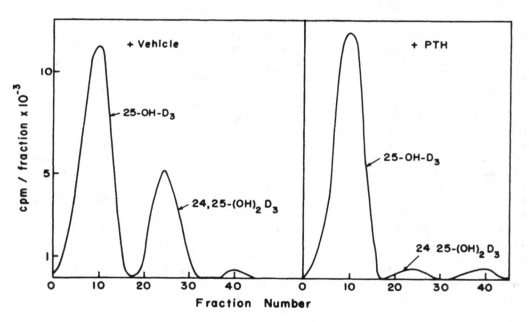

Figure 1. Suppression of renal $25-OH-D_3$-24-hydroxylase by parathyroid hormone. Young chicks were given intravenously 325 pmoles of $1,25-(OH)_2D_3$. Twenty-four hours later one-half of the chicks received 12.5 units of parathyroid hormone every 3 hours for 12 hours. Controls received the vehicle without the parathyroid hormone. The chicks were killed, their kidneys homogenized and the renal hydroxylases determined (14).

second section), we could examine the effect of the parathyroid
hormone on the renal 24-hydroxylase (14). The results shown in
Figure 1 demonstrate that short-term treatment with parathyroid
hormone suppresses the renal 24-hydroxylase without inducing the
renal 25-OH-D$_3$-1-hydroxylase. A more prolonged stimulation with
parathyroid hormone will, however, stimulate the renal 1-hydroxylase.
It, therefore, appears that the renal 25-OH-D$_3$-24-hydroxylase can
be regulated independent of the 25-OH-D$_3$-1-hydroxylase and furthermore it may be that the regulation of the 24-hydroxylase may be a
much more sensitive or the earlier event in the entire regulatory
phenomenon in response to parathyroid hormone.

The observation that the parathyroid hormone plays an important
role in the regulation of the 25-OH-D$_3$-1-hydroxylase led to the
idea that low calcium diets stimulate intestinal calcium absorption
by stimulating parathyroid hormone secretion through hypocalcemia
which in turn would stimulate production of 1,25-(OH)$_2$D$_3$. Increased
1,25-(OH)$_2$D$_3$ would then stimulate intestinal calcium absorption.
Thus it would appear that the hypocalcemic system involving the
parathyroid hormone and the renal production of 1,25-(OH)$_2$D$_3$ might
represent the long sought Nicolaysen endogenous factor (4, 15, 16).
To confirm this position we were able to demonstrate that the
administration of either exogenous 1,25-(OH)$_2$D$_3$ (17) or exogenous
parathyroid hormone (18) to parathyroidectomized animals eliminated
their ability to adapt their intestinal calcium absorption to
dietary calcium levels. Instead, animals were found to absorb
calcium at maximal rates independent of dietary calcium when
provided with sufficient amounts of 1,25-(OH)$_2$D$_3$ or exogenous
parathyroid hormone (see Figure 2).

REGULATION BY PHOSPHATE

It is well known that phosphate deprivation stimulates intestinal calcium absorption as demonstrated in several laboratories
(12, 19, 20). In the search for the mechanism whereby this intestinal calcium absorption could be stimulated by phosphate deprivation, we examined the question of whether the biosynthesis of 1,25-
(OH)$_2$D$_3$ might mediate this phenomenon inasmuch as we had shown that
1,25-(OH)$_2$D$_3$ specifically stimulates the intestinal phosphate
transport system of the ileum and jejunum (21). Tanaka et al.
demonstrated that phosphate deprivation markedly stimulates 1,25-
(OH)$_2$D$_3$ accumulation in blood and suppresses 24,25-(OH)$_2$D$_3$ accumulation even in thyroparathyroidectomized rats. It was, therefore,
possible to plot serum phosphorus concentration versus accumulation
of 1,25-(OH)$_2$D$_3$, demonstrating that serum inorganic phosphorus in
some manner independent of the parathyroid glands controls production of 1,25-(OH)$_2$D$_3$. Henry et al. (8) published a report in which
they claim a 0% phosphorus diet could not stimulate the renal

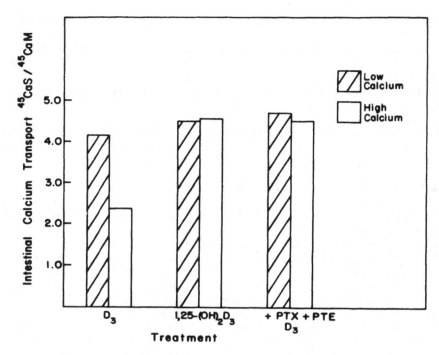

Figure 2. Elimination of intestinal adaptation to dietary calcium by exogenous parathyroid hormone and 1,25-(OH)$_2$D$_3$. Rats were maintained on either a .02% or 1.2% calcium diet for a total of 3 weeks. During the first week they were maintained in the vitamin D-deficient state. At that time they received either 650 pmoles of vitamin D$_3$ or 65 pmoles of 1,25-(OH)$_2$D$_3$ daily. In the parathyroid hormone experiment, the rats were thyroparathyroidectomized and supplemented with 650 pmoles of vitamin D$_3$ daily plus 40 units of parathyroid hormone every 8 hours. At the end of two weeks of such treatment all animals were killed and their intestinal calcium transport determined by the everted sac technique (17, 18).

25-OH-D$_3$-1-hydroxylase as measured in vitro. Upon close examination it became clear that it was not possible for them to have such a low phosphorus diet and instead their diets were probably .35% phosphorus. We, therefore, reexamined the question of phosphate depletion, this time utilizing the chicken where the 1-hydroxylase can be conveniently measured in vitro (22). The results shown in Table I demonstrate that phosphate depletion does in fact stimulate 5-fold the renal 25-OH-D$_3$-1-hydroxylase. In the same animals, one can show a marked stimulation of intestinal calcium absorption,

TABLE I: Stimulation of 25-OH-D$_3$-1-Hydroxylase by Phosphate Depletion in Chicks

Dietary Phosphorus (g%)	Serum Phosphorus (mg%)	1α-OH-ase (pmole 1,25-(OH)$_2$D$_3$/ 15 min/flask)	Calcium Absorption (%/15 min)
0.16	1.5	100	74
0.25	2.6	129	68
0.35	7.5	17	55
0.5	7.5	23	35
1.0	7.5	43	43

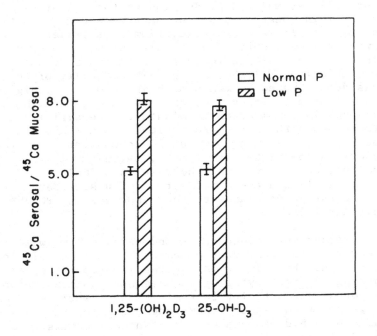

Figure 3. Failure of 1,25-(OH)$_2$D$_3$ to eliminate increased intestinal calcium transport brought about by phosphate depletion. Rats were maintained on a 0.3% or .02% phosphorus diet for three weeks. At one week, they received either 325 pmoles 25-OH-D$_3$ daily or 130 pmoles 1,25-(OH)$_2$D$_3$ daily. At the end of three weeks intestinal calcium transport was determined by the everted sac method (17).

however, the intestinal calcium absorption does not correlate
exactly with the level of renal $25-OH-D_3-1$-hydroxylase activity.
Furthermore, the administration of exogenous $1,25-(OH)_2D_3$ cannot
stimulate intestinal calcium absorption of normal phosphorus rats
to the level achieved by phosphate depletion, suggesting that
phosphate depletion has some effect in addition to stimulating the
$25-OH-D_3-1$-hydroxylase (17) (Figure 3). However, we would like to
emphasize that there is no doubt that phosphate depletion in birds
as well as other species does result in stimulation of the renal
$25-OH-D_3-1$-hydroxylase activity and thus accumulation of $1,25-$
$(OH)_2D_3$ in their tissues despite the claims to the contrary.

To complete the circuit of currently recognized regulators of
vitamin D metabolism, it has been claimed that calcitonin might
play a regulatory role (23). In the experiments of Galante et al.
(23), large amounts of calcitonin were injected into intact animals
and then the accumulation of radioactive $1,25-(OH)_2D_3$ from injected
radioactive $25-OH-D_3$ was assessed. The conclusion reached was that
calcitonin actually stimulated production of the $1,25-(OH)_2D_3$. We
have reexamined this question since we have been unable to find
evidence for calcitonin mediated regulation in a variety of experiments. We were able to confirm the results of Galante et al. in
which the injection of calcitonin to intact animals causes an
increased accumulation of $1,25-(OH)_2D_3$. The identity of this
substance was demonstrated by means of high resolution, high
pressure liquid chromatography (24, 25). However, when the animals
are thyroparathyroidectomized to eliminate the possibility of a
secondary response of the parathyroid glands to the hypocalcemia
brought about by the calcitonin, we could demonstrate no effect of
injected calcitonin on accumulation of $1,25-(OH)_2D_3$ in the rat
(25). Therefore, we believe that the results of Galante et al.
(25) involving calcitonin are a reflection of a secondary response
of the intact parathyroid glands to the hypocalcemia brought about
by the calcitonin injection.

At the International Congress of Endocrinology we will have an
extensive report on the role of the sex hormones in regulating the
renal hydroxylases. Briefly, female birds in preparation for egg
laying or during the egg laying cycle have high concentrations of
$25-OH-D_3-1$-hydroxylase activity in their kidneys whereas males of
comparable age under the same circumstances and fed the same diet
have virtually no 1-hydroxylase and substantial amounts of 24-
hydroxylase (26). Injection of estradiol to mature males will,
within 24 hours, suppress the 24-hydroxylase and markedly stimulate
the 1-hydroxylase (26) (Figure 4). Furthermore, immature animals
or castrates require both androgen and estradiol for this very
quick and dramatic response. There is no question that the sex
hormones play a major regulatory role on the vitamin D hydroxylases,
which may be of great significance in the genesis of metabolic
bone diseases affecting postmenopausal women.

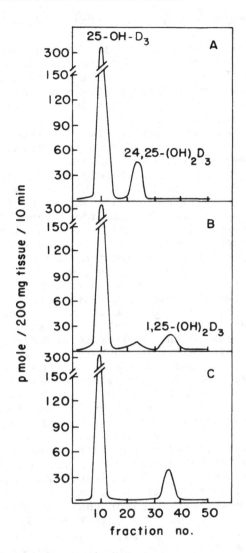

Figure 4. Stimulation of $25-OH-D_3-1$-hydroxylase by estrogen. Four-month old mature male or female quail were used. A) Mature male quail; B) Mature female quail in the egg laying process; C) Mature male quail 24 hours after a 5 mg injection of estradiol valerate. Kidneys were removed from appropriate quail, homogenized and the renal hydroxylases for $^3H-25-OH-D_3$ were determined. Note that following injection of 5 mg of estradiol, mature male quail kidney homogenates switched over from producing $24,25-(OH)_2D_3$ to $1,25-(OH)_2D_3$.

MECHANISM OF REGULATION OF THE RENAL 1-HYDROXYLASES

With the discovery of the regulation of the vitamin D hydroxylases in the kidney by the need for calcium and the need for phosphorus have come many attempts to elucidate the mechanisms involved.
These experiments have involved the addition of calcium and phosphorus to isolated mitochondrial preparations carrying out the
hydroxylation reactions, the addition of these ions and/or the
peptide hormones to isolated renal tubules, and etc. From the
massive amount of literature available in this area, one can
observe any result desired, either no effect or increased 1,25-
$(OH)_2D_3$ production or suppressed 1,25-$(OH)_2D_3$ production, etc.
These results are difficult to interpret because the regulation
which occurs in vivo requires many hours as has been emphasized in
the past (27). Because of the time considerations it is unlikely
that the physiolgic regulation involves ionic inhibition or activation of existing enzymes. However, we will leave the discussion of
these approaches to those who have carried them out, namely Professors
MacIntyre, Rasmussen and Norman. Instead, we have taken two different approaches. One approach has been an attempt to obtain a
tissue culture system which would be sensitive to the physiologic
regulators described from in vivo experiments. Unfortunately, we
have not yet succeeded in conclusively demonstrating a tissue
culture system which retains the ability to produce 1,25-$(OH)_2D_3$
for any degree of time in culture. We have, however, been able to
obtain monkey kidney cells and other isolated renal cell cultures
which carry out the 25-OH-D_3-24-hydroxylation reaction (D. Juan and
H. F. DeLuca, submitted for publication). In this system isolated
monkey kidney cells which have been grown for 4-5 days to confluency
in culture and then for an additional 4-5 days in serum free
medium are used. Monkey kidney cells retain the ability to produce
the 24,25-$(OH)_2D_3$ as identified by periodate sensitivity and by
cochromatography with authentic synthetic 24,25-$(OH)_2D_3$ on high
pressure liquid chromatography. When these monkey kidney cells are
subjected to synthetic human parathyroid hormone (1-34) (kindly
supplied by Dr. John Potts) it is clear that the ability to produce
24,25-$(OH)_2D_3$ is markedly suppressed (see Figure 5). However, even
when the 24-hydroxylase is suppressed, we have not yet been able to
observe the appearance of 1,25-$(OH)_2D_3$. This agrees with the in
vivo experiments in which the 24-hydroxylase appears to be the more
sensitive to the parathyroid hormone. Of some interest is the fact
that high ambient calcium concentration markedly stimulates production of the 24,25-$(OH)_2D_3$ in a direction comparable to that which
occurs in vivo. Finally, the same figure demonstrates that 1,25-
$(OH)_2D_3$ brings about a two-fold increase in the ability of the
monkey kidney cells to produce the 24,25-$(OH)_2D_3$. At the cellular
level, therefore, we can say that the parathyroid hormone appears
to function by suppressing the 24-hydroxylase, whereas 1,25-
$(OH)_2D_3$ enhances that activity. The effect of high calcium suggests

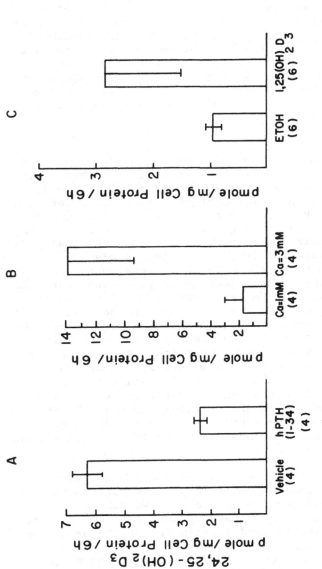

Figure 5. Suppression of 24,25-(OH)$_2$D$_3$ production $\underline{\text{in vitro}}$ by human (1-34) parathyroid hormone (A) and its stimulation or high ambient calcium concentration (B) or 1,25-(OH)$_2$D$_3$ (C) in isolated monkey kidney cells in culture. Kidney cells were isolated from Rhesus monkeys and grown to confluency on a chemically defined medium plus 10% fetal calf serum. They were then grown for an additional five days in serum-free chemically defined medium. The monkey kidney cells were then subjected to human parathyroid hormone (.05 units/ml) every 8 hours or the required calcium concentration or 65 pmoles of 1,25-(OH)$_2$D$_3$ every two days for a period of eight days. Six hours prior to extraction, 25 ng ^{3}H-25-OH-D$_3$ was administered to each culture. The culture medium and cells were extracted and chromatographed to reveal amount of ^{3}H-24,25-(OH)$_2$D$_3$.

that it can directly affect the renal $25-OH-D_3-24$-hydroxylase. It does not seem possible, however, that the effect of ambient calcium can account for the parathyroid hormone suppression since parathyroid hormone would be expected to increase cellular calcium (28). Recently we have been able to observe a stimulation of production of a $1,25-(OH)_2D_3$ like substance by 1-34 human parathyroid hormone, but have not yet been able to confirm that it is in fact $1,25-(OH)_2D_3$. Work is still in progress on the tissue culture systems and it may be that this system may allow a thorough study of the regulators of the renal hydroxylases at the cellular level with confidence that is not available with surviving segments of tissue.

Our other approach has been enzymological in nature in which we have been able to solubilize and isolate components of the renal $25-OH-D_3-1$-hydroxylase (29, 30). We have obtained the three components of the system. They are a NADPH flavoprotein called renal ferredoxin reductase, an iron sulfur protein called renal ferredoxin and a specific cytochrome P-450. The flavoprotein or ferredoxin reductase has been obtained only partially purified, but the ferredoxin itself has been obtained essentially pure and the renal cytochrome P-450 responsible for 1-hydroxylation is also only partially purified. When these three isolated components are combined with NADPH, $25-OH-D_3$ and molecular oxygen, excellent $1,25-(OH)_2D_3$ production occurs. If the cytochrome P-450 fraction is isolated from chickens given a source of vitamin D and high calcium diet, this fraction is inactive. On the other hand, the iron-sulfur protein fraction or the ferredoxin isolated from these animals remains active. These results suggest that it is the cytochrome P-450 component of the hydroxylase which is regulated. Of considerable interest is the fact that added calcium or alteration in phosphorus concentration of the reconstructed renal 1-hydroxylase system has little effect on the 1-hydroxylating activity. Thus if the ions regulate these hydroxylases they must act indirectly on other structural components of the mitochondria or on their synthesis and degradation.

At the present time, therefore, our results do not permit us to draw any conclusions regarding the molecular mechanisms whereby the renal $25-OH-D_3$ hydroxylases are regulated. We can certainly say, however, that 1) $1,25-(OH)_2D_3$ plays an important role in the regulation of its own metabolism and in stimulating the production of $24,25-(OH)_2D_3$; 2) the need for calcium which brings about parathyroid hormone secretion stimulates the renal $25-OH-D_3-1$-hydroxylase and suppresses the renal $25-OH-D_3-24$-hydroxylase; 3) the regulation of the renal $25-OH-D_3-1$-hydroxylase by hypocalcemia and parathyroid hormone secretion accounts for the Nicolaysen endogenous factor; 4) the need for phosphorus which brings about hypophosphatemia stimulates renal $25-OH-D_3-1$-hydroxylase and suppresses the renal $25-OH-D_3-24$-hydroxylase; however, in addition phosphate depletion stimulates intestinal calcium absorption by an unknown mechanism; 5) the regulation of the renal $25-OH-D_3-24$-hydroxylase may be the initial step in any of the regulation phenomenon described since conditions can be demonstrated where it is regulated without affecting $25-OH-D_3-1$-hydroxylase; 6) the sex hormones can have a dramatic effect on the renal $25-OH-D_3-1$-hydroxylase; and 7) the molecular mechanisms of the regulation of the renal hydroxylases remain unknown.

ACKNOWLEDGEMENT

Some of the original investigations reported in this presentation were supported by grant AM-14881 from the National Institutes of Health, contract E(11-1)-1668 from the U. S. Energy Research and Development Administration, and the Harry Steenbock Research Fund.

REFERENCES

1. DeLuca, H. F.: Vitamin D: the vitamin and the hormone. Fed. Proc. 33:2211, 1974.

2. Kodicek, E: The story of vitamin D, from vitamin to hormone. Lancet 1:325, 1974.

3. Boyle, I. T., Gray, R. W., and DeLuca, H. F.: Regulation by calcium of in vivo synthesis of 1,25-dihydroxycholecalciferol and 21,25-dihydroxycholecalciferol. Proc. Nat. Acad. Sci. USA 68:2131, 1971.

4. Boyle, I. T., Gray, R. W., Omdahl, J. L., and DeLuca, H. F.: Calcium control of the in vivo biosynthesis of 1,25-dihydroxy-vitamin D_3: Nicolaysen's endogenous factor. In "Endocrinology 1971" (S. Taylor, ed.). London: Wm. Heinemann Medical Books Ltd. 1972, p. 468.

5. Botham, K. M., Tanaka, Y., and DeLuca, H. F.: 25-Hydroxyvitamin D_3-1-hydroxylase. Inhibition in vitro by rat and pig tissues. Biochemistry 13:4961, 1974.

6. Holick, M. F., Schnoes, H. K., DeLuca, R. W., Gray, R. W., Boyle, I. T., and Suda, T.: Isolation and identification of 24,25-dihydroxycholecalciferol: a metabolite of vitamin D_3 made in the kidney. Biochemistry 11:4251, 1972.

7. Omdahl, J. L., Gray, R. W., Boyle, I. T., Knutson, J., and DeLuca, H. F.: Regulation of metabolism of 25-hydroxycholecalciferol by kidney tissue in vitro by dietary calcium. Nature New Biol. 237:63, 1972.

8. Henry, H. L., Midgett, R. J., and Norman, A. W.: Regulation
    of 25-hydroxyvitamin D_3-1-hydroxylase in vivo. J. Biol. Chem.
    249:7584, 1974.

9. Garabedian, M., Holick, M. F., DeLuca, H. F., and Boyle, I. T.:
    Control of 25-hydroxycholecalciferol metabolism by the para-
    thyroid glands. Proc. Nat. Acad. Sci. USA 69:1673, 1972.

10. Fraser, D. R., and Kodicek, E.: Regulation of 25-hydroxychole-
    calciferol-1-hydroxylase activity in kidney by parathyroid
    hormone. Nature New Biol. 241:163, 1973.

11. Tanaka, Y., and DeLuca, H. F.: The control of 25-hydroxyvitamin
    D metabolism by inorganic phosphorus. Arch. Biochem. Biophys.
    154:566, 1973.

12. Tanaka, Y., Frank, H., and DeLuca, H. F.: Intestinal calcium
    transport: stimulation by low phosphorus diets. Science 181:
    564, 1973.

13. Tanaka, Y., and DeLuca, H. F.: Stimulation of 24,25-dihydroxy-
    vitamin D_3 production by 1,25-dihydroxyvitamin D_3. Science 183:
    1198, 1974.

14. Tanaka, Y., Lorenc, R. S., and DeLuca, H. F.: The role of 1,25-
    dihydroxyvitamin D_3 and parathyroid hormone in the regulation of
    chick renal 25-hydroxyvitamin D_3-24-hydroxylase. Arch. Biochem.
    Biophys. 171:521, 1975.

15. Nicolaysen, R., Eeg-Larsen, N., and Malm, O. J.: Physiology of
    calcium metabolism. Physiol. Rev. 33:424, 1953.

16. Omdahl, J. L., and DeLuca, H. F.: Regulation of vitamin D
    metabolism and function. Physiol. Rev. 53:327, 1973.

17. Ribovich, M. L., and DeLuca, H. F.: The influence of dietary
    calcium and phosphorus on intestinal calcium transport in rats
    given vitamin D metabolites. Arch. Biochem. Biophys. 170:529,
    1975.

18. Ribovich, M. L., and DeLuca, H. F.: Intestinal calcium transport:
    parathyroid hormone and adaptation to dietary calcium. Arch.
    Biochem. Biophys., in press, 1976.

19. Carlsson, A.: Tracer experiments on the effect of vitamin D on
    the skeletal metabolism of calcium and phosphorus. Acta
    Physiol. Scand. 26:212, 1952.

20. Morrissey, R. L., and Wasserman, R. H.: Calcium absorption and calcium-binding protein in chicks on differing calcium and phosphorus intakes. Am. J. Physiol. 220:1509, 1971.

21. Chen, T. C., Weber, J. C., and DeLuca, H. F.: On the subcellular location of vitamin D metabolites in intestine. J. Biol. Chem. 245:3776, 1970.

22. Baxter, L. A., and DeLuca, H. F.: Stimulation of 25-hydroxy-vitamin D_3-1α-hydroxylase by phosphate depletion. J. Biol. Chem. 251:3158, 1976.

23. Galante, L., Colson, K. W., MacAuley, S. J., and MacIntyre, I.: Effect of calcitonin on vitamin D metabolism. Nature 238:271, 1972.

24. Jones, G., and DeLuca, H. F.: High-pressure liquid chromatography: separation of the metabolites of vitamins D_2 and D_3 on small-particle silica columns. J. Lipid Res. 16:448, 1975.

25. Lorenc, R., Tanaka, Y., DeLuca, H. F., and Jones, G.: Calcitonin and regulation of vitamin D metabolism. Endocrinology, in press, 1976.

26. Tanaka, Y., Castillo, L., and DeLuca, H. F.: Control of the renal vitamin D hydroxylases in birds by the sex hormones. Proc. Nat. Acad. Sci. USA, in press, 1976.

27. Ghazarian, J. G., Tanaka, Y., and DeLuca, H. F.: The biochemistry of the chick kidney mitochondrial 25-hydroxyvitamin D_3-1α-hydroxylase and its regulation. In "Calcium Regulating Hormones" (R. V. Talmage, M. Owen, and J. A. Parsons, eds.). Amsterdam: Excerpta Medica, 1975, p. 381.

28. Borle, A. B.: Calcium and phosphate metabolism. Ann. Rev. Physiol. 36:361, 1974.

29. Ghazarian, J. G., Jefcoate, C. R., Knutson, J. C., Orme-Johnson, W. H., and DeLuca, H. F.: Mitochondrial cytochrome P-450: a component of chick kidney 25-hydroxycholecalciferol-1α-hydroxylase. J. Biol. Chem. 249:3026, 1974.

30. Pedersen, J. I., Ghazarian, J. G., Orme-Johnson, N. R., and DeLuca, H. F.: Isolation of chick renal mitochondrial ferredoxin active in the 25-hydroxyvitamin D_3-1α-hydroxylase system. J. Biol. Chem., in press, 1976.

Interrelationships Between the Key Elements of the Vitamin D Endo-
crine System: 25-OH-D$_3$-1-Hydroxylase, Serum Calcium and Phosphorus
Levels, Intestinal 1,25(OH)$_2$D$_3$, and Intestinal Calcium Binding
Protein

Anthony W. Norman*, Ernest J. Friedlander and Helen Henry

Department of Biochemistry, University of California

Riverside, California 92502 USA

   Calcium and phosphorus homeostasis is exquisitely regulated
by the three hormones, calcitonin, parathyroid hormone, and
cholecalciferol (vitamin D$_3$). The most notable advance in our
understanding of the mechanism of action of vitamin D has been
the elucidation of the complex metabolic pathway which has evolved
to produce the biologically active form, 1,25-dihydroxyvitamin D$_3$
[1,25(OH)$_2$D$_3$]. Coupled with these developments concerning our
understanding of the metabolic pathway of conversion of vitamin D
into its active form, has been the realization that the mechanism
of action of the fat soluble vitamin D is in reality similar to
that of many of the classical steroid hormones, e.g. aldosterone,
testosterone, estrogen, hydrocortisone, and ecdysterone. It
should be noted that chemically vitamin D is in reality a steroid,
in particular a seco steroid. Seco steroids are those in which
one of the rings has undergone fission; in the instance of calciferol, this is ring B. It has been proposed (1,2) that vitamin D
may generate its characteristic physiological response (5) by its
ability to activate or stimulate the biochemical expression of
genetic information which ultimately leads to the synthesis of
functionally specialized proteins or the alteration of membrane
structure necessary for calcium absorption. In this regard, it
has been unequivocally established by Wasserman and colleagues
that one of the primary biological responses of vitamin D or its
active forms in the intestine is the generation of a specific
protein which has the capability of binding calcium in a highly
specific fashion (3). This protein has been termed vitamin D
dependent calcium binding protein (CaBP).

* This work was supported by United States Public Health Service
grants AM-09012 and AM-14,750.

Calciferol, which may either be ingested dietarily or produced
in the skin by a photochemical reaction, is first transported to
the liver, where it is hydroxylated at the 25 position.   25-
Hydroxy-vitamin D_3 [25-OH-D_3] is next transported to the kidney
where it further undergoes metabolism to produce either 1,25-
dihydroxyvitamin D_3 [1,25(OH)$_2$D3] or 24,25-dihydroxyvitamin D_3
[24,25(OH)$_2$D3].   These relationships are summarized in Figure 1.
The 1,25-(OH)$_2$D3 then proceeds by the circulatory system to its
various organs, primarily the intestine and bone where it interacts
and produces its characteristic physiological response.   The key
focal point in this endocrine pathway for production of the
biologically active form of vitamin D is the kidney.   The kidney
also has the potential in some species and under some physiological
circumstances to produce 24,25(OH)$_2$D3; the physiological role of
this steroid remains to be established.   The reader is referred
to Norman and Henry (4) and Coburn et al. (5) for the review of

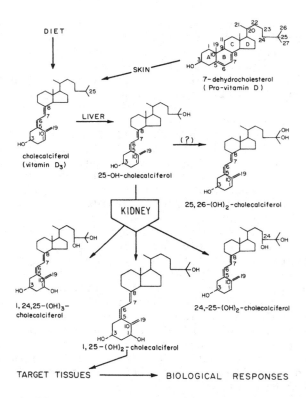

Figure 1.   Metabolic or endocrine pathway for the production of
the hormonally active form of vitamin D, 1,25(OH)$_2$D3.   The central
role of the kidney as it functions as an endocrine gland, related
to vitamin D metabolism, is apparent.

recent literature describing the general biochemical features and clinically relevant aspects of this vitamin D endocrine system.

What evidence is there to support the thesis that $1,25(OH)_2D_3$ is a hormone? It is not sufficient to just have a mode of action similar to that of other steroid hormones. A hormone is classically defined as being a systemic acting substance produced by specialized cells in response to a specific set of physiological stimuli or signals; very small amounts of the substance are then released into the circulation and transported to distal target organs where it interacts to elicit a set of specific physiological responses. It is the lack of these responses which usually generates indirectly the signal which results in the secretion of the hormone. Normally an endocrine system has a method of self regulation, i.e. once the physiological response which is produced by the presence of the hormone is manifested, there is an auto-regulation or homeostasis such that the secretion or production of the hormone is modulated or terminated. It is the purpose of this article to review recent experiments carried out in our laboratory which describe the homeostasis or autoregulation of the endocrine signals which are operative between the endocrine gland, the kidney, and its associated $25-OH-D_3-1$-hydroxylases or 24-hydroxylases and the intestine, where the production of CaBP is under the direct control of the presence of this steroid hormone.

The regulation of the renal production of $1,25(OH)_2D_3$ has been studied in the whole animal where the presence and absence of the peptide hormones, PTH, and calcitonin can be controlled by a surgical technique or hormone injection. Circulating levels of vitamin D and its metabolites and of calcium and phosphorus are affected by altering their quantities in the diet. It has been reported that both increased dietary calcium (6-8) and dietary phosphorus (8,9) reduced circulating and tissue levels of $1,25(OH)_2D_3$ from radioactively labeled vitamin D or 25-OH-D in chicks and rats. The effect of phosphorus was observed only in thyroparathyroidectomized rats (TPTX) (9). More recently, a radio-receptor assay has been employed by Brumbaugh and associates to measure unlabeled $1,25(OH)_2D_3$ (10); in these studies intact rats, as well as TPTX rats had reduced plasma levels of $1,25(OH)_2D_3$ when dietary phosphorus was increased. Henry et al. (11) found the specific activity of the renal 25-OH-D-1-hydroxylase to be inversely related to dietary and serum calcium, but was unrelated to dietary serum or renal tissue phosphorus levels. An interesting feature of most of the foregoing studies has been the observation that in the presence of vitamin D or one of its metabolites, a decrease in the production or appearance in blood or tissue of $1,25(OH)_2D_3$ is accompanied by an increase in the production or appearance of $24,25(OH)_2D_3$. DeLuca and colleagues (8,9) have repeatedly pointed out this apparent reciprocal relationship.

Parathyroid hormone has been implicated by a number of studies as a stimulatory hormone for the production of $1,25(OH)_2D_3$ by the kidney. Parathyroidectomy of vitamin D-deficient chicks has been observed by Henry et al. (11) as well as by Fraser and Kodicek (12) to result in a marked fall in 1-hydroxylase activity as measured under conditions in vitro. Others, however, have reported an effect of parathyroidectomy on 1-hydroxylase levels only in the presence of dietary vitamin D_3. Interestingly, parathyroid extract was capable of maintaining 1-hydroxylase levels in chicks a few days old (12), but was reported to have no effect on 1-hydroxylation in intact two-week old chicks (13). In rats, thyroparathyroidectomy led to a decrease in plasma levels of $1,25(OH)_2D_3$ (14) which is overcome by the administration of parathyroid extract or feeding a diet low in phosphorus content. Favus et al. made the interesting observation (15) that adaptation of intestinal calcium absorption to differing levels of dietary calcium is capable of occuring in TPTX rats, as well as their sham-operated controls. Further, in spite of the reduced plasma levels of $1,25(OH)_2D_3$, the amount of the steroid localized in the intestine was similar in both the sham and TPTX animals. In contrast, Seymour and DeLuca (16) concluded that the hypoparathyroid animal cannot synthesize appreciable quantities of $1,25(OH)_2D_3$. Haussler et al. (17) have reported lower than normal levels of $1,25(OH)_2D_3$ in hypoparathyroid human patients, and somewhat higher than normal levels associated with hyperparathyroidism. In contrast to the above results suggesting the parathyroid hormone plays a role, but not necessarily an absolute one, in promoting the renal production of $1,25(OH)_2D_3$, Galante et al. (18,19) have reported that PTH inhibits and calcitonin stimulates $1,25(OH)_2D_3$ production in vivo. Clearly, the roles of these two peptide hormones in the regulation of vitamin D metabolism have not yet been clearly defined.

Another potential regulator of $1,25(OH)_2D_3$ production is vitamin D or one of its metabolites. The observation that renal 1-hydroxylase levels are inversely correlated with the vitamin D status of the animal has been made by Henry et al. (11,20), as well as by others (12,21). $1,25(OH)_2D_3$ is as effective as the parent vitamin in lowering enzyme concentration in the kidney (11,22). These observations have led to the hypothesis that $1,25(OH)_2D_3$ may decrease its own production by reducing PTH secretion. In this regard, it may be pertinent that we have recently shown that tritiated $1,25(OH)_2D_3$ is rapidly and specifically accumulated by the parathyroid glands in a fashion somewhat to that shown previously to occur in the intestine (23).

An alternative approach to the problem of elucidation of the mechanism of regulation of production of $1,25(OH)_2D_3$ has been to carry out experiments employing isolated mitochondria. These subcellular organelles are then exposed to a variety of environmental conditions which may either stimulate or inhibit the production of

1,25(OH)$_2$D$_3$. As indicated above, modulation of the renal production of 1,25(OH)$_2$D$_3$ by the prevailing mineral status (i.e. serum
calcium or serum or phosphorus) of the organism may be suggested as
a functional regulatory mechanism for this steroid hormone. Henry
and Norman (20,24) reported the inhibition of the l-hydroxylase by
low calcium concentrations (10^{-5}-10^{-4} M); similar observations have
also been reported by other investigators (12,21). It has also
been reported, however, (25) that calcium has no effect on the rate
of l-hydroxylation. Still other investigators have observed that
in mitochondria previously depleted of calcium by extensive washing
with EGTA, the addition of increasing concentrations of calcium
back to the medium, first stimulates and then at higher concentrations, inhibits l-hydroxylation (26,27). Whether there is a physiologically significant basis for any of these observations remains
to be established.

The effects of phosphate on l-hydroxylation have been less
widely investigated than those of calcium, but with no more agreement in results or interpretation. Henry and Norman (24) have reported a 50% inhibition of l-hydroxylation by 5 mM phosphate in the
absence of added calcium and, as with calcium, NADPH-supported
hydroxylation is as sensitive to phosphate inhibition as is that
supported by malate. Colston et al. (28) reported that phosphate
has no effect in the absence of added calcium and reversed the
inhibitory effect of calcium when both ions were present together.
Bikle et al. (29) reported calcium-enhanced phosphate stimulation
of l-hydroxylation when the pH of the incubation mixture was less
than 7.0. These authors suggested in general terms that the l-
hydroxylation process may be regulated by a complex interaction of
calcium, phosphate, and hydrogen ions.

In this regard, while it appears to be generally agreed that
the "calcium demand" of the organism, i.e. a lowered serum calcium
level and associated elevation of circulating levels of PTH, may
result in an increased production of 1,25(OH)$_2$D$_3$, there is no
general agreement as to the consequences of "phosphate demand",
i.e. lowered the serum phosphorus level. Baxter and DeLuca have
recently reported that feeding chicks a low phosphorus diet for a
prolonged period of time resulted in a marked increase in enzyme l-
hydroxylase activity, relative to chicks fed a normal phosphorus
diet. This result supplemented the earlier observation of Tanaka
and DeLuca (9) who had indicated that a lowered renal inorganic
phosphate level stimulated the conversion of 25-OH-D$_3$ to 1,25(OH)$_2$D$_3$
as measured by chromatographic evaluation of circulating levels of
vitamin D metabolites. Both these results were contrary to the
earlier reports of Henry et al. (11), who measuring initial reaction
velocities of the 25-OH-D$_3$-l-hydroxylase activities, could find no
evidence in support of the concept that lowered serum phosphorus
might stimulate or elevate this activity. Therefore, the question
of whether the increased accumulation of 1,25(OH)$_2$D$_3$ in blood and

tissues reported by Tanaka and DeLuca, because of phosphate deprivation, is the result of increased 25-OH-D_3-1-hydroxylase activities
remained unresolved.

A related and very important question concerns determination
of whether the increased biosynthesis of 1,25(OH)$_2D_3$ can account
for the increased calcium absorption brought about by low phosphorus
intakes (31,32) or whether the phosphorus effect is subsequent to
the renal production of 1,25(OH)$_2D_3$. For example Bar and Wasserman
(33) found that chicks fed dehydrotachysterol as an analog of
1,25(OH)$_2D_3$ showed an increased intestinal absorption of calcium

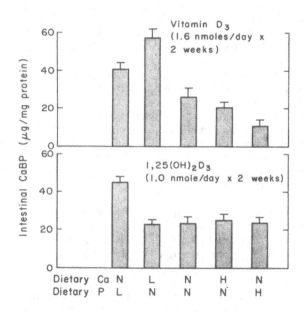

Figure 2. Differential production of intestinal calcium binding
protein (CaBP) after daily administration of vitamin D_3 or
1,25(OH)$_2D_3$. Groups of six-eight chicks, 14 days old, were raised
on the indicated experimental diets for an additional 2 weeks, over
which time they received 1.6 nmoles/day of vitamin D_3 (upper panel)
or 1.0 nmole/day of 1,25(OH)$_2D_3$ (lower panel). Analysis of the
diets indicated that the percent calcium was L = 0.11%, N = 0.7%,
H = 1.2%. Intestinal CaBP was evaluated by the radialimmunodiffusion technique. Errors shown are the standard error of the mean.

when fed low phosphorus diets. Furthermore exogenous $1,25(OH)_2D_3$
eliminated adaptation of intestinal calcium transport to low calcium
diets, while it did not eliminate the stimulation of intestinal
calcium transport by low phosphorus diets (32).

     In Figure 2 is shown the differential response in chicks in
terms of their steady state levels of intestinal calcium binding
protein (CaBP) as a function of whether they were fed vitamin D_3
or $1,25(OH)_2D_3$ over a period of two weeks. It should be clearly
evident that in the presence of dietary vitamin D (top panel) diets
with low calcium as well as a low phosphorus content, result in the
production of significantly elevated levels of CaBP. On the basis
of this data one might postulate that this stimulation of CaBP by
low Ca or low P diets is the result of regulatory signals on the
kidney-1-hydroxylase system, but as shown in the bottom panel of
Figure 2, this is not a tenable thesis. Under circumstances where
the kidney is short-circuited, i.e. in the presence of daily administration of $1,25(OH)_2D_3$, there would be no possibility of regulation of the 1-hydroxylase in a meaningful sense. Under these
circumstances, there is no adaptation of CaBP in response to low
dietary Ca levels, while there is evident a significant stimulation
of synthesis of CaBP in the presence of diets with a low phosphorus
content. Thus, the possibility exists that there is a two-fold
effect of phosphate deprivation, one which may be manifest in
stimulating renal enzyme activity and one which may be effected
through low phosphate induced stimulus of either the delivery of
$1,25(OH)_2D_3$ to the intestine or its subsequent interaction with the
receptors therein, which somehow both lead to an enhanded production of CaBP.

     As shown in Figure 3, the phosphate induced stimulation of
CaBP was not dependent upon the dose of $1,25(OH)_2D_3$ administered.
Shown in Figure 3 is a dose response study where increasing amounts
of $1,25(OH)_2D_3$ were administered daily to chicks fed a variety of
dietary levels of Ca and P. Thus, the dramatic stimulation of the
steady state level of intestinal CaBP by phosphate deprivation and
the striking absence of the stimulation of steady state levels of
intestinal CaBP by calcium depletion in the presence of a wide
range of administered dose of $1,25(OH)_2D_3$ was clearly apparent. An
intriguing problem for the future is to identify the basis for the
mechanism for the phosphate deprivation of $1,25(OH)_2D_3$ stimulated
CaBP.

     The prime focus of the remainder of this chapter is to address
the question of how perturbations in circulating levels of serum
calcium and/or phosphorus may modulate the renal production of
either $1,25(OH)_2D_3$ or $24,25(OH)_2D_3$. The general experimental
protocol employed for these studies was to take groups of 6-12, 14
day old vitamin D-deficient chicks, and place them on diets ranging
in calcium content from 0.1-2.1% and/or 0.15-1.1% phosphorus, and

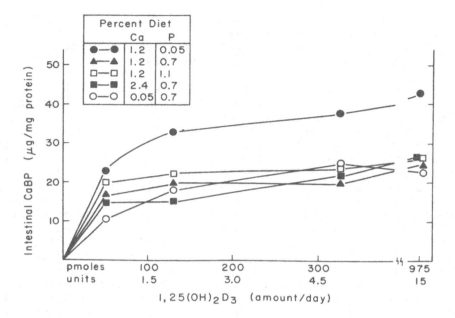

Figure 3.   Relationship between varying dietary Ca and P levels on the production of intestinal calcium proten (CaBP) after $1,25(OH)_2D_3$ administration.   Groups of 6-8 chicks, 14 days old, were raised on the indicated diet for another two weeks and received the indicated levels of $1,25(OH)_2D_3$ daily.   Intestinal CaBP was evaluated by the radialimmodiffusion technique.

to administer on a daily basis 1.62 nmoles (25 IU) of $1,2-^3$H-vitamin D_3/day for a two week period of time.   It was presumed that over this two week interval all birds would adapt to the particular level of calcium and phosphorus they were receiving in their diet, and would therefore ultimately be in a steady state situation.   At the end of this period of time, all birds were killed, and individual values of the specific activity of the 25-OH-D_3-1-hydroxylase and 25-OH-D_3-24-hydroxylase activity were carried out under in vitro conditions, as previously described by Henry and Norman (20); this method determines the initial reaction velocity of the enzyme activity.   Also, for each bird, individual levels of serum calcium and phosphorus were obtained by standard techniques, as well as an individual determination of the CaBP level by the technique of radialimmunodiffusion, which employed a specific antibody prepared to chick intestinal calcium binding protein.   In addition for each

group of 6-8 birds, the distribution of vitamin D and its metabolites
in the blood and intestinal mucosa, were evaluated by chromatography
on 1x80 cm columns of Sephadex LH-20. Thus, through this experimental protocol it is possible to correlate the specific activity
of both renal enzyme activities, the 1α and 24- hydroxylases, the
serum Ca and P levels with the intestinal levels of 1,25(OH)$_2$D$_3$ and
CaBP. These relationships are discussed in detail in the following
paragraphs.

Figure 4 shows the relationship between changing serum calcium
levels and the corresponding level of the 25-OH-D$_3$-1-hydroxylase.
There is a highly significant inverse correlation, such that as
serum calcium falls, the specific activity of the 1-hydroxylase

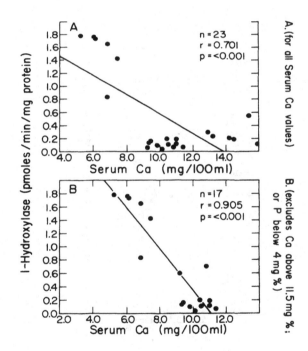

Figure 4. Relationship between specific activity of the 25-OH-D$_3$-
1-hydroxylase and circulating serum calcium levels. Groups of 6-8
chicks, 14 days old, were fed diets ranging from 0.21-2.1% calcium,
0.11-1.1% P, and received daily for two weeks 1.62 nmoles of vitamin
D$_3$. (A) Includes all 1-hydroxylase values for all serum calcium
determinations; (B) Excludes 1-hydroxylase values for serum Ca
above 11.5 mg/100 ml or P below 4 mg/100ml.

rises dramatically. It should be noted, however, that in the
population of birds which received vitamin D daily for two weeks,
the enzyme activity present in those birds receiving a calcium
depleted diet (i.e. had a serum calcium below 7.0 mg/100 ml) is
only approximately 1/3 of the specific activity that a vitamin D-
deficient chick would have (see Henry et al. Reference 11). This
inverse relationship is significantly increased when the 1-hydroxy-
lase values corresponding to chicks with serum calciums above
11.5 mg/100 ml are excluded; the slope is more than doubled in
comparison to when the entire population is evaluated.

    In Figure 5, a similar analysis is shown for the relationship
between the renal 25-OH-D$_3$-1-hydroxylase and circulating serum

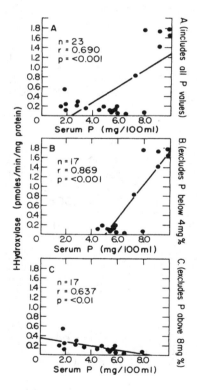

Figure 5. Relationship between specific activity of 25-OH-D$_3$-1-
hydroxylase and circulating serum phosphorus levels. Groups of 6-
8 chicks, 14 days old, were fed diets ranging in Ca from 0.2-2.1%,
and 0.15-1.1% P, and received daily for two weeks 1.6 nmoles of
vitamin D$_3$. (A) Includes 1-hydroxylase for all serum P values; (B)
Excludes 1-hydroxylase values for serum P below 4 mg/100 ml; (C)
Excludes 1-hydroxylase values for serum P above 8 mg/100 ml.

values for phosphorus. Panel A shows the relationship for the 1-hydroxylase for all values of serum P, while panel B excludes 1-hydroxylase values with a serum P below 4 mg/100 ml and in panel C 1-hydroxylase values are excluded for serum P values above 8 mg/100 ml. It should be noted upon inspection of panel A that the population of 1-hydroxylase values for the complete population of serum P values falls into three distinct subsets, those occurring between 4-8 mg/100 ml and those above 7 mg/100 ml. Thus when the total population is subdivided as shown in panels B and C, one can obtain highly significant but completely opposite correlations between 1-hydroxylase levels and the circulating level of serum phosphorus. Under circumstances where serum phosphorus exceeds 5 mg/100 ml, there is a direct correlation between the steady state level of the $25-OH-D_3-1$-hydroxylase and the phosphorus level, while as shown in panel C when serum P ranges from 1.5 to 8 mg/100 ml there is a modest inverse correlation between the 1-hydroxylase level and the corresponding serum P value. An important problem is to place this modest dependency on serum phosphorus, shown in Figure 5, and the striking dependency upon serum calcium, as shown in Figure 4, into the appropriate physiologic framework or set of circumstances.

In view of the results of Boyle et al. (17) suggesting an inverse relationship between the circulating levels of $1,25(OH)_2D_3$ and $24,25(OH)_2D_3$ which they reported on the basis of chromatographic evaluation of plasma levels of these metabolites, it was of importance in the foregoing studies to also evaluate the steady state level of the renal $25-OH-D_3-24$-hydroxylase activities. This was possible by utilization of appropriate Sephadex-LH-20 columns which separate the radioactive peak of $24,25(OH)_2D_3$ from both $1,25(OH)_2D_3$ and $25-OH-D_3$. The results of these studies are presented in Figure 6. Figure 6-A shows the relationship between the 24-hydroxylase and the circulating level of serum calcium for all groups of chicks. First, it should be noted that the steady state level of the 24-hydroxylase is markedly lower than that for the $25-OH-D_3-1$-hydroxylase shown in Figures 4 and 5. Secondly, it is apparent that there is no significant correlation between changes in the circulating levels of serum calcium and the 24-hydroxylase steady state level. Shown in panels B and C of Figure 5 is a similar evaluation of the relationship between steady state $25-OH-D-24$-hydroxylase and circulating values of serum phosphorus. As shown in panel B, there was also no correlation between the 24-hydroxylase and the entire population of serum P values; however, as shown in panel C, when the 24-hydroxylase values correspond to the serum P above 7 mg/100 ml were excluded, there was a modest inverse correlation between serum P and this enzyme activity. These results would appear to cast major doubt upon the participating of the renal 24-hydroxylase in modulated endocrine activities pertaining to calcium and phosphorus homeostasis. Under the circumstances of a vitamin D-replete animal, this enzyme does not undergo

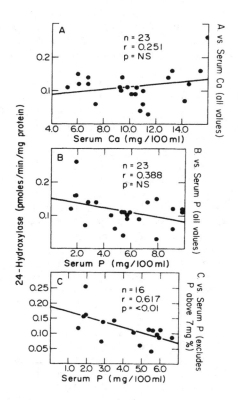

Figure 6. Relationship between specific activity of 25-OH-D$_3$-24-hydroxylase and circulating levels of serum calcium or phosphorus. Groups of 6-8 chicks, 14 days old, were fed diets ranging from 0.21-2.1% calcium and 0.15-1.1% P and received daily for two weeks, 1.6 nmoles of vitamin D$_3$. (A) 24-Hydroxylase values for all serum calcium values; (B) 24-Hydroxylase values for all serum P values; (C) Excludes 24-hydroxylase values for serum P above 7 mg/100 ml.

any significant change in its steady state activities; the only striking change apparent in the 24-hydroxylase is its complete absence in a vitamin D-deficient animal (7,11).

Norman and Henry (4) have previously postulated a correlation between the "calcium demand" of the organism and the steady state level of both intestinal CaBP and the renal 25-OH-D-1-hydroxylase. Thus one might anticipate that under circumstances of increased "calcium demand" there would be elevated levels of the 1-hydroxylase which would in turn result in elevated production of CaBP.

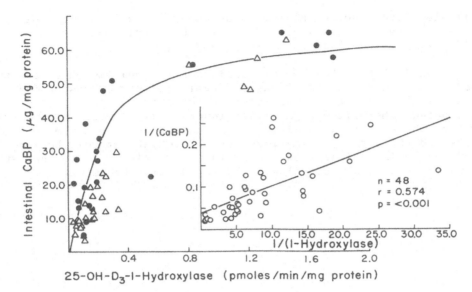

Figure 7. Relationship between intestinal calcium binding protein (CaBP) and steady state levels of renal 25-OH-D₃-1-hydroxylase levels. Groups of 6-8 chicks, 14 days old, were fed diets ranging from 0.2-2.1% Ca and 0.15-1.1% P and received daily for two weeks 1.6 nmoles of vitamin D₃. After sacrifice, the specific activity of the 25-OH-D₃-1-hydroxylase and the level of intestinal CaBP was determined individually for each bird. Data in main panel are plotted as rectangular hyperbola, while the inset panel presents the same data plotted in a double reciprocal fashion.

Shown in Figure 7 is the quantitative relationship between the steady state level of the renal 1-hydroxylase and corresponding steady state levels of intestinal CaBP which result in birds fed diets with a wide range of CaBP levels. The results appear to follow the hyperbolic curve of a substrate-enzyme mediated-product relationship. Thus as shown in the inset to Fig. 7 a plot of 1/CaBP versus 1/1-hydroxylase yields a highly significant linear relationship. The intercept of the line on the ordinate indicates the maximal amount of CaBP which might be obtained, in this instance a value of 60-75 μg/mg protein. The specific activity of the 1-hydroxylase which is capable of producing the half-maximal value of CaBP is approximately 0.2 pmoles/minute/mg protein. From inspection of Figure 4-B, it can be seen that this specific activity corresponds to a serum calcium of ca. 10 mg/100 ml; thus under normal steady state circumstances, when there is adequate dietary calcium

available, normal serum calcium values of 9-10 mg/100 ml can be
maintained <u>via</u> this low level of renal 1-hydroxylase and this
"half-maximal amount" of intestinal CaBP.

Shown in Figure 8 is an evaluation of the relationship between
steady state intestinal $1,25(OH)_2D_3$ levels and the corresponding
circulating levels of serum calcium or phosphorus. As might be
anticipated, there is a significant inverse relationship with serum
calcium, while there is a direct relationship between serum phosphorus and the corresponding level of $1,25(OH)_2D_3$ steroid hormone
bound to the intestinal tissue. It is interesting to note that at
the normal serum calcium value of 10 mg/100 ml, the amount of

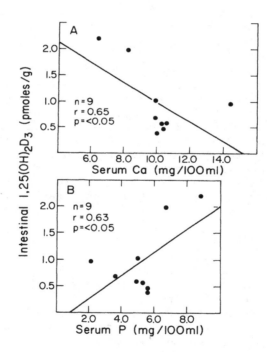

Figure 8. Relationship between intestinal levels of $^3H-1,25(OH)_2D_3$
and circulating levels of serum Ca and P. Groups of 6-8 chicks, 14
days old, were fed diets ranging in composition from 0.2-2.1% Ca
and 0.15-1.1% P, and received daily for two weeks, 1.6 nmoles of
$1,2-^3H$-vitamin D3. Metabolite concentrations were evaluated <u>via</u>
Sephadex LH-20 chromatography and are corrected for tritrum loss.
(A) Intestinal $1,25(OH)_2D_3$ for all serum calcium values; (B)
Intestinal $1,25(OH)_2D_3$ for all serum P values.

1,25(OH)$_2$D$_3$ bound to the intestinal mucosa is approximately one-half its maximal attainable value, i.e., under normal-calcemic circumstances, the animal is regulated at its midpoint value.

Figures 9 and 10 respectively show the correlation between the intestinal calcium-binding protein and circulating steady state levels of serum P or serum Ca. In each instance when the values of intestinal calcium-binding protein are evaluated for the entire population of either serum P (9-A) or serum Ca (Figure 10), there is no significant correlation. Upon inspection of these two panels, however, it should be apparent that the populations of serum P and serum Ca divide themselves into three subsets. Accordingly, as

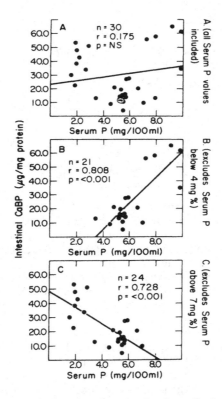

Figure 9. Relationship between intestinal calcium binding protein (CaBP) and circulating levels of serum phosphorus. Groups of 6-8 chicks, 14 days old, were fed diets ranging in composition from 0.2-2.1% Ca and 0.15-1.1% P, and received daily for two weeks, 1.6 nmoles of vitamin D3. (A) Values of CaBP are reported for all serum P below 4 mg/100 ml; (C) Excludes CaBP values for serum P determinations above 7 mg/100 ml. Intestinal CaBP was determined by quantitative radialimmunodiffusion assay.

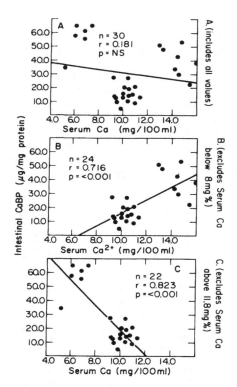

Figure 10. Relationship between intestinal calcium binding protein
(CaBP) and circulating levels of serum calcium. Groups of 6-8
chicks, 14 days old, were fed diets ranging from 0.2-2.1% Ca and
0.15-1.1% P and received daily, for two weeks, 1.6 nmoles of vitamin
D_3. (A) Includes CaBP values for all serum Ca determinations; (B)
Excludes CaBP values for serum Ca values below 8 mg percent; (C)
Excludes CaBP values for serum calcium values of 11.8 mg percent.

shown in Figures 9-B and 9-C as well as 10-B and 10-C, there are
dramatic but opposite relationships apparent between the values of
intestinal calcium CaBP and either P or serum Ca. As shown in
Figure 10-B there is a highly significant positive correlation
between intestinal CaBP and serum P for values of serum P above
4 mg/100 ml while in marked contrast, there is a highly significant
inverse correlation between intestinal CaBP and serum P for serum P
values below 8 mg/100 ml. Similarly, as shown in Figure 10-B,
there is a positive correlation between intestinal CaBP and serum
Ca values above 8 mg/100 ml, while there is a highly significant
inverse correlation between intestinal CaBP and serum Ca values
when they are below 11.5 mg/100 ml. It would seem significant that
the intersection of the two regression lines for the positive and
inverse correlations for both serum Ca and serum P is at the normo-

calcemic value for calcium of 10 mg/100 ml and 5-6 mg/100 ml P.
Thus when the animal is able to achieve normal serum calcium of
10 mg/100 ml and normal serum P of 5-6 mg/100 ml there is a corresponding steady state level of intestinal CaBP of approximately
20 µg/mg of protein. Under these circumstances, then, the animal
has a large capacity for further elevation in intestinal CaBP in
the event that some dietary stress is induced or there is some
depletion of either serum Ca or P via other physiological circumstances.

    Shown in Figure 11 (panels A and B) is a summary of our current
understanding of calcium and phosphorus homeostasis as pertains to
regulation of the kidney levels of 25-OH-D$_3$-1-hydroxylase and 25-
OH-D$_3$-24-hydroxylase (panel A) and the steady state relationships
between intestinal levels of CaBP which are endocrinologically
linked to the circulating levels of serum Ca and serum P.   In terms

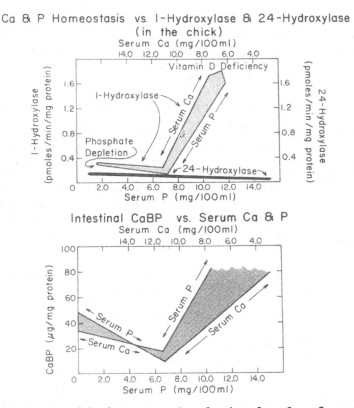

Figure 11. Relationship between circulating levels of serum calcium
and phosphorus versus (upper panel) steady state levels of 25-OH-D-
1-hydroxylase and 25-OH-D-24-hydroxylase and (lower panel) intestinal levels of calcium binding protein (CaBP).

of the renal 1-hydroxylase, <u>it is quite apparent that the dominant factor in its regulation is the circulating serum Ca level</u>; under circumstances where serum Ca falls, there is a sharp rise in the enzymatic capability for production of $1,25(OH)_2D_3$ which can produce, as the animal becomes increasingly vitamin D-deficient, a 10-20 fold increase in the enzymatic capability for production of the steroid hormone $1,25(OH)_2D_3$. There is, however, a modest yet quite significant capability for stimulation of the 1-hydroxylase activity under circumstances of dietary phosphate depletion; however, this capability, in comparison to the dominant effects of serum calcium, seems of questionable physiological significance. It should be recalled from Figure 2 that phosphate depletion may play a more important role in the actual binding of $1,25(OH)_2D_3$ to the intestinal mucosal tissue. This fact is also apparent in panel B of Figure 11 which summarizes the relationships of changing serum Ca and serum P values for the steady state levels of intestinal CaBP. Once again, it would appear that the downward perturbation of serum Ca values is capable of inducing a more dramatic elevation of intestinal CaBP than is a downward perturbation of serum phosphorus. However, it should also be apparent by comparison of panel A and panel B of Figure 11 that phosphate depletion is capable of exerting a relatively greater effect on the intestinal level of CaBP than it is upon the renal 24-OH-D-1-hydroxylase.

Thus in summary, we have been able to carry out a quantitative evaluation of many of the key elements of the vitamin D endocrine system. In particular, we have focused on quantitative relationships which govern the regulation of the renal production of $1,25(OH)_2D_3$ and $24,25(OH)_2D_3$ in concert with the "calcium demand" and "phosphorus demand" of the animal. This has involved an analysis of the enzymatic activity of the kidney as an endocrine gland from the point of view of its production of these two steroids, as well as an analysis of the specific protein product, CaBP, that one of these hormones, $[1,25(OH)_2D_3]$, is capable of inducing in a prime vitamin D target tissue, the intestine.

Acknowledgements: We are indebted to Ms. J. E. Bishop and Ms. P. A. Roberts for unflagging technical assistance.

1. Norman, A. W.: Actinomycin D and the response to vitamin D. Science 149:184, 1965.
2. Zull, J.E., Misztal, C., and DeLuca, H.F.: On the relationship between vitamin D action and actinomycin-sensitive processes. Proc. Nat. Acad. Sci. (US) 55: 177, 1966.
3. Wasserman, R. H.: The vitamin D-dependent calcium-binding protein, in, H. F. DeLuca and J. W. Suttie (eds.) The Fat-Soluble Vitamins, Univ. of Wisconsin Press, p. 21, 1969.
4. Norman, A. W., and Henry, H.: 1,25-Dihydroxylcholecalciferol- a hormonally active form of vitamin D_3, in, R. O. Greep (ed.) Recent Progress in Hormone Research 30:431, 1974.

5. Henry, H., and Norman, A. W.: Presence of renal 25-hydroxy-vitamin D-1-hydroxylase in species of all vertebrate classes. Comp. Biochem. Physiol. 50:431, 1975.

6. Omdahl, J. L., Gray, R. W., Boyle, I. T., Knutsen, J., and DeLuca, H. F.: Regulation of metabolism of 25-hydroxycholecal-ciferol by kidney tissue in vitro by dietary calcium. Nature New Biol. 237:63, 1972.

7. Boyle, I. T., Gray, R. W., and DeLuca, H. F.: Regulation by calcium of in vivo synthesis of 1,25-dihydroxycholecalciferol and 21,25-dihydroxycholecalciferol. Proc. Nat. Acad. Sci. US 68:2131, 1971.

8. Edelstein, S., Harell, A., Bar, A., and Hurwitz, S.: The functional metabolism of vitamin D in chicks fed low-calcium and low-phosphorus diets. Biochim. Biophys. Acta 385:438, 1975.

9. Tanaka, Y., and DeLuca, H. F.: The control of 25-hydroxyvita-min D metabolism by inorganic phosphorus. Arch. Biochem. Biophys. 154:566, 1973.

10. Hughes, M. R., Brumbaugh, P. F., Haussler, M. R., Wergedal, J. E., and Baylink, D. J.: Regulation of serum $1\alpha,25$-dihydroxy-vitamin D_3 by calcium and phosphate in the rat. Science 190:578, 1975.

11. Henry, H. L., Midgett, R. J., and Norman, A. W.: Regulation of 25-hydroxyvitamin D_3-1-hydroxylase, in vivo. J. Biol. Chem. 249:7584, 1974.

12. Fraser, D. R., and Kodicek, E.: Regulation of 25-hydroxychole-calciferol-1-hydroxylase activity in kidney by parathyroid hormone. Nature New Biol. 241:163, 1973.

13. Tanaka, Y., Lorenc, R. S., and DeLuca, H. F.: The role of 1,25 dihydroxyvitamin D_3 and parathyroid hormone in the regulation of chick renal 25-hydroxyvitamin D_3-24-hydroxylase. Arch. Biochem. Biophys. 171:521, 1975.

14. Garabedian, M., Holick, M. F., DeLuca, H. F., and Boyle, I. T.: Control of 25-hydroxycholecalciferol metabolism by parathyroid glands. PNAS 69:1673, 1972.

15. Favus, M. J., Walling, M. W., and Kimberg, D. V.: Effects of dietary calcium restriction and chronic thyroparathyroidectomy on the metabolism of [^{3}H]25-hydroxyvitamin D_3 and the active transport of calcium by rat intestine. J. Clin. Invest. 53:1139, 1974.

16. Seymour, J. L., and DeLuca, H. F.: Action of 25-hydroxydihy-drotachysterol3 on calcium metabolism in normal and thyropara-thyroidectomized rats. Endocrinology 94:1009, 1974.

17. Haussler, M. R.: Vitamin D_3: metabolism, mode of action, and assay of circulating hormonal form, in, A. W. Norman, K. Schaefer, H.-G. Grigoleit, D. vonHerrath, and E. Ritz (eds.), Vitamin D and Problems Relating to Uremic Bone Disease. Walter de Gruyter, p. 25, 1975.

18.   Galante, L., Colston, K., MacAuley, S., and MacIntyre, I.:
      Effect of parathyroid extract on vitamin D metabolism. The
      Lancet 7, 985, 1972.

19.   Galante, L., Colston, K. W., MacAuley, S. J., and MacIntyre,
      I.: Effect of calcitonin on vitamin D metabolism. Nature
      238:271, 1972.

20.   Henry, H. L., and Norman, A. W.: Studies on calciferol
      metabolism. IX. Renal 25-hydroxy-vitamin D_3-1-hydroxylase.
      Involvement of cytochrome P450 and other properties. J. Biol.
      Chem. 249:7529, 1974.

21.   Horiuchi, N., Suda, T., and Sasaki, S.: Direct involvement
      of vitamin D in the regulation of 25-hydroxycholecalciferol
      metabolism. FEBS Letters 43(3):353, 1974.

22.   Tanaka, Y., and DeLuca, H. F.: Stimulation of 24, 25-di-
      hydroxy-vitamin D_3. Science 183:1198, 1974.

23.   Henry, H. L., and Norman, A. W.: Studies on the mechanism
      of action of calciferol. VII. Localization of 1,25-dihydroxy-
      vitamin D_3 in chick parathyroid glands. Biochem. Biophys.
      Res. Commun. 62:781, 1975.

24.   Henry, H. L., and Norman, A. W.: Studies on calciferol
      metabolism. XIII. Regulation of 25-hydroxy-vitamin D_3-1-
      hydroxylase in isolated renal mitochondria. Arch. Biochem.
      Biophys. 172:582, 1976.

25.   Chazarian, J.G., and DeLuca, H. F.: 25-Hydroxycholecalcif-
      erol-1-hydroxylase: A specific requirement for NADPH and a
      hemoprotein component in chick kidney mitochondria. Arch.
      Biochem. Biophys. 160:63, 1974.

26.   Suda, T., Horiuchi, N., Sasaki, S., Ogata, E., Izawa, I.,
      Nagata, W., and Kimura, S.: Direct control by calcium of
      25-hydroxycholecalciferol-1-hydroxylase activity in chick
      kidney mitochondria. Biochem. Biophys. Res. Commun. 54:512,
      1973.

27.   Horiuchi, N., Suda, T., Sasaki, S., Ogata, E., Izawa, I.,
      Sano, Y., and Shimazawa, E.: The regulatory role of calcium
      in 25-hydroxycholecalciferol metabolism in chick kidney in
      vitro. Arch. Biochem. Biophys. 171, 540, 1975.

28.   Colston, K. W., Evans, I. M. A., Galante, L., MacIntyre, I.,
      and Moss, D. W.: Regulation of vitamin D metabolism: factors
      influencing the rate of formation of 1,25-dihydroxycholecal-
      ciferol by kidney homogenates. Biochem. J. 134:817, 1973.

29. Bikle, D. D., Murphy, E. W., and Rasmussen, H.: The ionic control of 1,25-dihydroxyvitamin D_3 synthesis in isolated chick renal mitochondria. J. Clin. Invest. 55:299, 1975.

INFLUENCE OF PHOSPHATE DEPLETION ON THE BIOSYNTHESIS AND CIRCULATING LEVEL OF 1α,25-DIHYDROXYVITAMIN D

M. Haussler, M. Hughes, D. Baylink*, E. T. Littledike[†],
D. Cork, and M. Pitt
Arizona Medical Center, Tucson, AZ, *V.A. Hospital,
Seattle, WA, and [†]National Animal Disease Laboratory,
Ames, IA.

Vitamin D_3 is metabolized in the liver to 25-hydroxyvitamin D_3 (25-OH-D_3) and then in the kidney to 1α,25-dihydroxyvitamin D_3 (1α,25-(OH)$_2D_3$). The action of vitamin D_3 to mobilize calcium and phosphate from intestine and bone is thought to be mediated by the 1α,25-(OH)$_2D_3$ metabolite and therefore this sterol is considered to be the hormonal form of vitamin D (1). 1α,25-(OH)$_2D_3$ qualifies as a mineral regulating hormone based upon observations that its biosynthesis appears to be regulated by the calcium and phosphorus status of animals (2) and its biochemical action on target tissues such as intestine resembles the functioning of classic steroid hormones in their respective target organs (3). Thus 1α,25-(OH)$_2D_3$ stimulates intestinal calcium absorption through a mechanism involving transport of the hormone to the cell nucleus by a cytoplasmic receptor protein, enhancement of nuclear RNA synthesis and ultimate induction of functional proteins such as calcium binding protein (4,5,6).

The key regulated step in the formation of 1α,25-(OH)$_2D_3$ from the parent vitamin is the renal 1α-hydroxylation of 25-OH-D_3 (7). This is the rate limiting reaction in the production of 1α,25-(OH)$_2D_3$ and the renal 1α-hydroxylase (1α-OHase) enzyme has become the focal point for investigations of the dietary, humoral, and pathologic conditions which affect the biosynthesis and secretion of 1α,25-(OH)$_2D_3$. Formation of the 1α,25-(OH)$_2D_3$ hormone from 25-OH-D_3 by the 1α-OHase appears to be regulated by calcium (8), parathyroid hormone (PTH) (9,10), phosphate (10,11) and the vitamin D status of the animal (7,12). Evidence suggests that hypocalcemia stimulates PTH secretion which in turn increases the production of 1α,25-(OH)$_2D_3$ at the kidney (9,10). Thus PTH, rather than calcium, may be the dominant modulator of the 1α-OHase with respect to calcium homeostasis. The finding of abnormally low circulating $1\alpha,25-(OH)_2D$ in patients with hypoparathyroidism (13) and pseudo-hypoparathyroidism (14) and elevated plasma levels of $1\alpha,25-(OH)_2D$ in cases of primary hyperparathyroidism (15) is consistent with the concept of PTH functioning as a primary modulator of $1\alpha,25-(OH)_2D$ synthesis. Further confirmation of this notion has come from experiments in parathyroidectomized chicks (16,17).

There is agreement (7,12,17) that vitamin D-deficiency enhances renal 1α-OHase activity, at least in chicks, and that the enzyme activity is suppressed by treatment of the animals with vitamin D_3 or $1\alpha,25-(OH)_2D_3$. Most likely, it is the consequence of $1\alpha,25-(OH)_2D_3$ action, namely increased serum calcium and decreased circulating PTH and perhaps augmented serum phosphate which attenuate the 1α-OHase enzyme activity.

Although homeostatic control of the 1α-OHase by calcium (via PTH) and by vitamin D metabolites is generally accepted, the situation of the phosphate-$1\alpha,25-(OH)_2D_3$ regulating system is more controversial. $1\alpha,25-(OH)_2D_3$ is a phosphate mobilizing hormone in gut, bone, and perhaps kidney (2), but whether phosphate can in turn control $1\alpha,25-(OH)_2D_3$ formation is still an unsettled question. In the rat, chronic phosphate deprivation stimulates the conversion of injected radioactive $25-OH-D_3$ to $1\alpha,25-(OH)_2D_3$ (11) and elicits a five-fold increase in the absolute circulating concentration of the $1\alpha,25-(OH)_2D_3$ hormone (10). In both studies in the rat, this adaptive enhancement of $1\alpha,25-(OH)_2D_3$ was independent of the presence of the parathyroid or thyroid glands (10,11). These data suggest that hypophosphatemia, per se, or some factor associated with phosphate depletion, has a direct positive influence on the 1α-OHase enzyme. On the other hand, a study by Henry et al. (17) in the chick indicated that animals raised on a low phosphate diet did not have elevated renal 1α-OHase activities as measured in vitro. A more recent study by Baxter and DeLuca (18) in chicks suggests that low dietary phosphate elicits a five-fold increase in the activity of the 1α-OHase.

The present studies were designed to further examine the possible interrelationship between phosphate depletion and the biosynthesis of $1\alpha,25-(OH)_2D_3$. In order to determine the effects of phosphate deprivation and its possible interplay with the better characterized calcium-PTH-$1\alpha,25-(OH)_2D_3$ homeostatic system, either 1α-OHase activity was monitored by standard enzymatic assay or total plasma $1\alpha,25-(OH)_2D$ was measured via radioreceptor assay. Studies were carried out in chicks, rats, pigs, and in humans with certain disorders of calcium and phosphate metabolism.

EFFECTS OF DIETARY VARIATIONS ON CHICK 1α-OHase

To investigate the influence of dietary restriction of calcium, phosphorus, and vitamin D on the renal 1α-OHase enzyme, the growing chick was chosen as an experimental animal. Other than the obvious ease of dietary manipulation in this species, the chick was selected because it is the only animal where the 1α-OHase is readily quantitated in kidney homogenates via in vitro enzyme assay techniques. Since serum calcium and phosphorus are reciprocally related and in turn governed by vitamin D status, dietary calcium variation was studied under conditions of constant phosphorus intake and, conversely, phosphorus was modulated during constant calcium intake in a second experiment. In both experiments involving mineral changes, half of the animals were supplemented with vitamin D_3 and the other half maintained on vitamin D-deficient diets. All chicks were one week old when placed on the test diets and were kept on these diets for three additional weeks prior to sacrifice. At the termination of the experiment the following measurements were made: 1) body weight, 2) plasma calcium and plasma phosphorus (Autoanalyzer), 3) radiographic appearance of bone, and 4) renal 1α-OHase activity. Radiographs of the tibiae and femurs were obtained using a Senograph X-Ray Unit (Keleket/CGR). This machine has a stationary molybdenum anode with a focal spot of 0.7 mm and a beryllium window for X-ray filtration. DuPont Cronex NDT industrial X-ray film in an X-ray exposure holder was used. Radiographic technique was 35 mA, 35 kV with a 2-4 sec exposure. The FFD was 17 inches with the extremity placed directly against the film pack. Films were developed over 4 min in an automatic Kodak X-O-Mat with GAF chemicals at a temperature of 91 F. 1α-hydroxylase assays were performed on kidney homogenates exactly as described by Tucker et al. (7). A 9% homogenate of kidney in 0.3 M sucrose was prepared and 0.4 ml was added to 9.6 ml of a phosphate buffer, pH 7.4, containing magnesium and a NADPH regenerating system. The reaction was initiated by adding 65 pmoles of 25-OH[26(27)-methyl-$^3H_2$]D_3 (final concentration 6.5 x 10^{-9} M) in 50 μl of ethanol and was allowed to proceed under air for 20 min at 37 C. Preliminary experiments were done to show that the reaction was linear with respect to time (up to 20 min) and enzyme (up to 0.4 ml homogenate). After completion of the reaction, the sterols were extracted with methanol-chloroform (2:1, v/v) and separated by chromatography on 1 x 15 cm Sephadex LH-20 columns as described elsewhere (10). Data are expressed as femtomoles of $1\alpha,25$-$(OH)_2[^3H]D_3$ product formed per min per mg of homogenate protein.

Calcium and Vitamin D Modulation

Table 1 indicates data on the final body weight and serum ion concentrations of chicks grown on various levels of dietary calcium.

Table 1. Summary of final body weight, plasma calcium, and phosphorus concentrations from chicks treated with various levels of dietary calcium for three weeks.

Diet	Treatment	Final Body Weight (g)	Plasma Calcium* (mg/100 ml)	Plasma Phosphorus* (mg/100 ml)
Low Calcium (0.2%)	D-deficient	111	5.5 ± .1	5.3 ± .3
	+D$_3$ (6 IU/day)	178	9.2 ± .1	6.1 ± .2
Standard Rachitogenic (0.7%)	D-deficient	136	6.3 ± .2	5.0 ± .5
	+D$_3$ (6 IU/day)	270	10.5 ± .1	6.4 ± .1
High Calcium (3.0%)	D-deficient	220	10.6 ± .2	2.2 ± .2
	+D$_3$ (6 IU/day)	192	10.4 ± .2	5.5 ± .5

*Average of 5 chicks ± S.E.M.

Either low (0.2%), standard (0.7%), or high (3.0%) calcium diets were fed to vitamin D-deficient or vitamin D-supplemented (+D$_3$) chicks for three weeks. Growth was retarded by excluding vitamin D at all dietary calcium levels except the high calcium diet. Optimal growth was seen in chicks raised on the standard calcium level and in the presence of vitamin D.

Plasma calcium values were normal (i.e., 10-11 mg per 100 ml) in the +D$_3$-standard calcium dieted chicks and in both D-deficient and +D$_3$ chicks raised on the high calcium diet, while all other groups exhibited significant hypocalcemia. Plasma phosphorus was only slightly suppressed by vitamin D deficiency except in the case of D-deficient-high calcium chicks, which had severe hypophosphatemia (2.2 mg/100 ml). This hypophosphatemia was created by the combination of a vitamin D lack and high dietary calcium. Thus, both plasma calcium and phosphorus were normal only in two groups of animals: 1) +D$_3$-standard calcium diet and 2) +D$_3$-high calcium diet. Since both ions must be present in optimal concentrations to elicit normal bone calcification, adequate bone development would be expected only in those two groups of chicks. Bone integrity, density, and pattern of calcification were assessed radiographically. Figure 1 illustrates the radiographic appearance of bone of representative chicks raised on the various levels of dietary calcium and vitamin D used in the present study. All chicks deficient of vitamin D$_3$, regardless of dietary calcium, exhibited classic rachitic lesions and showed

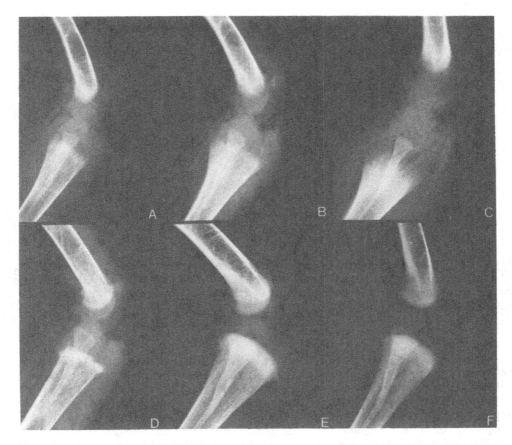

<u>Figure 1</u>. Radiographic appearance of knees from chicks fed various levels of dietary calcium. Pictured in the top row are lateral projections of knees from chicks raised on D-deficient diets with different amounts of calcium: A) 0.2%, B) 0.7%, and C) 3.0%. Shown in the bottom row are radiographs from +D$_3$ chicks with various levels of dietary calcium: D) 0.2%, E) 0.7%, and F) 3.0%.

severely uncalcified metaphyseal regions (Figure 1A-C). Rachitic changes were alleviated by vitamin D treatment only in the standard (Figure 1E) or high calcium (Figure 1F) dieted chicks. +D$_3$ chicks raised on the low calcium diet (Figure 1D) retained rachitic-like bones with a wide growth plate and uncalcified epiphyseal area. Therefore, normally calcified bones by radiographic criteria were seen only in the chicks which had normal plasma concentrations of calcium and phosphorus.

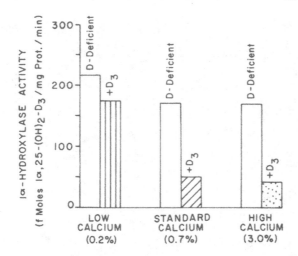

<u>Figure 2</u>. Comparison of renal 1α-OHase activity in rachitic and +D₃ chicks raised on several levels of calcium in the diet. All numbers are representative assays on a pooled kidney homogenate from five animals per group.

In order to relate the dietarily induced changes in plasma ions and bone integrity in these chicks with the activity of the renal 1α-hydroxylase enzyme, at the termination of the dietary calcium experiment kidneys were removed from all animals and assayed for the enzyme. Figure 2 illustrates 1α-OHase enzyme activities in all six groups of chicks in question. Highest activities occurred in the D-deficient-low calcium chicks, but all D-deficient groups displayed high enzyme activities (170-220 fmoles/mg protein/min). +D₃-low calcium chicks also had 1α-OHase activities which were extremely high and comparable to D-deficient values. Two groups of animals, +D₃-standard calcium and +D₃-high calcium yielded 1α-OHase activities which were suppressed to normal levels of 25-50 fmoles/mg protein/min.

Thus, 1α-OHase induction occurred in all cases except the animals which had totally normal plasma ions and bone development. In other words, there is a strict correlation between normal bone development and the level of 1α-OHase enzyme. Any condition such as hypocalcemia or hypophosphatemia which prevents the proper calcification of bone and leads to rachitic changes also causes the induction of the 1α-OHase. Whether the trigger for induction of the 1α-OHase is low plasma ion concentration (calcium or phosphorus) or whether there is a direct message to the kidney enzyme from the uncalcified bone remains to be determined. Yet, it is likely that hypocalcemia is signaling the enhancement of the 1α-OHase via increases in PTH secretion, since PTH is a known positive effector of the kidney enzyme (9,10,16,17).

Phosphorus and Vitamin D Modulation

Since plasma phosphorus level is implicated as a controlling factor for the 1α-OHase enzyme, alterations in serum phosphorus concentrations were created in vitamin D-deficient and vitamin D-supplemented (+D$_3$) chicks by dietary variations in phosphorus. D-deficient or +D$_3$ chicks were raised on three levels of dietary phosphorus: Low (0.1%), standard (0.5%), or high (3.0%). Dietary level of calcium was held constant at 0.7% in all diets varying in phosphorus content. Growth rate was determined over a three week period on the test diets and at the end of the experiment, terminal values were obtained for body weight, plasma calcium and phosphorus, radiographic appearance of bones, and renal 1α-OHase. The data from this experiment appear in Table 2 and Figures 3 and 4.

Growth was severely impaired by exclusion of vitamin D and the most striking lack of growth was seen in both D-deficient and +D$_3$ chicks raised on high phosphorus diets. Plasma calcium values were normal only in 2 groups of animals: +D$_3$-low phosphorus diet and +D$_3$-standard phosphorus diet. All D-deficient animals were very

Table 2. Summary of final body weight, plasma calcium, and phosphorus concentrations from chicks treated with various levels of dietary phosphorus for three weeks.

Diet	Treatment	Final Body Weight (g)	Plasma Calcium* (mg/100 ml)	Plasma Phosphorus* (mg/100 ml)
Low Phosphorus (0.1%)	D-deficient	165	7.5 ± .7	3.5 ± .5
	+D$_3$ (6 IU/day)	233	10.0 ± .5	5.2 ± .4
Standard Rachitogenic (0.5%)	D-deficient	155	4.9 ± .2	6.0 ± .7
	+D$_3$ (6 IU/day)	230	10.6 ± .3	6.8 ± .3
High Phosphorus (3.0%)	D-deficient	87	5.3 ± .5	13.9 ± .1
	+D$_3$ (6 IU/day)	128	6.1 ± .4	13.9 ± .1

*Average of 5 chicks ± S.E.M.

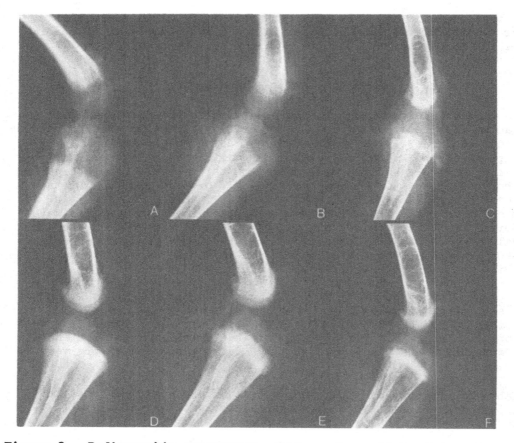

Figure 3. Radiographic appearance of knees from chicks fed various levels of dietary phosphorus. Pictured in the top row are lateral projections of knees from chicks raised on D-deficient diets with different amounts of phosphorus: A) 0.1%, B) 0.5%, and C) 3.0%. Shown in the bottom row are radiographs from +D$_3$ chicks with various levels of dietary phosphorus: D) 0.1%, E) 0.5%, F) 3.0%.

hypocalcemic as were the +D$_3$ high phosphorus dieted chicks. High dietary phosphate is a known cause of hypocalcemia, and the mechanism of this effect is related to the constant ion product for calcium and phosphate.

Plasma phosphorus levels were very low in the D-deficient-low phosphorus dieted chicks and extremely high in all chicks raised on the high phosphorus diet. Plasma phosphorus was slightly depressed in the +D$_3$-low phosphorus group (Table 2). Thus, only two groups of chicks had near normal circulating levels of both calcium and phosphorus, namely the +D₃-low and +D₃-standard phosphorus dieted animals, and only these two groups of animals would be expected to have normal bone development. This notion is verified by radiographic examination of the bones (Figure 3). Extensive uncalcified epiphyseal plates are seen in all D-deficient groups (Figure 3A-C). Rachitic-like lesions are also apparent in the +D₃-high phosphorus bones (Figure 3F).

1α-OHase enzyme activities in the chicks raised on various levels of phosphorus are depicted in Figure 4. As was seen in the previous experiment of varying calcium in the diet, all D-deficient chicks have very high enzyme activities (i.e., 150-250 fmoles/mg protein/min). However, the D-deficient low phosphorus animals have the most striking enhancement of enzyme activity, suggesting that low plasma phosphorus (_per se_) may be a potent inducer of the 1α-OHase. Among the +D₃ groups, the high phosphorus dieted chicks also exhibited a high enzyme activity, either because of the hypocalcemia created by high phosphorus levels or the resulting rachitic bones. Normal (suppressed) 1α-OHase levels were present in the two groups having normal calcium, phosphorus, and bone development (+D₃-low and +D₃-standard phosphorus). Also of interest in Figure 4 is the fact that the +D₃-low phosphorus animals, which had the "best" calcified bones (Figure 3D), yield the most suppressed levels of renal 1α-OHase.

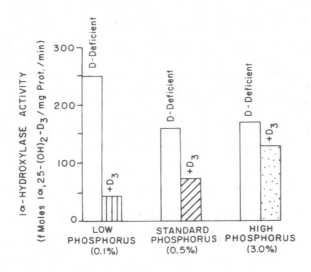

Figure 4. Comparison of renal 1α-OHase activity in rachitic and +D₃ chicks raised on several levels of phosphorus in the diet. All numbers are representative assays on a pooled kidney homogenate from five animals per group.

Thus the present experiment further supports the concept that animals with uncalcified bones will have enhanced activity of 1α-OHase. Conversely, healthy bones lead to a suppression of the enzyme activity to normally low levels. It is suggested that uncalcified bone may be elaborating a chemical message which in turn stimulates and/or induces the renal 1α-hydroxylase. Of course another possible connection between bone integrity and the renal enzyme could be via plasma ion levels. Thus, hypocalcemia or hypophosphatemia could independently lead to improperly formed bones and enhancement of kidney 1α-hydroxylase activity. Therefore, it does appear that the kidney can respond to either hypocalcemia or hypophosphatemia to increase the production of the hormonal form of vitamin D. However, high plasma phosphorus, per se, does not act as a classic "feedback inhibitor" of $1\alpha,25\text{-}(OH)_2D_3$ synthesis since 1α-OHase levels are highly induced in $+D_3$-high phosphorus chickens (Figure 4).

Unfortunately, our study in the chick does not resolve the conflicting experiments of Henry et al. (17) and Baxter and DeLuca (18). The data illustrated in Figure 4 for phosphate deprived $+D_3$ chicks correspond more closely to the results of Henry et al. (17) with no apparent elevation of the 1α-OHase in low-phosphorus $+D_3$ chicks. However, we used a diet (19) similar to that of Henry et al. (17) and obtained comparable levels of serum phosphorus. Baxter and DeLuca (18) were able to obtain much more marked hypophosphatemia in their $+D_3$ chicks and, under these conditions, observed a dramatic increase in the 1α-OHase activity. Nevertheless, in the present study, we did obtain independent evidence for hypophosphatemic stimulation of the 1α-OHase in vitamin D-deficient chicks (Figure 4). Also, when severe hypophosphatemia was produced by high calcium diets in vitamin D-deficient chicks (Table 1), the 1α-OHase was markedly elevated even though plasma calcium was normal (Table 1, Figure 2). Moreover, we have shown that there exists a striking relationship in which either hypocalcemia, hypophosphatemia, or rachitic bone is able to signal the activation of the renal enzyme producing a sterol hormone which functions to mediate calcium and phosphate absorption and ultimately reverse bone decalcification.

CIRCULATING $1\alpha,25\text{-}(OH)_2D$ IN PHOSPHATE DEPRIVED RATS AND PIGS

Another approach to examining the effects of hypophosphatemia on $1\alpha,25\text{-}(OH)_2D$ biosynthesis is to measure the total circulating concentration of the sterol hormone under conditions of dietary phosphate restriction. As with all hormones, the blood level of $1\alpha,25\text{-}(OH)_2D$ probably most directly correlates with the biologic status of the animal with respect to vitamin D, calcium, and phosphorus metabolism. $1\alpha,25\text{-}(OH)_2D$ was monitored in rat and pig blood by the specific radioreceptor assay originally described by Brumbaugh et al. (20) and modified more recently by Hughes et al. (21). The

assay employs the chick intestinal cytosol receptor and classic competitive protein binding techniques to quantitate $1\alpha,25$-$(OH)_2D$.
Bound and free hormone are separated by virtue of the association
of the hormone-cytosol receptor complex with intestinal chromatin
and millipore filtration methodology. The assay has a minimum sensitivity of 17 pg and is a valid procedure for measuring serum or
plasma $1\alpha,25$-$(OH)_2D$ concentrations of as low as 1 ng/dl. The receptor system is equally sensitive to $1\alpha,25$-$(OH)_2D_3$ and $1\alpha,25$-$(OH)_2D_2$
- meaning that all measured levels represent total $1\alpha,25$-$(OH)_2D$ (21).
Assays are routinely performed in triplicate with a 10-15% interassay
variation and biological samples require purification through three
successive columns (Sephadex LH-20, silicic acid, and Celite; 50-75%
final yield) prior to radioreceptor assay. The assay has been vali-
dated by showing undetectable levels of $1\alpha,25$-$(OH)_2D$ in rachitic
chicks (20) and in anephric patients (22). Further clinical validi-
fication includes a demonstration of normal $1\alpha,25$-$(OH)_2D$ levels in
anephric subjects receiving successful renal transplants (1,22) and
elevated $1\alpha,25$-$(OH)_2D$ in cases of primary hyperparathyroidism (15).
Moreover, the normal human $1\alpha,25$-$(OH)_2D$ concentration as measured
by radioreceptor assay (2.1-4.5 ng/dl) has been confirmed by bio-
assay (23) and a recently devised competitive binding method (24).

    We have previously reported that placing weanling rats on a low
phosphorus diet for two weeks causes a five-fold adaptive enhancement of circulating $1\alpha,25$-$(OH)_2D$ (10). In order to characterize the
mechanism of this adaptive increase, we measured serum $1\alpha,25$-$(OH)_2D$
as a function of time of dietary phosphorus restriction in thyroparathyroidectomized (TPTX) rats. Figure 5 illustrates that serum

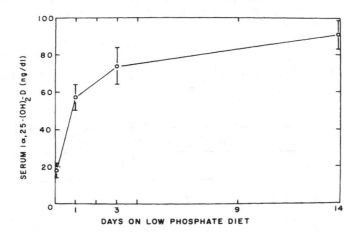

Figure 5. Time course of increased circulating $1\alpha,25$-$(OH)_2D$ in TPTX
weanling rats placed on a low phosphorus diet. Dietary phosphorus
was 0.04% and calcium was 0.6%. The experiment was carried out
exactly as described by Hughes et al. (10).

$1\alpha,25-(OH)_2D$ increases surprisingly rapidly, with almost a three-fold stimulation within one day of low dietary phosphorus. These data suggest that the rat is dramatically sensitive to phosphate depletion and the rapidity of the effect on $1\alpha,25-(OH)_2D$ intimates a possible direct positive influence of low circulating phosphate on the renal 1α-OHase enzyme. Since TPTX rats were used, these data further demonstrate that calcium and phosphorus hormones such as PTH and calcitonin are not involved in this response, but other hormonal factors are not ruled out. Detailed studies of the 1α-OHase in isolated systems are required to elucidate the biochemical mechanism of the low phosphate effect on $1\alpha,25-(OH)_2D$ production.

In order to verify the concept of phosphorus depletion-mediated enhancement of circulating $1\alpha,25-(OH)_2D$ in another animal, the pig was chosen for study. Table 3 summarizes data from pigs placed on a low phosphorus diet for up to five weeks. During this period, plasma phosphorus levels fell from approximately 6 mg/dl to 3-4 mg/dl. Concomitantly, plasma $1\alpha,25-(OH)_2D$ rose markedly, with the maximum elevation being three to five times control (0 weeks) values. Again, neither parathyroidectomy (PTX) nor thyroparathyroidectomy (TPTX) had any influence on the low phosphorus effect on plasma $1\alpha,25-(OH)_2D$. Therefore, based upon studies in both rats and pigs, phosphate depletion apparently accelerates the formation (or retards the degradation) of $1\alpha,25-(OH)_2D$ and this phenomenon may provide a means for environmental adaptations in animals. Phosphate depletion also could have influences on calcium and phosphate metabolism independent of these observed modulations of circulating $1\alpha,25-(OH)_2D$ (25,26). However, of great significance is the possibility that humans possess an analogous adaptive mechanism relating phosphate to circulating $1\alpha,25-(OH)_2D$ and that this mechanism may be aberrant in certain disorders of mineral metabolism.

Table 3. Circulating $1\alpha,25-(OH)_2D$ concentration in pigs placed on a low phosphate diet for 0 - 5 weeks.

Group	Plasma $1\alpha,25-(OH)_2D$ (ng/dl)*		
	0 weeks	3 weeks	5 weeks
Intact	9.3 ± 0.6	20.7 ± 3.4	31.1 ± 5.5
PTX	8.0 ± 0.3	16.5 ± 2.3	28.1 ± 1.5
TPTX	11.3 ± 0.7	21.5 ± 1.5	45.5 ± 4.4

*Average of 3 pigs $\pm$ S.E.M.

HUMAN HYPOPHOSPHATEMIC DISORDERS

Hypophosphatemia was noted in the classic descriptions of both idiopathic hypercalciuria (27) and vitamin D-resistant rickets (28) and yet these disorders have been controversial in terms of parathyroid hormone involvement. However, work by Arnaud et al. (29) clearly suggests that PTH is normal in untreated vitamin D-resistant rickets. Also, data from Pak et al. (30) indicate that PTH is slightly suppressed in absorptive hypercalciuria. These two maladies then provide us with cases of phosphate depletion in humans without concomitant hyperparathyroidism, a situation similar to phosphate depletion of rats and pigs (Figure 5, Table 3). Table 4 summarizes $1\alpha,25-(OH)_2D$ levels in eighteen cases of idiopathic hypercalciuria compared with 18 age-matched control subjects. The sterol hormone is significantly elevated in these cases and the findings are striking when we consider that these patients were relatively hypoparathyroid (31).

These results suggest a possible chain of events which result in idiopathic hypercalciuria. The primary lesion may be a renal leak of phosphate (Baylink, unpublished). The resulting hypophosphatemia then stimulates the production of $1\alpha,25-(OH)_2D$ and an augmented intestinal calcium absorption occurs. Either a transient increase in blood calcium or enhanced circulating $1\alpha,25-(OH)_2D$ (or both) may then feedback inhibit the secretion of PTH (32) to cause relative hypoparathyroidism. The combination of aberrantly high plasma $1\alpha,25-(OH)_2D$ and low PTH creates an ideal situation for stimulated absorption of calcium from the intestine and decreased renal tubular reabsorption of calcium - all of which results in hypercalciuria and renal stone disease. Whether or not these events comprise the pathophysiology of idiopathic hypercalciuria, the

Table 4. Circulating $1\alpha,25-(OH)_2D$ in patients with idiopathic hypercalciuria.

Group	No.	Plasma phosphorus (mg/dl $\pm$ S.D.)	Plasma $1\alpha,25-(OH)_2D$ (ng/dl $\pm$ S.D.)
Normal	18	3.7 ± 0.3	3.3 ± 0.8
Idiopathic Hypercalciuria	18	2.9 ± 0.6*	5.2 ± 1.9*

*Significantly different from normal, $P < 0.001$

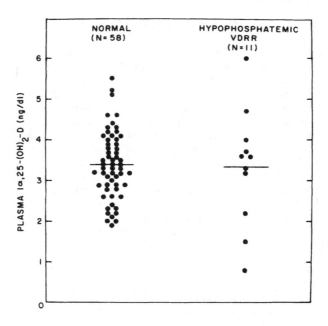

<u>Figure 6</u>. Circulating 1α,25-(OH)$_2$D in familial hypophosphatemic
rickets. The average plasma phosphorus values in the 11 patients
with VDRR was 2.0 mg/100 ml (normal = 3.5-4.5). Several of the
patients were undergoing therapy with phosphate and large doses of
vitamin D$_2$ when sampled.

present data support the concept that hypophosphatemia in humans
leads to enhanced circulating 1α,25-(OH)$_2$D. The fact that phosphate
depletion of normal humans causes increased calcium absorption and
hypercalciuria (33) is consistent with this concept but measurement
of plasma 1α,25-(OH)$_2$D in such phosphate deficient humans is necessary for absolute confirmation of this mechanism.

Marked hypophosphatemia occurs in X-linked vitamin D-resistant
rickets and the primary lesion in this disorder is thought to be a
deficient phosphate conservation at the kidney (34). However, as is
seen in Figure 6, these patients have normal circulating concentrations of 1α,25-(OH)$_2$D. If the principle of low phosphate stimulation
of plasma 1α,25-(OH)$_2$D is correct, and it is borne out in the case
of mild hypophosphatemia of idiopathic hypercalciuria (Table 4),
then the severe phosphate deficiency of vitamin D-resistant rickets
should be associated with dramatic increases in 1α,25-(OH)$_2$D as
observed in rats and pigs (Figure 5, Table 3). Thus, either the low
phosphate theory is contradicted in vitamin D-resistant rickets or,

more likely, this inherited disorder involves a defect in the ability of the renal 1α-hydroxylase to respond to the low phosphate signal. The fact that 1α,25-(OH)$_2$D$_3$ is ineffective therapeutically when administered to patients with vitamin D-resistant rickets (35) is puzzling, but circulating 1α,25-(OH)$_2$D$_3$ was not measured to ensure that the doses raised blood levels of the hormone. Recently, Rasmussen et al. (36) have successfully treated familial hypophosphatemic rickets with a combination of oral phosphate and large doses of 1α-hydroxyvitamin D$_3$. The synthetic 1α-hydroxyvitamin D$_3$ is efficacious because it is efficiently and rapidly converted to the 1α,25-(OH)$_2$D$_3$ hormone (37). Based upon these observations, it is possible that the etiology of familial hypophosphatemic rickets involves a genetic lesion leading to a single renal tubular defect which is manifested both as an inability to resorb phosphate and unresponsiveness of the 1α-OHase to normal stimuli such as hypophosphatemia.

CONCLUSION

In addition to vitamin D-deficiency, hypocalcemia and hyperparathyroidism, phosphate depletion appears to augment renal 1α-OHase enzyme activity. When vitamin D is available in the diet, phosphate deprivation elicits a dramatic increase in the total circulating level of its hormonal metabolite. Since 1α,25-(OH)$_2$D avidly mobilizes phosphate from such sites as intestine, a new hormonal loop in the regulation of phosphate has been illuminated. Further experimentation into the relationship between phosphate and 1α,25-(OH)$_2$D should improve our understanding of human maladies such as renal stone disease and familial hypophosphatemic rickets.

ACKNOWLEDGMENTS

This study was supported by PHS grants AM 15781, AM 09096, and DE 02600. M. Hughes is supported on PHS training grant GM 01982.

REFERENCES

1. Haussler, M. R.: Vitamin D: mode of action and biomedical applications. Nutr. Rev. 32:257, 1974.
2. DeLuca, H. F.: Vitamin D: the vitamin and the hormone. Fed. Proc. 33:2211, 1974.
3. O'Malley, B. W. and Schrader, W. T.: The receptors of steroid hormones. Sci. Amer. 234:32, 1976.
4. Brumbaugh, P. F. and Haussler, M. R.: Specific binding of 1α,25-dihydroxycholecalciferol to nuclear components of chick intestine. Jour. Biol. Chem. 250:1588, 1975.

5. Zerwekh, J. E., Lindell, T. J., and Haussler, M. R.: Increased intestinal chromatin template activity. Influence of $1\alpha,25$-dihydroxyvitamin D_3 and hormone-receptor complexes. Jour. Biol. Chem. 251:2388, 1976.

6. Emtage, J. S., Lawson, D.E.M., and Kodicek, E.: Vitamin D-induced synthesis of m-RNA for calcium binding protein. Nature 246:100, 1973.

7. Tucker, G., Gagnon, R. E., and Haussler, M. R.: Vitamin D_3-25-hydroxylase: tissue occurrence and apparent lack of regulation. Arch. Biochem. Biophys. 155:47, 1973.

8. Boyle, I. T., Gray, R. W., and DeLuca, H. F.: Regulation by calcium of in vivo synthesis of 1,25-dihydroxycholecalciferol and 21,25-dihydroxycholecalciferol. Proc. Natl. Acad. Sci., U.S.A. 68:2131, 1971.

9. Garabedian, M., Holick, M. F., DeLuca, H. F., and Boyle, I. T.: Control of 25-hydroxycholecalciferol metabolism by parathyroid glands. Proc. Natl. Acad. Sci., U.S.A. 69:1673, 1972.

10. Hughes, M. R., Brumbaugh, P. F., Haussler, M. R., Wergedal, J. E., and Baylink, D. J.: Regulation of serum $1\alpha,25$-dihydroxyvitamin D_3 by calcium and phosphate in the rat. Science 190:578, 1975.

11. Tanaka, Y. and DeLuca, H. F.: The control of 25-hydroxyvitamin D metabolism by inorganic phosphorus. Arch. Biochem. Biophys. 154:566, 1973.

12. Cork, D. J., Haussler, M. R., Pitt, M. J., Rizzardo, E., Hesse, R. H., and Pechet, M. M.: 1α-Hydroxyvitamin D_3: a synthetic sterol which is highly active in preventing rickets in the chick. Endocrinol. 94:1337, 1974.

13. Brumbaugh, P. F., Haussler, D. H., Bressler, R., and Haussler, M. R.: Radioreceptor assay for $1\alpha,25$-dihydroxyvitamin D_3. Science 183:1089, 1974.

14. Drezner, M. K., Neelon, F. A., Haussler, M., McPherson, H. T., and Lebovitz, H. E.: 1,25-Dihydroxycholecalciferol deficiency: the probable cause of hypocalcemia and metabolic bone disease in pseudohypoparathyroidism. Jour. Clin. Endocrinol. Metab. 42:621, 1976.

15. Haussler, M. R., Bursac, K. M., Bone, H., and Pak, C.Y.C.: Increased circulating $1\alpha,25$-dihydroxyvitamin D_3 in patients with primary hyperparathyroidism. Clin. Res. 23:322A, 1975.

16. Fraser, D. R. and Kodicek, E.: Regulation of 25-hydroxychole-calciferol-1-hydroxylase activity in kidney by parathyroid hormone. Nature New Biol. 241:163, 1973.

17. Henry, H. L., Midgett, R. J., and Norman, A. W.: Regulation of 25-hydroxyvitamin D_3-1-hydroxylase in vivo. Jour. Biol. Chem. 249:7584, 1974.

18. Baxter, L. A. and DeLuca, H. F.: Stimulation of 25-hydroxy-vitamin D_3-1α-hydroxylase by phosphate depletion. Jour. Biol. Chem. 251:3158, 1976.

19. McNutt, K. W. and Haussler, M. R.: Nutritional effectiveness of 1,25-dihydroxycholecalciferol in preventing rickets in chicks. Jour. Nutr. 103:681, 1973.

20. Brumbaugh, P. F., Haussler, D. H., Bursac, K. M., and Haussler, M. R.: Filter assay for 1α,25-dihydroxyvitamin D$_3$. Utilization of the hormone's target tissue chromatin receptor. Biochemistry 13:4091, 1974.

21. Hughes, M. R., Baylink, D. J., Jones, P. G., and Haussler, M. R.: Radioligand receptor assay for 25-hydroxyvitamin D$_2$/D$_3$ and 1,25-dihydroxyvitamin D$_2$/D$_3$: application to hypervitaminosis D. Jour. Clin. Invest. 58:61, 1976.

22. Haussler, M. R., Baylink, D. J., Hughes, M. R., Brumbaugh, P. F., Wergedal, J. E., Shen, F. H., Nielsen, R. L., Counts, S. J., Bursac, K. M., and McCain, T. A.: The assay of 1α,25-dihydroxy-vitamin D$_3$: physiologic and pathologic modulation of circulating hormone levels. Clin. Endocrinol. (supplement) 5:151S, 1976.

23. Hill, L. F., Mawer, E. B., and Taylor, C. M.: Determination of plasma levels of 1,25-dihydroxycholecalciferol in man. Vitamin D and Problems Related to Uremic Bone Disease (ed. by A. W. Norman, K. Schaefer, H. G. Grigoleit, D. V. Herrath, and E. Ritz), pp. 755-762. Walter Gruyter, Berlin, 1975.

24. Eisman, J. A., DeLuca, H. F., and Kream, B. E.: Intestinal 1,25-dihydroxyvitamin D$_3$ binding protein: use in a competitive binding assay. Fed. Proc. 35:1718 abstr., 1976.

25. Ribovich, M. L. and DeLuca, H. F.: The influence of dietary calcium and phosphorus on intestinal calcium transport by rats given vitamin D metabolites. Arch. Biochem. Biophys. 170:529, 1975.

26. Steel, T. H. and DeLuca, H. F.: Influence of dietary phosphorus on renal phosphate reabsorption in the parathyroidectomized rat. Jour. Clin. Invest. 57:867, 1976.

27. Albright, F., Henneman, P. H., Benedict, P. H., and Forbes, A. P. Idiopathic hypercalciuria. Proc. of the Royal Soc. of Med. 46:1077, 1953.

28. Albright, F., Butler, A. M., and Bloomberg, F.: Rickets resistant to vitamin D therapy. Amer. Jour. of Diseases of Children 54:529, 1937.

29. Arnaud, C., Glorieux, F., and Scriver, C. R.: Serum parathyroid hormone in X-linked hypophosphatemia. Science 173:845, 1971.

30. Pak, C.Y.C., Ohata, M., Lawrence, E. C., and Snyder, W.: The hypercalciurias. Causes, parathyroid functions and diagnostic criteria. Jour. Clin. Invest. 54:387, 1974.

31. Shen, F., Baylink, D. J., Nielson, R., Hughes, M. R., and Haussler, M. R.: Increased serum 1,25-dihydroxycholecalciferol in patients with idiopathic hypercalciuria. Clin. Res. 23:423A, 1975.

32. Chertow, B. S., Baylink, D. J., Wergedal, J. E., Su, M.H.H., and Norman, A. W.: Decrease in serum immunoreactive parathyroid hormone in rats and in parathyroid hormone secretion in vitro by 1,25-dihydroxycholecalciferol. Jour. Clin. Invest. 56:668, 1975.

33. Dominquez, J. H., Gray, R. W., and Lemann, J.: Accelerated 25-hydroxyvitamin D metabolism during dietary phosphate deprivation in humans. Clin. Res. 23:420A, 1975.

34. Glorieux, F. H., Scriver, C. R., Reade, T. M., Goldman, H., and Roseborough, A.: Use of phosphate and vitamin D to prevent dwarfism and rickets in X-linked hypophosphatemia. New Engl. Jour. Med. 287:481, 1972.

35. Brickman, A. S., Coburn, J. W., Kurokawa, K., Bethune, J. E., Harrison, H. E., and Norman, A. W.: Actions of 1,25-dihydroxy-cholecalciferol in patients with hypophosphatemic, vitamin D-resistant rickets. New Engl. Jour. Med. 289:495, 1973.

36. Rasmussen, H., Anast, C., Parks, J., Haussler, M., Lane, J., and Pechet, M.: $1\alpha(OH)D_3$ in treatment of hypophosphatemic rickets. Clin. Res. 24:486A, 1976.

37. Zerwekh, J. E., Brumbaugh, P. F., Haussler, D. H., Cork, D. J., and Haussler, M. R.: 1α-Hydroxyvitamin D_3: an analog of vitamin D_3 which apparently acts by metabolism to $1\alpha,25$-dihydroxy-vitamin D_3. Biochemistry 13:4097, 1974.

THE REGULATION OF VITAMIN D METABOLISM

K.W. Colston, P.J. Butterworth*, I.M.A. Evans, and
I. MacIntyre
Endocrine Unit, Dept. Chemical Pathology, Royal Post-
graduate Medical School, London W12 OHS, *Department
Biochemistry, Chelsea College, London SW3

INTRODUCTION

It is now firmly established that vitamin D_3 (cholecalciferol)
must first be converted to more active forms by a series of hydroxylations before exerting its characteristic effects on calcium
metabolism. The first hydroxylation takes place predominantly in
the liver where cholecalciferol is converted to 25-hydroxycholecal-
ciferol (25 OH D_3), the major circulating form of the vitamin (1).
A second hydroxylation takes place only in the kidney; 25 OH D_3 is
hydroxylated by a mitochondrial enzyme system either in position I
to form 1,25 dihydroxycholecalciferol (1,25(OH)$_2$D$_3$) (2), the most
active metabolite of vitamin D_3 known. An alternative step hydroxy-
lates 25 OH D_3 in position 24 to produce 24,25 dihydroxycholecalciferol (24,25 (OH)$_2$D$_3$), a less active metabolite (3).
Many factors have been suggested as regulators of the renal
metabolism of 25 OH D_3, the most prominent being the serum calcium
concentration (4), renal phosphate levels (5), parathyroid hormone
and feedback regulation by vitamin D_3 itself. The role of parathyroid hormone is unclear, since it has been shown both to depress
and to stimulate renal 25 OH-1-hydroxylase activity, depending on
the experimental conditions used (6-9). The precise mechanisms by
which many of these factors exert their effects at a subcellular
level remains to be clarified. However, the feedback regulation of
vitamin D metabolism has been studied in more detail and is described
below. 1,25 dihydroxycholecalciferol has been shown to depress
1-hydroxylase levels and induce the appearance of 24-hydroxylase
activity in vitamin D deficient chicks. Furthermore, this effect
of 1,25(OH)$_2$D$_3$ is mediated via a nuclear process involving changes
in total gene transcription.

All the mentioned effects can be considered as "long term" regulators since their effects take hours or days to become apparent. It is likely that one further regulatory mechanism is the modulation of the activity of existing enzyme molecules through a direct interaction with Ca^{++} and Pi ions. Such a system would offer an "immediate" as opposed to a "long term" means of control. The location of the hydroxylases in mitochondria, organelles known for their ability to accumulate Ca and thereby control cytosolic Ca^{++} would ensure that the enzymes sense changes in Ca^{++} within the cytosol.

There have been several attempts to study the direct effect of Ca^{++} and Pi ions on the activity of the 25 OH D_3-hydroxylase in isolated chick mitochondria in vitro, but the reports emerging from these studies are conflicting in that some show a stimulation of enzyme activity with increasing Ca^{++} concentration and some a decrease. The disparity of the findings can probably be accounted for, in part, by the different conditions prevailing, since isolated mitochondrial experiments need to be carefully designed so that any observed changes in enzyme activity are not solely the result of a change in mitochondrial integrity through swelling or alterations in intramitochondrial pH.

METHODS

Preparation of Mitrochondria

One-day old chicks (Orchin Farm, Great Missenden, Bucks) were maintained on a vitamin D deficient diet (Ca 0.3%, Pi 0.5%) for 3 weeks. Chicks were then killed by decapitation and the kidneys immediately removed and placed in ice-cold medium (200 mM sucrose; 15 mM Tris-acetate buffer pH 7.4 supplemented with 2 mM EGTA) that had been depleted of oxygen by gassing with nitrogen for 2 hours. The tissue was homogenized in the buffer and the mitochondrial fraction was then isolated by conventional methods. The mitochondria were then washed twice with the Tris acetate buffer containing 10 mM EGTA and finally with the Tris acetate buffer alone. The isolated mitochondria were then suspended in approximately 5 ml of the Tris acetate buffer containing 1 mg/ml bovine serum albumin to give a concentration of mitochondrial protein of 15-30 mg per ml. The anaerobic conditions and presence of EGTA allow a depletion of intramitochondrial Ca^{++}.

Aliquots (0.1 ml) of the mitochondrial suspension were preincubated for 10 min at 37°C in a total volume of 1.5 ml buffer (15 mM Tris acetate pH 7.4, 1.9 mM Mg Cl_2, 200 mM sucrose, 5 mM sodium succinate). In some experiments $CaCl_2$ or $Na_2 HPO_4$ was added to the required concentration as stated in "Results". The substrate (26,27-methyl-3H-25(OH)D_3) obtained from the Radiochemical Centre, Amersham, Bucks., with a specific activity of 10 Ci/mmol, 6/25 pmol per incubate, was added in 5 µl ethanol. After a further 10 min incubation the reaction was stopped by the addition of 4.5 ml methanol/chloroform 2:1 v/v. Samples were then extracted, chromatographed and counted as previously described (11).

RESULTS AND DISCUSSION

The mitochondria prepared as described were found to be coupled.

Figure 1 shows the effect of added $CaCl_2$ on 1-hydroxylase activity in intact mitochondria. The response to calcium was biphasic. Addition of increasing concentration of Ca^{++} up to 0.117 mM caused a marked decrease in enzyme activity, more than 50%

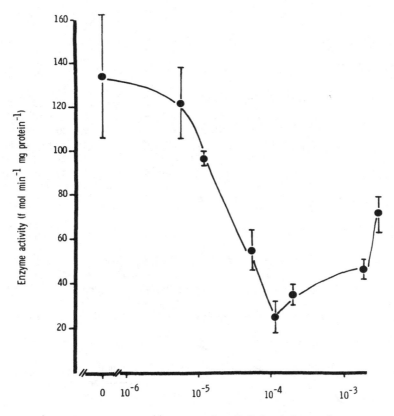

Initial Ca^{++} concentration (M) in incubating medium

Fig 1. Effect of increasing Ca^{++} concentration on 1-hydroxy-
lase activity in isolated kidney mitochondria. The
incubation medium contained 200 mM sucrose, 15 mM
Tris acetate buffer pH 7.4, 5 mM sodium succinate and
1.9 mM $MgCl_2$ with 2.9 mg mitochondrial protein. The
substrate concentration was 15 pmol per 1.5 ml incubate.

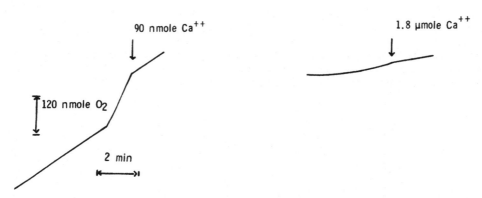

Fig 2a and 2b.   Effect of Ca^{++} on the respiration of chick
                  kidney mitochondria. The incubation medium
                  consisted of 200 mM sucrose, 15 mM Tris ace-
                  tate buffer, pH 7.4, 4 mM Na$_2$ succinate and
                  3 mg of mitochondrial protein in a total volume
                  of 2.5 ml. Ca^{++} was added in a pulse at the
                  point shown. The oxygen consumption was
                  measured polarographically.

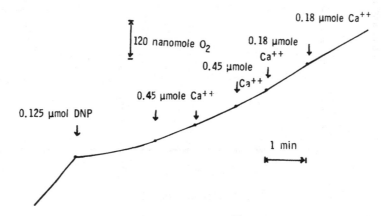

Fig 2c.   Effect of higher levels of Ca^{++} on the respiration of
           chick kidney mitochondria. The conditions were simi-
           lar to those in Fig 2a, except that the total volume
           of the incubation medium was 4.4 ml containing 6.2 mg
           of mitochondrial protein.

inhibition was seen with 0.058 mM added CaCl$_2$. At higher concentrations of Ca^{++} a reversal of this inhibition was seen. Furthermore, this reversal of inhibition by Ca^{++} ions did not seem to be dependent upon an exogenous supply of NADPH, (Fig 1).

The inhibition of 1-hydroxylase activity with 0.058 mM Ca^{++} was not due to a change in mitochondrial integrity since respiration was not inhibited following uptake of Ca^{++} (Fig 2a). In contrast, respiration was stimulated transiently by the pulse of Ca^{++}, as expected (10). However, with the higher levels of Ca^{++} associated with reversal of enzyme inhibition, mitochondria showed a disturbance in respiration following Ca^{++} uptake (Fig 2b). This inhibition of respiration was relieved by the addition of the uncoupler DNP (Fig 2c).

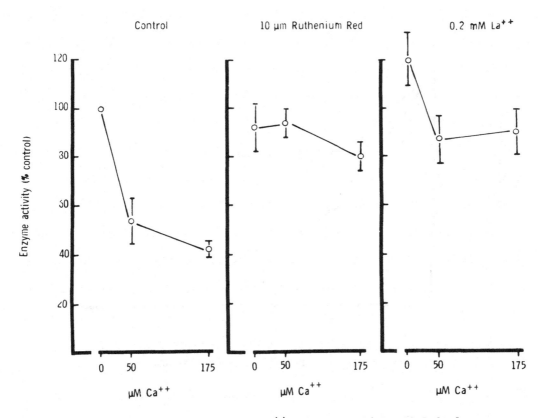

Fig 3.   Effect of increasing Ca^{++} concentration of 1-hydroxy-
         lase activity in isolated mitochondria.

         The incubation medium contained 2.9 mg mitochondrial
         protein. The substrate concentration was 15 pmol per
         1.5 ml incubate.

Further evidence of the involvement of mitochondrial levels of
Ca^{++} on 1-hydroxylase activity was obtained with experiments using
inhibitors of Ca^{++} uptake. Both LaCl$_3$ (0.2 mM) and ruthenium red
(10 μM) prevented the inhibition of 1-hydroxylase activity induced
by Ca^{++} (Fig 3).

The inhibition of enzyme activity with low concentrations of
Ca^{++} was found to be modified, but not completely reversed, when
Pi was present in the incubation medium (Fig 4). Higher levels of
Pi alone had an inhibitory effect on the enzyme (Fig 5). The level
of mitochondrial Ca^{++} concentration would seem to be an important
modulator of 1-hydroxylase activity. The inhibition of enzyme
activity occurs at initial concentrations of calcium in the incubation medium which are very low (0.058 mM) and this effect may well

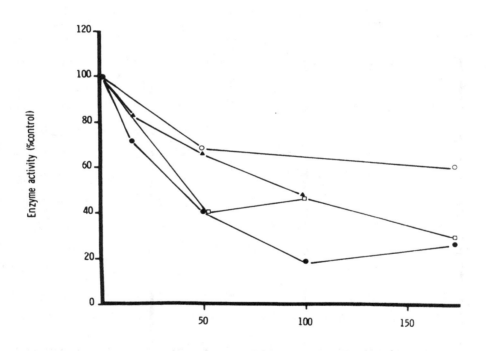

Initial concentration (μM) Ca^{++} in incubation medium

Fig 4.   Effect of Ca^{++} and Pi on 1-hydroxylase activity.

● zero Pi   ☐ 0.01 mM Pi   ▲ 0.3 mM Pi   o 1.0 mM Pi

Enzyme activities are expressed as a percentage of control. Zero Ca^{++} for each Pi concentration equals 100%.
Incubation conditions were similar to those described
previously.

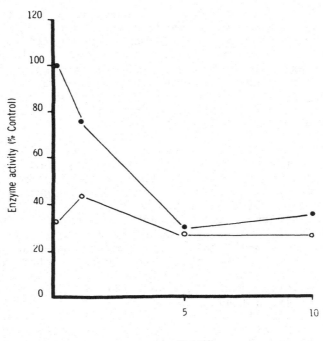

Fig 5. Effect of Pi on 1-hydroxylase activity in the presence
and absence of Ca++. Activities are expressed as percentage of control (zero Ca++ zero Pi) levels. Incubation conditions were similar to those described
previously.

● no added Ca++
O 60 μM added Ca++

have physiological significance. Furthermore, uptake of these
amounts of Ca++ (29 nmol Ca++ per mg mitochondrial protein) does
not cause mitochondrial damage as assessed by respiration studies.
Our studies with the inhibitors LaCl3 and ruthenium red confirm
that this Ca++ associated inhibition of enzyme activity is dependent
upon uptake of Ca++ by the mitochondria.

In vivo, it is improbable that Ca++ can be accumulated by
mitochondria without a simultaneous uptake of Pi (12). Thus, the
results of the studies of the inhibition of the hydroxylase by Ca++
ions in the presence of Pi may be a realistic guide to the nature
of any "direct" regulation by Ca++ ions. Simultaneous uptake of
Ca++ and Pi may result in storage of some of the Ca++ in an insoluble

form that is unable to interact with the enzyme and so the inhibition is relieved. On the other hand, some kind of interaction between Pi and the hydroxylase that lessens the sensitivity of Ca^{++} cannot be ruled out. In any event, the presence of Pi appears to buffer, to some extent, the hydroxylase activity against wide fluctuations in Ca^{++} concentration. This phenomenon could be of physiological significance. Since the hydroxylase activity seems to be inhibited by Pi in the absence of Ca^{++}, it is likely that this anion can have a regulatory role in addition to that of buffering Ca^{++} inhibition.

Thus, the changes in intracellular levels of Ca^{++} and Pi ions and the uptake of these ions by renal mitochondria may provide a means of short term regulation of vitamin D metabolism. As already mentioned, a number of other factors have been suggested as long term modulators of $1,25(OH)_2D_3$ production.

One such mechanism is the feedback regulation of vitamin D metabolism. In states of vitamin D deficiency there is a marked increase in the activity of the renal 1-hydroxylase enzyme (7,13). When chicks are reared on a vitamin D deficient diet from the day of hatching there is a marked enhancement of renal 1-hydroxylase activity after 4 days coinciding with a virtual disappearance of 24-hydroxylase activity (14).

In contrast, administration of physiological doses of vitamin D_3 causes a marked inhibition of 1-hydroxylase activity and an appearance of 24-hydroxylase activity (6,15). These changes in enzyme activities were apparent 2-3 days after treatment. More rapid effects have been seen with equivalent doses of the natural kidney hormone $1,25(OH)_2D_3$ but the fastest and most pronounced changes in renal hydroxylase activities are produced by large doses of this steroid (Table 1). Thus, 62.5 nmol (25 µg) $1,25(OH)_2D_3$ induces the appearance of 24-hydroxylase and a concomitant disappearance of 1-hydroxylase activity at 9 hr.

TABLE 1

Treatment (no:birds)		1-hydroxylase	24-hydroxylase
Ethanol	(4)	69.90 ± 8.16	3.05 ± 1.17
62.5 nmol $1,25(OH)_2D_3$	(4)	17.00 ± 5.20	36.2 ± 3.64

Effect of synthetic $1,25(OH)_2D_3$ on renal 1- and 24-hydroxylase enzyme activities at 9 hr.

Enzyme activities are expressed as mean (± S.E.M.) f mol dihydroxy metabolite produced min^{-1} mg $protein^{-1}$ with 3 replicate estimations of enzyme activity per bird.

TABLE 2

Treatment (no:birds)		1-hydroxylase	24-hydroxylase
Control	(3)	30.23 ± 5.76	6.94 ± 1.91
125 nmol 1,25(OH)$_2$D$_3$	(3)	1.38 ± 1.37	30.45 ± 3.54
1,25(OH)$_2$D$_3$ actinomycin D	(3)	26.32 ± 4.61	11.2 ± 0.84
Actinomycin D	(3)	19.38 ± 5.31	8.5 ± 0.89

Effect of actinomycin D (400 nmol per bird) on the induction of
24-hydroxylase activity by 1,25(OH)$_2$D$_3$ (125 nmol per bird).

Renal 1- and 24-hydroxylase activities were assayed 9 hr after
1,25(OH)$_2$D$_3$ administration and are expressed as mean (± S.E.M.)
f mol dihydroxy metabolite produced min^{-1} mg protein^{-1}. Actinomycin D was given intravenously in 5 equal doses (total dose 400
nmol) beginning 30 min before administration of 1,25(OH)$_2$D$_3$.

TABLE 3

Treatment (no:birds)		1-hydroxylase	24-hydroxylase
Control	(3)	44.63 ± 5.93	2.13 ± 1.14
1,25(OH)$_2$D$_3$	(3)	6.94 ± 2.66	27.00 ± 4.45
1,25(OH)$_2$D$_3$ + α-amanitin	(3)	32.61 ± 6.00	1.44 ± 0.99
α-amanitin	(3)	22.13 ± 4.44	1.63 ± 0.65

Effect of α-amanitin (100 nmol) on the induction of 24-hydroxylase
activity by 1,25(OH)$_2$D$_3$ (125 nmol).

Renal 1- and 24-hydroxylase activities were assayed 9 hr after
1,25(OH)$_2$D$_3$ administration and are expressed as mean (± S.E.M.)
f mol dihydroxy metabolite produced min^{-1} mg protein^{-1}. α-Amanitin
was given intravenously in a single dose 30 min before administration of 1,25(OH)$_2$D$_3$.

The relatively slow changeover from 1- to 24-hydroxylase activity following 1,25(OH)$_2$D$_3$ treatment would imply that this effect
is not simply one of product inhibition but may indicate an initiation of some cellular process such as new protein synthesis. This
hypothesis is supported by studies using inhibitors of transcription.

Treatment with actinomycin D, which inhibits transcription by
binding to the DNA template, abolished both the appearance of 24-

hydroxylase activity and the disappearance of l-hydroxylase activity in response to $1,25(OH)_2D_3$ (Table 2). Similarly, α-amanitin, which inhibits messenger RNA synthesis by its action on RNA polymerase II, also prevents the change in renal enzyme activities 9 hr after administration of $1,25(OH)_2D_3$ (Table 3).

More recent studies have shown that $1,25(OH)_2D_3$ may exert its effect on the renal hydroxylase enzymes via changes in gene transcription. $1,25(OH)_2D_3$ has been shown to cause an immediate and sensitive decrease of RNA I and II polymerase activities (14). This rapid inhibition of RNA polymerase II activity by $1,25(OH)_2D_3$ is similar to the effects seens with other steroid hormones, notably the action of progesterone on the chick oviduct (15). This experimental data is consistent with the view that vitamin D regulates its own metabolism in a feedback manner and that it exerts its effects, as do other steroid hormones, by a nuclear effect involving changes in gene transcription. Such a nuclear feedback control would explain how the kidney responds to the prevailing vitamin D status of the animal.

Thus, variation in the amount and type of renal enzyme with intake of vitamin D may prove to be an important factor in the physiological regulation of vitamin D metabolism.

REFERENCES

1. J.W. Blunt, H.F. DeLuca, and H.K. Schnoes: 25-Hydroxycholecalciferol. A biologically active metabolite of vitamin D_3. Biochemistry 7, 3317-3322, 1968.
2. E. Kodicek, and D.R. Fraser: Regulation of 25-hydroxycholecalciferol-1-hydroxylase activity in kidney by parathyroid hormone. Nature:New Biology, 241:163-166, 1973.
3. M.F. Holick, H.K. Schnoes, and H.F. DeLuca: Isolation and identification of 24,25-dihydroxycholecalciferol, a metabolite of vitamin D_3 made in the kidney. Biochemistry 11:4251-4255, 1972.
4. I.T. Boyle, R.W. Gray, and H.F. DeLuca: Regulation by calcium of in vivo synthesis of 1,25-dihydroxycholecalciferol and 21, 25 dihydroxycholecalciferol. Proceedings of the National Academy of Science of the USA 63:2131-2134, 1971.
5. Y. Tanaka, and H.F. DeLuca: Control of 25-hydroxy vitamin D metabolism by inorganic phosphorus. Arch Biochem and Biophys 154:566-574, 1973.
6. L. Galante, K.W. Colston, I.M.A. Evans, P.G.H. Byfield, E.W. Matthews, and I. MacIntyre: The regulation of vitamin D metabolism. Nature 244:438-440, 1973.
7. D.R. Fraser, and E. Kodicek: Regulation of 25-hydroxy-cholecalciferol-1-hydroxylase activity in kidney by parathyroid hormone. Nature:New Biology 241:163-166, 1973.

8. M. Garabedian, M.F. Holick, H.F. DeLuca, and I.T. Boyle: Control of 25-hydroxycholecalciferol metabolism by parathyroid glands. Proceedings of the National Academy of Science of the USA 69:1673-1976, 1972.

9. L. Galante, S.J. MacAuley, K.W. Colston, and I. MacIntyre: Effect of parathyroid extract on vitamin D metabolism. Lancet i, 985:988, 1972.

10. E. Carafoli, K. Malmstrom, M. Capano, E. Sigel, and M. Crompton: Mitochondria and the regulation of cell calcium. In Contraction and Secretion, pp. 53-64, North Holland Co., 1975.

11. K.W. Colston, I.M.A. Evans, L.S. Galante, I. MacIntyre, and . D.W. Moss: Regulation of vitamin D metabolism: factors influencing the rate of formation of 1,25 dihydroxy-cholecalciferol by kidney homogenates. Biochem J 134:617-820, 1973.

12. C. Carafoli, K. Malmstrom, E. Sigel, and M. Crompton: The regulation of intracellular calcium. Clin Endo 5:suppl, 49-59S, 1976.

13. I. MacIntyre, K.W. Colston, and ImM.A. Evans: The regulation of vitamin D metabolism. Proceedings of the XIth European Symposium on Calcified Tissues, Denmark (in press)

14. I. MacIntyre, K.W. Colston, I,M.A. Evans, and T.C. Spelsberg: Manuscript in preparation, 1976.

15. T.C. Spelsberg, and R.F. Cox: Biochemica Biophysica Acta (in press) 1976.

16. I.M.A. Evans, K.W. Colston, L.S. Galante, and I. MacIntyre: Feedback regulation of 25-hydroxycholecalciferol metabolism by vitamin D_3. Clinical Science and Molecular Med 48:227-230, 1975.

Phosphate Transport and
Phosphate in Disease States

PHOSPHATE TRANSPORT BY ISOLATED RENAL AND INTESTINAL PLASMA MEMBRANES

R. Kinne, W. Berner, N. Hoffmann and H. Murer

Max-Planck-Institut fur Biophysik

Frankfurt (Main), Germany

Studies of luminal and contraluminal membranes isolated from epithelial cells have contributed markedly to our understanding of the molecular mechanisms, the driving forces and the sequence of events involved in transcellular transport of solutes (1). They were extended recently to investigate the properties of phosphate transport systems in renal and intestinal brush border and basal-lateral plasma membrane vesicles (2,3). The investigations revealed that both in the renal proximal tubule and in the small intestine the luminal membranes but not the contraluminal membranes contain a sodium-phosphate cotransport system. This suggests that the driving force for the transcellular phosphate movement is derived from the sodium gradient present and maintained across the brush border membrane. The importance of the sodium cotransport system for the active phosphate reabsorption in the proximal tubule is further indicated by the fact that parathyroid hormone (PTH), which decreases the phosphate reabsorption in the renal proximal tubule also reduces the capacity of the sodium-phosphate cotransport system in isolated renal brush border microvilli (4).

Separation of luminal and contraluminal membranes of renal proximal tubule and small intestine.

The general approach used in the studies on the transport properties of luminal and contraluminal membranes of epithelial cells is composed of the following steps. First the epithelial cells are segregated from each other and from the interstitium, when they are disrupted and a membrane fraction is prepared by differential centrifugation in which the luminal and contraluminal regions of the cellular envelope are enriched whereas the content of other cellular organelles is reduced compared to the starting material.

The membranes are then separated from each other by free flow
electrophoresis (5,6) (or density gradient centrifugation (7)) and
transformed into membrane vesicles into which uptake of solutes is
studied by a rapid filtration method (8).

Phosphate transport by renal plasma membrane vesicles

Figure 1 shows the uptake of phosphate into luminal and cotran-
luminal plasma membrane vesicles isolated from rat proximal tubule.
In the brush border membrane vesicles phosphate uptake in the
presence of sodium shows an overshoot - the intravesicular concentration transiently exceeds the concentration in the incubation
medium - and is inhibited by arsenate. Replacement of sodium by
potassium reduces the initial uptake to 25% of the uptake observed
in the presence of sodium and abolishes the inhibitory effect of
arsenate. So in isolated brush border membrane vesicle uptake of
phosphate can be demonstrated which has the same general properties
such as sodium dependence (9) and inhibition by arsenate (10) as
the transepithelial transport in the proximal tubule.

In the basal-lateral plasma membranes, however, the phosphate uptake is sodium independent, thus the sodium-dependent phosphate
transport system seems to be located exclusively in the luminal
membrane of the proximal tubule.

As shown in Figure 2 sodium exerts a dual effect on the phosphate
transport in the brush border. In the presence of a sodium chloride
concentration difference across the brush border membrane, a transient accumulation of phosphate inside the vesicles to a concentration exceeding the concentration in the incubation medium is
observed. In the absence of a sodium gradient, the overshoot
disappears but the intial rate of phosphate uptake is still about
4 times higher than in the presence of potassium. These findings
firstly indicate that the driving force for the overshoot is provided by the electrochemical potential difference of sodium across
the brush border membrane. Secondly they provide evidence for a
direct interaction of sodium with the transport system probably
involving a sodium-phosphate cotransport system. Such a cotransport system should not only show stimulation of phosphate uptake
by sodium but also a stimulation of sodium flux by phosphate. As
demonstrated in Figure 3 indeed addition of phosphate to vesicles
preequilibrated with sodium stimulates sodium uptake and leads to
a transient accumulation of sodium inside the vesicles; a finding
which renders additional support to the postulated presence of a
sodium-phosphate cotransport system.

Since phosphate is an anion which at physiological pH is present
as primary and as secondary phosphate, it was of interest to determine which anion species is transported preferentially.

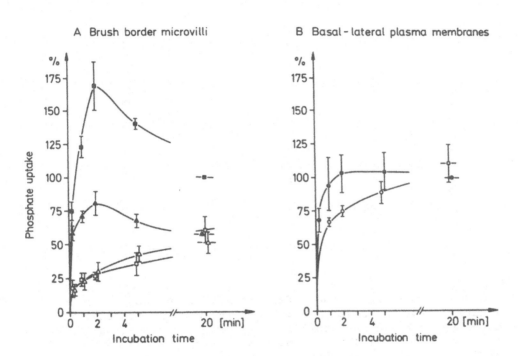

Figure 1 – Uptake of inorganic phosphate by brush border membrane vesicles (A), and by basal-lateral plasma membrane vesicles (B) isolated from rat renal cortex. The vesicles contained 100 mM mannitol and 10 mM Tris - HEPES (N-2-hydroxyethylpiperazine-N'-2-ethane sulfonic acid) pH 7.4 and were incubated in a medium containing in addition 1 mM phosphate (^{32}P-labelled) and 100 mM NaCl (■, ●) or 100 mM KCl (◻, ○). (▲) represents the uptake in the sodium medium in the presence of 5 mM arsenate, (△) the uptake in the presence of potassium and arsenate. Redrawn from Hoffmann et al. (2).

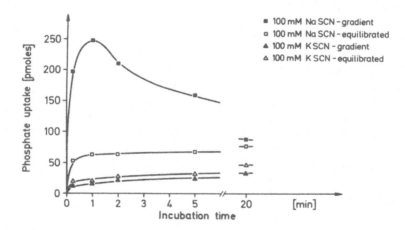

Figure 2 – Comparison of the effect of sodium and potassium on the phosphate uptake by isolated brush border membrane vesicles under gradient and non-gradient conditions. For studies of uptake under cation gradient conditions the membranes were preincubated for 1 h at 25°C in mannitol Tris-HEPES buffer, and the uptake was determined in a medium containing 100 mM mannitol, 20 mM Tris-HEPES, pH 7.4, and 100 mM NaSCN (■ -■) or 100 mM KSCN (▲ - ▲), respectively. For non-gradient conditions the buffer used for the preincubation con-tained in addition 100 mM NaSCN (□ -□) or 100 mM KSCN (Δ - Δ), respectively. Intravesicular space as determined by the amount of D-glucose present in the vesicles after 20 min was identical under all 4 incubation conditions.

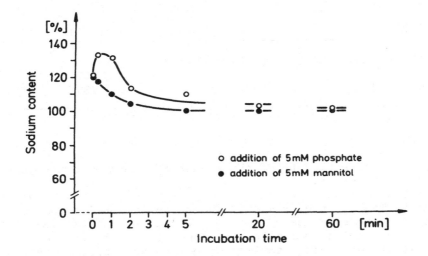

Figure 3 - Phosphate induced sodium accumulation in isolated renal brush border membrane vesicles. The membranes were incubated for 1 h at 25°C in a solution containing 100 mM mannitol, 5 mM Tris-HEPES, pH 7.4, 95 mM KSCN and 5 mM ^{22}NaSCN. At zero time 30 µl of a solution containing 5 mM Tris-HEPES, 95 mM KSCN and 5 mM phosphate (o—o) or 5 mM mannitol (●—●) were added to 150 µl of the membrane suspension. The values are expressed as percent of the new equilibrium reached after 60 min of incubation.

Table 1

Uptake of inorganic phosphate
by isolated brush border membrane vesicles.

Influence of medium pH

pH in the incubation medium	Intestinal brush border	Renal brush border
	in % of uptake at pH 7.4	
6.00	188	58
7.40	100	100
8.00	48	135

Therefore the effect of pH of the incubation medium on the phosphate uptake was determined.

As shown in Table I the uptake of phosphate by renal brush border membranes in the presence of 100 mM NaCl almost doubles when the pH of the incubation medium is increased from pH 6 to pH 8. This might indicate - if other actions of pH on the transport system can be excluded - that the secondary phosphate is the anion species which is transported predominantly.

It was found in addition (Fig. 4) that the phosphate uptake depends in a nonhyperbolic fashion on the ambient sodium concentration. Kinetic analysis of the sodium dependence showed that the curves easily fit to an equation where the interaction of two sodium ions with the transport system is assumed (2). Thus the results on pH dependence and sodium dependence of the phosphate transport by renal brush border membrane vesicles would suggest that secondary phosphate is transferred together with two sodium ions which results in an electroneutral transfer of sodium and phosphate across the membrane. This assumption is supported by the results obtained in studies where the electrical potential difference across the brush border membrane (membrane potential) was altered by artificially imposed diffusion potentials (11). As demonstrated in Table II alterations of the membrane potential do not substantially alter the rate of phosphate uptake whereas striking changes are observed in the "electrogenic" (11) glucose-sodium cotransport.

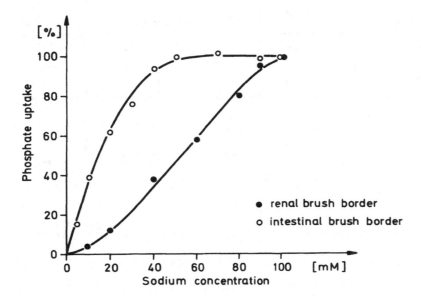

Figure 4 - Influence of sodium on the phosphate uptake by isolated renal (●—●) and intestinal (o—o) brush border membrane vesicles. The incubation medium contained 100 mM mannitol, 20 mM Tris-HEPES, pH 7.4, 1 mM phosphate (renal brush borders) or 0,1 mM phosphate (intestinal brush borders) and the sodium concentrations indicated in the figure. Sodium was replaced by choline. Uptake measured after 15 seconds has been corrected for the uptake obtained in a sodium-free medium and is expressed as percent of the transport observed in the presence of 100 mM NaCl. Redrawn from Hoffmann et al. (2) and Berner et al (3).

TABLE II

Influence of Membrane Potential on Phosphate and Glucose
Uptake by Isolated Brush Border Membrane Vesicles

Salt gradient (medium>vesicles) (100 mM salt)	Membrane potential (relative to NaCl gradient)	Phosphate uptake		D-glucose uptake
		Intestinal brush border	Renal brush border	Intestinal brush border
		(in % of uptake in the presence of NaCl)		
NaSCN	inside negative	96.8	112	370
NaCl	0	100	100	100
Na$_2$SO$_4$	inside positive	106	87	65.4

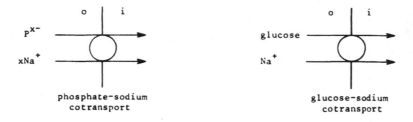

phosphate-sodium
cotransport

glucose-sodium
cotransport

Phosphate transport by intestinal plasma membranes.

Table II depicts one important observation on the phosphate transport by intestinal brush border, namely that it is also predominantly electroneutral. This already suggests that phosphate is
transported via a cotransport system together with positively
charged molecules. Indeed as shown in Figure 4 the uptake of phosphate by intestinal brush border membranes depends on the presence
of sodium in the incubation medium. Contrary to the renal transport system, however, a hyperbolic saturation curve is obtained
for the sodium dependence which points to a one to one interaction
between the transport system and sodium. Furthermore as indicated
in Table I intestinal brush border membranes take up phosphate
more rapidly at pH 6 than at pH 8. Taking together, electroneutra-
lity, simple saturation kinetics for sodium and increased uptake
at low pH, the results would lead to the assumption that in the
intestinal brush border membrane a sodium-phosphate cotransport
system is operating which catalyses the electroneutral transfer of
one sodium ion and and one primary phosphate across the membrane
(3). The preferential transport of the primary phosphate is one
of the peculiarities of the intestinal transport system compared

to the renal transport system, another - depicted in Table III - is the 130 fold lower maximal velocity of the system in the intestinal membranes. Further properties such as the affinity for phosphate, arsenate and sodium are quite similar in both systems (Table III).

TABLE III

Properties of Phosphate Transport Systems in Renal and Intestinal Brush Border Membranes

	Renal Brush Border	Intestinal Brush Border
K_m (phosphate)	0.8×10^{-4}M	1.1×10^{-4}M
V_{max} (phosphate)	10 nmoles/mg x 15 sec	0.08 nmoles/mg x 15 sec
K_i (arsenate)	11×10^{-4}M	3.4×10^{-4}M
K_m (sodium)	60×10^{-3}M	27×10^{-3}M
Probable mode of transfer	secondary phosphate with two sodium ions	primary phosphate with one sodium ion

K_m and V_{max} for phosphate and K_i for arsenate were determined at pH 7.4 in the presence of a 100 mM NaCl gradient, K_m for sodium was measured at pH 7.4 and 1 mM P_i for the renal and 0.1 mM P_i for the intestinal brush border membranes.

Mode of transcellular phosphate transport in renal proximal tubule and small intestine.

From the above described results and conclusions a general scheme for the transcellular transport of phosphate across the renal and intestinal epithelium can be derived (Fig. 5). At the luminal cell pole phosphate enters the cell together with sodium via electro-neutral sodium-phosphate-cotransport systems, thereby the concentration difference for sodium across the brush border membrane provides the driving force for an intracellular accumulation of phosphate. At the contraluminal cell pole sodium-independent transport systems are located which facilitate the exit of phosphate along its chemical and electrical gradient. This scheme classifies the active phosphate absorption in the small intestine and in the renal proximal tubule as secondary active transport, where the

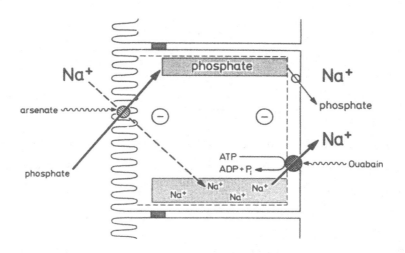

Figure 5 - Schematic representation of the transport systems and
driving forces involved in active phosphate transport by the renal
proximal tubule and the small intestine. Transport of phosphate
occurs from the left to the right and involves: electroneutral
cotransport with sodium across the luminal membrane (⏀) and
intracellular accumulation driven by the concentration difference
of sodium (Na; < Na_O) and sodium-indenpendent - probably carrier
mediated - efflux across the contraluminal cell membrane (⏀) following the electro-chemical potential difference for phosphate.
The low intracellular sodium concentration is maintained by the
action of the Na-K-ATPase (⏀) located in the basal-lateral
plasma membranes. The inhibition of phosphate transport by arsenate
and by sodium depletion takes place at the luminal cell membrane;
the inhibition of phosphate transport by ouabain can be explained
by the assumption that due to an inhibition of Na-K-ATPase the
intracellular sodium concentration increases and therefore the
driving force for the luminal entry of phosphate via the sodium-
phosphate cotransport system is diminished.

active transport of sodium is linked by flux coupling to the movement of phosphate across the cell.

Hormonal regulation of the phosphate transport system in renal brush border membranes.

Parathyroid hormone is known to decrease - besides other actions -
the reabsorption of phosphate in the proximal tubule. In recent
studies from our laboratory it was demonstrated that two membrane
bound systems - the PTH-sensitive adenylate cyclase and a cAMP-
dependent protein kinase - probably involved in the chain of events
which comprises the hormone action, are distributed unevenly in
the plasma membrane evelope of the proximal tubular cell (12,13).
The adenylate cyclase is confined almost exclusively to the basal-
lateral plasma membranes (12), whereas the cAMP stimulated self-
phosphorylating system is more concentrated in the luminal membrane
(13). The latter result suggested that PTH might exert its action
by altering the state of phosphorylation of membrane components
which in turn might result in a change of the transport properties
of the luminal membrane.

This hypothesis is supported by the results shown in Fig. 6, where
the phosphate transport capacity of brush border membranes isolated
from normal rats is compared to the transport capacity of brush
border membranes isolated from rats which received i.m. 30 USP
parathyroid hormone (Para-Thormone (P-20), Eli Lilly, Indianopolis,
USA) one hour before sacrifice. Treatment of the animals with PTH
reduces the initial rate of phosphate uptake by brush border membranes and the overshoot by $\sim 40\%$. Kinetic analysis reveals that
only "V_{max}" of the initial uptake is reduced, the "K_m" of the
system for phosphate remains unchanged (4). It should be noted that
this increase in transport is not observed for the sodium-independent phosphate uptake by the brush borders, for the sodium-dependent D-glucose uptake nor for the sodium uptake of the vesicles.
Thus a specific reduction of the sodium-dependent phosphate transport seems to be brought about by PTH; this reduction in transport
capacity of the luminal membrane for phosphate could easily explain the PTH provoked inhibition of phosphate reabsorption in the
proximal tubule. The reason for the although smaller but still
significant inhibition of isotonic fluid absorption and glucose
transport by PTH in the proximal tubule remains still unclear.
The above reported results would suggest that intracellular events
or events taking place at the contraluminal membrane are involved
in the expression of these phenomena.

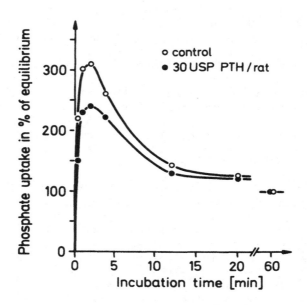

Figure 6 – Effect of parathyroid hormone (PTH) on the phosphate
uptake by isolated renal brush border membrane vesicles. Control
rats received 0.3 ml 0.2% phenol in aqueous solution i.m. 1 h before sacrifice, PTH rats received 0.3 ml of Para-Thormone (Eli
Lilly, 100 USP/ml). The brush border membranes were isolated
according to Booth and Kenny (14) and phosphate uptake was studied
in a medium containing 100 mM mannitol, 20 mM Tris-HEPES, pH 7.4,
0.1 mM phosphate and 100 mM NaCl. The results are expressed as
percent of the uptake observed after 60 minutes (equilibrium).
Treatment of the animals with PTH results in a reduced initial
rate of uptake and in a diminished overshoot.

REFERENCES

1. Kinne, R.: Membrane-molecular aspects of tubular transport. In MTP International Review of Science. Kidney and Urinary Tract Physiology. Vol II, Ed. K. Thurau, London: Butterworths, Baltimore, Univ. Park Press (in press).

2. Hoffman, N., Thees, M., Kinne, R.: Phosphate transport by isolated renal brush border vesicles. Pflugers Arch. 362:147-156, 1976.

3. Berner, W., Kinne, R., Murer, H.: Phosphate transport into brush border membrane vesicles isolated from rat small intestine. Biochem. J. (submitted for publication).

4. Evers, C., Murer, H., and Kinne, R.: Unpublished observations.

5. Heidrich, H.G., Kinne, R., Kinne-Saffran, E., and Hannig, K.: The polarity of the proximal tubule cell in rat kidney: Different surface charges for the brush-border microvilli and plasma membranes from the basal infoldings. J. Cell. Biol. 54:232-245, 1972.

6. Murer, H., Hopfer, U., Kinne-Saffran, E., Kinne, R.: Glucose transport in isolated brush-border and lateral-basal plasma-membrane vesicles from intestinal epithelial cells. Biochim. Biophys. Acta 345:170-179, 1974.

7. Murer, H., Ammans, E., Biber, J., and Hopfer, U.: The surface membrane of the small intestinal epithelial cell. I. Localization of adenylcyclase. Biochim. Biophys. Acta 433:509-519, 1976.

8. Hopfer, U., Nelson, K., Perrotto, J., Isselbacher, K.J.: Glucose transport in isolated brush border membrane from rat small intestine. J. Biol. Chem. 248:25-32, 1973.

9. Baumann, K., de Rouffignac, C., Roinel, N., Rumrich, G., and Ullrich, K.J.: Renal phosphate transport: Unhomogeneity of local proximal transport rates and sodium dependence. Pflugers Arch. 356:287-297, 1975.

10. Ginsburg, J.M., Lotspeich, W.D.: Interrelations of arsenate and phosphate transport in the dog kidney. Amer. J. Physiol. 205:707-714, 1963.

11. Murer, H., Hopfer, U.: Demonstration of electrogenic Na$^+$-dependent D-glucose transport in intestinal brush border membranes. Proc. Natl. Acad. Sci. USA 71:484-488, 1974.

12. Shlatz, L.I., Schwartz, I.L., Kinne-Saffran, E., and Kinne, R.: Distribution of parathyroid hormone-stimulated adenylate cyclase in plasma membranes of cells of the kidney cortex. J. Membrane Biol. 24:131-144, 1975.

13. Kinne, R., Shlatz, L.J., Kinne-Saffran, E., and Schwartz, I.L.: Distribution of membrane-bound cyclic AMP-dependent protein kinase in plasma membranes of cells of the kidney cortex. J. Membrane Biol. 24:145-159, 1975.

14. Booth, A.G., and Kenny, A.J.: A rapid method for the preparation of microvilli from rabbit kidney. Biochem. J. 142:575-581, 1974.

DIPHOSPHONATES

MODE OF ACTION AND CLINICAL APPLICATIONS

H. Fleisch, D. Fast, R. Rizzoli, U. Trechsel
and J.-P. Bonjour
Department of Pathophysiology, University of
Berne, Berne, Switzerland

Introduction

This paper will review the current knowledge of the mode
of action of diphosphonates on calcium and phosphate
metabolism and of the clinical application of these
compounds. The relation with inorganic phosphate will
be emphasized. In view of the space available no references will be given, the reader being referred to
two recent reviews (1,2).

The development of the "phosphonate concept" came from
previous studies on inorganic pyrophosphate. Observations in the early 1960's showed that human plasma and
urine contain substances which inhibit the precipitation of calcium phosphate from solution. One of these
inhibitors was isolated and identified as inorganic
pyrophosphate. Pyrophosphate was then found to have
various physical-chemical effects on calcium phosphate
salts, such as the ability to bind to apatite crystals,
to inhibit crystal growth and crystal aggregation, to
inhibit transformation from amorphous calcium phosphate
into its crystalline phase and to inhibit crystal dissolution. Similar inhibitory properties on calcium carbonate have actually been used in industry to prevent
scaling in water installations. Later pyrophosphate was
found to prevent various types of experimental soft
tissue calcification when administered parenterally to
animals. Bone mineralization, however, was blocked only

in tissue culture but not in living animals. These results and the fact that pyrophosphate is present in
plasma, urine, saliva, bone and teeth led to the hypothesis that this compound had a role in the regulation
of calcium deposition and dissolution in vivo, protec-
ting soft tissues from mineralization and regulating
the entry and exit of calcium and phosphate in bone.
The local concentration of pyrophosphate would be regulated by the pyrophosphatases, such as the alkaline,
neutral, or acid phosphatases, all of which have been
suggested to be involved in calcification and bone metabolism.

If such a concept is correct the question arises as to
whether some diseases of calcium metabolism are due to
disturbances in pyrophosphate metabolism. The most obvious disease is hypophosphatasia, which is characterized by deficient mineralization and in which increased
plasma and urinary levels of pyrophosphate have been
described. Whether an abnormality of pyrophosphate exists in other types of rickets is debatable. The same
is true for the role of pyrophosphate in the pathophysiology of urinary stones, although pyrophosphate has
been found to be decreased in certain groups of patients
with stones and increased by administration of orthophosphate, a procedure which is now widely used in therapy to prevent formation of urinary calcium stones. Finally, pyrophosphate might be involved in joint disorders, since its concentration has been found to be increased in some of these diseases. One of them is
pseudogout (chondrocalcinosis), a condition in which
calcium pyrophosphate crystals deposit in synovial membranes, articular cartilage and periarticular tissues
and cause arthropathy.

All these studies lead to the possibilities that conden-
sed phosphates might be used therapeutically. However,
they were found to be rapidly destroyed when injected
and broken down in the gastrointestinal tract when given
orally. Thus these compounds did not appear very promising for therapeutical use. The only exception was their
use in skeletal scintigraphy, in which pyrophosphate is
linked to the γ-emitting isotope ^{99m}technetium. The
technetium in this condition acquires the characteristics
of pyrophosphate and rapidly enters bone and binds to
the mineral. Technetium-Sn-PPi is now used routinely as
a bone scanning agent, particularly for detecting tumor

deposits and bone diseases.

It was therefore necessary to find other agents with similar effects to pyrophosphate but which would be resistant to enzymatic destruction. The diphosphonates,
closely related in structure to pyrophosphate but possessing P-C-P bonds instead of P-O-P bonds, appeared to
fulfil these requirements.

Physical-chemical Effects

The diphosphonates' effects on the behaviour of calcium
salts in vitro are very similar to those of pyrophosphate. Thus at concentrations as low as 10^{-6} M they inhibit the precipitation of calcium phosphate from solution,
the growth and the aggregation of existing crystals and
also block the transformation of amorphous calcium phosphate into hydroxyapatite. Furthermore they also inhibit crystal dissolution and stimulate disaggregation.
They were also shown to act on other crystals, such as
brushite and calcium oxalate. All these effects are
probably explained by their very strong affinity to the
crystal surface.

Biological Effects

Diphosphonates have been found, like pyrophosphate, to
inhibit various experimental calcifications such as aortic and kidney calcification induced by vitamin D and
skin calcification induced by dihydrotachysterol. Other
types of calcification such as that accompanying magnesium deficiency, experimental arthritis in rats, or that
occuring in spontaneous osteoarthritis in mice are also
inhibited. Finally, disodium ethane-1-hydroxy-1,1-di-
phosphonate (EHDP) inhibits the development of dental
calculus in rats when applied topically. In contrast
to pyrophosphate, however, diphosphonates are effective
whether administered by mouth or parenterally. There
is a close correlation between the ability of individual
diphosphonates to inhibit crystal growth in vitro and
their effect in vivo. The major structure required
seems to be the P-C-P bond, compounds containing P-C-C-P
or single C-P bonds being generally ineffective.

Certain diphosphonates, especially EHDP, when given at

high doses lead to the appearance of unmineralized tissue in bone and cartilage. In growing animals this results in an X-ray picture which is similar to classical rickets. However histologically, at least in the chick, the two conditions differ greatly. Indeed while the cartilage from vitamin D-deficient birds shows an accumulation of proliferating cells, the cartilage from the EHDP-treated animals consists mainly of hypertrophic cells. It seems, therefore, that vitamin D deficiency leads to an impairment of cell differentiation whereas EHDP causes just an inhibition of mineralization. The effect of EHDP on mineralization is reversed when administration is discontinued. The dose required to impair bone mineralization varies according to species, the duration of treatment and the route of administration. Roughly it appears at doses of about 1 mg P/kg day given parenterally. The simpliest explanation for these effects is that EHDP prevents the formation of apatite crystals by a physical-chemical effect. However other modes of action, for example by impairing the functioning of extracellular vesicles, cannot be disregarded. It is interesting that dichloromethane diphosphonate (Cl_2MDP), although it is a good inhibitor of mineralization in vitro, has no effect even at much larger concentrations than EHDP on bone and cartilage mineralization. This difference is not yet explained but might have important implications in the therapeutical application of the diphosphonates.

As shown in numerous studies, the diphosphonates also inhibit bone resorption. Thus they prevent the resorption induced by parathyroid hormone (PTH) or lipopolysaccharides in mouse calvaria in tissue culture. In vivo they partially prevent the increase in calcemia induced by PTH in thyroparathyroidectomized rats. When given to new-born mice they impair bone remodelling, and the skeleton eventually resembles that of grey-lethal osteopetrotic mice. In young rats they lead to an inhibtion of bone resorption, which can be detected by microradiography, by histology and by ^{45}Ca kinetic techniques. Finally, the inhibition of resorption can be shown in experimental models of osteoporosis in rats in which bone loss is induced by nerve section producing immobilization of a hind limb. In all these models Cl_2MDP has always been much more effective than EHDP. This difference between the two compounds is difficult to explain by the physical-chemical mechanism since in vitro

EHDP is much more powerful in inhibiting crystal dissolution than Cl_2MDP.

Cellular Effects

This as well as other differences in the effects of the
two compounds suggested that some of the effects, especially those on bone resorption, could not be explained
just by their physical-chemical actions and that they
possibly had cellular effects. This proved to be true.
In vitro phosphonates have been shown to be powerful
inhibitors of acid phosphatase, acid pyrophosphatase
and other lysosomal enzymes. Interestingly there was
a correlation between these effects and the effect in
vivo on the inhibition of bone resorption. An inhibition was also described for adenyl cyclase. However
in tissue culture, doses of diphosphonates which inhibit bone resorption had no effect on production of
cyclic AMP. In cell culture Cl_2MDP, and to a lesser
degree EHDP, were found to increase cellular glycogen
and to inhibit glucose consumption and lactate production. These effects occurred in cartilage cells, in
fibroblasts and in cells obtained from calvaria. Finally diphosphonates have been found to inhibit the release
of calcium from mitochondria from kidney either when
added in vitro or when given in vivo. It could well be
that some of these mechanisms are important in the final effect of these compounds in vivo. Thus for example the inhibition in lactic acid production could
explain the inhibition of bone resorption. The reason
the diphosphonates act only on bone and not on other
tissues would be due to their property to be adsorbed
on crystal surfaces. Only in bone would they be in
concentrations high enough to act on cells.

Diphosphonates Used as a Tool to Study Calcium and Phosphate Metabolism

It has been suggested many years ago that a link exists
between the need of the bone for calcium and calcium
absorption in the gut. In view of their direct effect
on bone, diphosphonates seemed to be an excellent tool
to study this link. Indeed low amounts of EHDP have
been shown to induce a positive calcium balance in rats
because of an inhibition of bone resorption while high

amounts were shown to decrease the balance because of
the inhibition of mineralization. With Cl_2MDP only bone
resorption was inhibited. These results were found to
correlate surprisingly well with the intestinal absorption of calcium. Thus the low dose of EHDP increased
absorption while the high dose of EHDP was associated
with a decrease. This change appeared to be specific
for calcium and was associated with a reduction in
calcium-binding protein and calcium-stimulated ATPase
in the intestinal mucosa. These results and the fact
that the inhibitory effect could be reversed by low doses of 1,25-dihydroxycholecalciferol (1,25-$(OH)_2D_3$) suggested an effect on vitamin D metabolism. This proved
to be correct. Indeed the low doses of EHDP led to increased accumulation of 1,25-$(OH)_2D_3$ in the gut, but
high doses to a decrease in the production of this metabolite. Since the effect in mineralization is not
corrected by 1,25-$(OH)_2D_3$ and since the histological
appearance of the epiphyseal plate under EHDP is different from that of vitamin D deficiency, it seems likely
that the course of the event is an inhibition of the mineralization by EHDP which then decreases 1,25-$(OH)_2D_3$
synthesis by a mechanism unknown up to now.

This interpretation is also supported by the recent result
that EHDP has no effect on the hydroxylase when added in
vitro to tubules of quails. Furthermore the inhibitory
effect seen in vivo is greatly reduced in birds fed a low
calcium diet. Of interest from the regulatory aspect is
the finding that the stimulation of the 1-hydroxylation
by renal tubules in vitro produced by feeding the quails
a low Ca diet was present in EHDP-treated animals. However stimulation due to a low P diet was not only inhibited by EHDP, but actually reversed. Thus it appears
that EHDP affects the regulatory mechanism by which
1,25-$(OH)_2D_3$ synthesis is linked to phosphate.

Diphosphonates have also been used to investigate phosphate homeostasis. It is well known that while the intestine plays a very important role in regulating calcium balance this seems less true for phosphate. Thus
a change in the dietary phosphate does not lead to a
significant change in the fractional absorption in the
gastrointestinal tract such that the absorbed phosphate
is proportional to the intake. However some regulation
of the absorption exists. Thus after administration of
EHDP in doses which inhibit the 1,25-$(OH)_2D_3$ synthesis,

phosphate absorption is somewhat decreased, this decrease being corrected by the administration of 1,25-(OH) D_3.
These results agree with data showning that vitamin D or 1,25-
(OH)2D3 stimulates phosphate absorption. It is, however, puzzling
that the reduction of absorption under EHDP corresponds astonish-
ingly well to the reduction of skeletal uptake induced by the
diphosphonate.

It has been recently shown that altering the phosphate
in the diet dramatically changes the capacity of reabsorption of the kidney. The effect is largely independent of PTH. This adaptory mechanism actually appears
to be at least 30 times more active than that involving
PTH. It seems therefore that there is a regulation which
adapts the handling of the kidney to the intake of phosphate in order to satisfy the needs of the body. Micropuncture studies have shown that his mechanism is probably located in the proximal tubule and in the terminal
nephron. If this concept is correct the decrease of
uptake of phosphate by the bone induced by EHDP should
lead to similar changes in renal handling. Studies presented in this meeting show that this is indeed the
case and that under EHDP the renal fractional excretion
of phosphate increases drastically.

Metabolism of the Diphosphonates

Diphosphonates unlike pyrophosphate are not destroyed
in the gastrointestinal tract and are absorbed intact.
The site is uncertain but occurs, at least in chicks,
in the ileum. The absorption of EHDP varies according
to the species but usually is between 1 and 10 % of the
oral dose. However the absorption can vary more than
10 fold from one individual to another within one species, being higher in younger animals than in older
ones. approximately half of the absorbed dose goes into bone,
the rest being excreted into the urine. The renal clearance
of EHDP and Cl2MDP is high and, at least in rats, exceeds that of
of inulin indicating the existence of a secretory pathway. This
pathway does not seem to involve the classical ones for organic
acids and bases. In man the clearance is similar to that of
inulin.

The major part of the retained fraction accumulates in
bone, only very small amounts being retained by soft
tissues.

Clinical Studies

The various experimental studies with diphosphonates naturally led to the suggestion that these compounds might be useful in therapy of various disorders of calcium metabolism. Until now only EHDP has been tried in humans and this only in a limited number of diseases.

Like pyrophosphate, diphosphonates are now widely used as bone scanning agents for diagnostic purposes. The basis for this application is their strong affinity for hydroxyapatite as well as the fact that they pass rapidly from blood into bone, shown both in tissue culture and in vivo. The well recognized advantages of the γ-emitting isotope ^{99m}technetium are utilized by linking this compound to the pyrophosphate or EHDP. Thus the technetium takes the characteristics of these compounds and accumulates in the skeleton and other calcified sites. The complex has been found to be very efficient in identifying increased skeletal turnover, for example in Paget's disease, and for detecting bone tumors and recently for localizing and evaluating heart infarctions. ^{99m}technetium compounds offer distinct advantages over ^{18}F and ^{87}Sr and are replacing them in clinical practice.

Naturally it has been tried to make use of the striking effect on calcium phosphate deposition. Several studies have shown that EHDP, when applied topically, can reduce dental calculus formation in man and recently this compound has been added to toothpastes. This finding is potentially important in relation to dental health since calculus is thought to predispose people to the development of periodontal disease and tooth loss.

EHDP has been studied in various types of ectopic calcification. Most studies have dealt with myositis ossificans progressiva, a congenital disorder characterized by formation of ectopic bone in muscle. Since no double-blind study was made, a clear cut conclusion is difficult. It appears nevertheless that EHDP has no effect in reversing pre-existing lesions, but seems to slow down the progress of the disease. Other types of disseminated ectopic calcifications, such as those associated with dermatomyositis or calcinosis universalis, appear unaltered by the administration of EHDP. However a definite answer is difficult to give since most

of these diseases show spontaneous exacerbations and
remissions. On the other hand, in a double-blind study,
EHDP was shown to inhibit the ectopic calcification occuring around the hip after total hip replacement, at
least as long as the drug was given. When the drug was
stopped mineralization did occur but the mobility of
the treated patients was improved over those not receiving the drug.

The inhibition by diphosphonates of crystal growth and
aggregation of apatite, brushite, and calcium oxalate
in vitro, as well as a study on rats in vivo, raised the
possibility that diphosphonates might inhibit stone formation. Preliminary clinical trials suggested that EHDP
may indeed be able to reduce the rate of production of
stones containing calcium in man, but only at relatively high doses which are known to affect the skeleton.
The question therefore arises as to whether any benefit
in stone diseases is larger than possible negative effects on the skeleton.

In view of the action of the diphosphonate on bone resorption various studies have dealt with the possible
effect of EHDP in osteoporosis. While the drug seems
to slow down bone loss during immobilization after spinal injuries the results are less promising in postmenopausal or senile osteoporosis. However since Cl_2MDP
is much more powerful in reducing bone resorption without inhibiting mineralization, trials should be again
made with this drug in the future.

The most extensive and most promising results have been
with Paget's diseases. Indeed EHDP is a very effective
agent for reversing the raised plasma alkaline phosphatase and urinary hydroxyproline associated with increased bone turnover in this disease. It also corrects
the abnormalities in skeletal scans and in ^{45}Ca kinetics.
The results are dose-dependent and normal values can be
achieved within three months of the treatment. Interestingly the biochemical suppression of the disease can
last for more than two years after stopping the drug.
A double-blind study has suggested that there is also a
dose-dependent response of the clinical symptoms. Morphologically EHDP has been shown to reduce the number
of osteoblasts and osteoclasts which are too numerous in
this disease. Furthermore the bone formed under EHDP
seems to return to the normal laminar type. Diphospho-

nates have an advantage over calcitonin in that they can
be given by mouth rather than by parenteral administration and that their effect lasts after stopping the
treatment.

The clinical studies have until now not revealed any
significant toxic effect. The main side effect is the
inhibition of normal mineralization which is seen when
the compound is given orally at a dose above 10 mg/kg
daily. Morphological studies showed the appearance of
increased osteoid tissue in adults, and in children
radiological signs of rickets as well as muscle weakness
have been described. All these signs disappear rapidly
after discontinuation of the treatment. In a few patients pathological fractures have occurred.

Another side effect of EHDP is the rise of plasma phosphate often to high levels. This change which appears
after 24 hours already but reaches its maximum only after 2 - 3 weeks is associated with a change in the renal handling of phosphate with a fall in the fractional
excretion of phosphate and a rise in the Tm/GFR. The
mechanism of these alterations remains unclear. It is
not induced by a secondary hypoparathyroidism, since
other signs of this disease such as low plasma calcium
and diminished tubular reabsorption of calcium are not
seen and since PTH levels in blood are normal. It is
also interesting that this hyperphosphataemia has not
been found in any other animal species studied so far.
Further studies on this effect may uncover new aspects
of phosphate metabolism.

Summary

Compounds containing P-O-P bonds (e.g. inorganic pyrophosphate) or P-C-P bonds (diphosphonates) share the
property of being able to inhibit both the formation,
aggregation and dissolution of calcium phosphate crystals in vitro. They also inhibit formation and aggregation of calcium oxalate in vitro.

Pyrophosphate is present in body fluids and in mineralized tissues and may have a physiological function in
regulating calcification and bone turnover. Abnormalities in the metabolism of pyrophosphate may be important
in the development of some human diseases notably hypo-

phosphatasia, urinary stones, and pseudogout.

Diphosphonates inhibit ectopic calcification, and slow down bone resorption and bone turnover in several experimental systems in vivo. These effects are probably due to not only their physical-chemical properties but also to cellular effects. These compounds have been useful agents in studying various aspects of the regulation of calcium phosphate and vitamin D metabolism. In clinical studies EHDP is effective against ectopic calcification after total hip replacement, against dental calculus and in disorders of increased bone resorption such as Paget's disease. Finally ^{99m}technetium complexes of EHDP, pyrophosphate and other polyphosphates have recently been used successfully as bone scanning agents, and after myocardial infarctions.

Acknowledgements

This work has been supported by the Procter and Gamble Company, USA, and by the Swiss Foundation for Scientific Research (grant No. 3.121.73).

References

1. Russell, R.G.G., and Fleisch, H.: Pyrophosphate and diphosphonates in skeletal metabolism. Clin.Orthop. Rel.Res. 108: 241, 1975.

2. Fleisch, H., and Russell, R.G.G.: Experimental and clinical studies with pyrophosphate and diphosphonates. In: Calcium Metabolism and Bone in Renal Disease (David, D.S., ed.), John Wiley & Sons Inc., New York, in press.

MECHANISM OF RENAL ACTION OF PARATHYROID HORMONE

Kiyoshi Kurokawa

University of Southern California School of Medicine

2025 Zonal Avenue, Los Angeles, California

Parathyroid hormone (PTH) is a major hormone involved in the maintenance of calcium and phosphorus homeostasis. The two major target organs for this peptide hormone are bone and kidney. In this communication, we briefly review our knowledge on the mechanisms of actions of PTH on the kidney, and by doing so we could envision some insight into the mechanisms of action of PTH on bone, since some of the basic hormone-cell interaction may be similar. For those who are interested, two recent review articles (1,2) are available discussing in detail the various aspects of PTH-kidney relationship. The present discussion will be limited to the acute effects of PTH on the kidney.

In response to PTH, three immediate changes take place in renal cells. These are: 1) the activation of membrane-bound adenylate cyclase with a rise in intracellular cyclic AMP levels; 2) changes in the distribution of intracellular calcium ion (Ca^{++}) and 3) alterations in the levels of certain intermediary metabolites in vivo, and the stimulation of renal gluconeogenesis in vitro.

Studies on the possible role of adenylate cyclase-cyclic AMP system as a mediator of PTH action were pioneered by Chase and Aurbach (3,4). Their observations can be summarized as follows: 1) the intravenous infusion of PTH into parathyroidectomized (PTX) rats induces an immediate and marked increase in cAMP in renal tissue and in urine which proceeds the phosphaturic response; 2) urinary cAMP excretion is lower in PTX rats than in rats with intact parathyroid glands; 3) infusion of $CaCl_2$ into rats with intact parathyroid glands reduces urinary cAMP excretion; and 4) PTH activates adenylate cyclase of the renal cortex in vitro. Also, the systemic infusion of dibutyryl cAMP in rats and dogs increases phosphate excretion similar to that produced by PTH (5). Furthermore, Agus et al (6) using micropuncture techniques found

that the administration of PTH or dibutyryl cyclic AMP reduced
the proximal tubular reabsorption of phosphorus, calcium and
sodium. All these observations are consistent with the notion that
at least the first step in some of the renal actions of PTH is
mediated through the activation of renal cortical adenylate cyclase.

Effects of PTH on Ca metabolism of renal cells have been
studied extensively by Borle (6). He has shown that PTH, but not
cAMP, stimulates Ca^{++} uptake by renal cell, and both PTH and cAMP
enhance the efflux of radiocalcium from renal cell prelabelled
with radiocalcium. Kinetic analysis of data indicates that PTH
increases Ca^{++} entry into cell probably by its direct action on
the plasma membrane and the cAMP formed intracellularly augments
the efflux of Ca^{++} from mitochondria into the cell cytosol. Thus,
the net effect of PTH is to increase cytosolic Ca^{++} level. This
effect of cAMP on the mitochondria membrane is of critical importance since the Ca^{++} flux across the mitochondrial membrane is one
order of magnitude greater than the Ca^{++} flux across the plasma
membrane on which PTH has a direct action. Thus, an increase
only in Ca^{++} influx across the plasma membrane by PTH could not
raise the cytosolic Ca^{++} concentration effectively, since Ca^{++}
entering the cell is immediately taken up and sequestered by
mitochondria.

Rasmussen and his colleagues (7-9) studied the effects of PTH
on renal cell metabolism both in vivo and in vitro. Their data
could be summarized as follows: 1) both PTH and cAMP induced a
Ca^{++}-dependent stimulation of renal gluconeogenesis in vitro, 2)
PTH stimulated cAMP production by renal cell both in the presence
and absence of Ca^{++} but, in the latter condition, there was no
associated enhancement of renal gluconeogenesis, 3) the in vitro
measurements of the metabolite profile and the rates of glucose
production by renal cortical tubules from several substrates demonstrates that either an increase in Ca^{++} concentration in the
incubation medium or the addition of PTH or cAMP to the medium
with a fixed Ca^{++} concentration enhances renal gluconeogenesis.
This occurs due to the activation of phosphoenolpyruvate carboxy-
kinase and the inhibition of pyruvate kinase both cytosolic enzymes, and the activation of α-ketoglutarate dehydrogenase, a
mitochondrial enzyme, 4) in the absence of Ca^{++}, PTH does not
cause a significant change in metabolite profile, despite a similar
rise in cell cAMP, and 5) an increase in phpsphate concentration
in the incubation medium suppresses renal gluconeogenesis despite
an increase in total calcium content of renal cell. These observations led these investigators to conclude that a rise in Ca^{++}
in cell cytosol is the major intracellular messenger for the PTH-
stimulated renal gluconeogenesis and the hormone induced alterations in renal intermediary metabolism. These interpretations
further supported by the work of Borle described above.

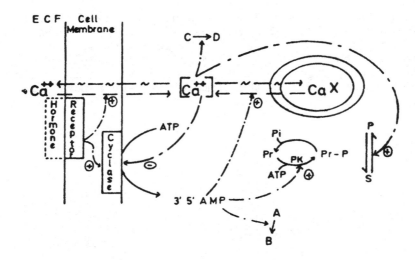

Fig. 1. Schematic model for the cellular mechanism of
         action of parathyroid hormone. See text for detail.
         The figure was reproduced from reference 10 with the
         permission of the authors and the publisher.

        Based on these observations, Rasmussen et al have proposed the
following scheme for the cellular mechanism of action of PTH (10,
Figure 1). The interaction of PTH with its receptor located in the
outside of plasma membrane leads to two simultaneous events, an activation of the membrane-bound adenylate cyclase and an increase in
calcium uptake. The rise in cell cAMP has at least two effects, an
activation of protein kinases leading to the phosphorylation of
specific proteins and an increase in calcium efflux from mitochondria.
The increase in Ca^{++} in cytosol activates Ca^{++}-dependent enzymes and
inhibits adenylate cyclase, the latter process being a negative feedback loop in these cellular events. Since the changes in Ca^{++} in
cytosol are of extreme importance for PTH action, factors which may
affect cAMP and Ca^{++} in cell cytosol would have significant effects
on cellular response to PTH. These include the concentration of
hydrogen ion and phosphorus (9).
        Further relationship between calcium, cAMP and PTH is illustra-
ted in Figure 2. This clearly indicates that an initial rise in
cell cAMP in response to PTH is not influenced by Ca^{++} concentration
in the incubation medium, while the changes in cell cAMP following
the initial burst seem dependent on Ca^{++}-concentration in the incubation medium. Moreover, the longer preincubation of renal tubule
cells in high Ca^{++} medium or in the Ca^{++}-free medium does not alter
the initial rises in cell cAMP in response to PTH (Figure 3). It
is likely that during the longer preincubation period the cell
cytosolic Ca^{++} would be maintained significantly higher in tubule

cells preincubated in the medium containing 2.0 mM calcium than those
in Ca^{++}-free medium (7). Thus, these data strongly suggest that the
inhibition of PTH-induced rises in cAMP is not simply due to a higher
cytosolic Ca^{++}, but due to some Ca^{++}-and PTH-dependent processes
occurring in the proximity of adenylate cyclase. Similar hormone-
induced unresponsiveness to the hormone has been reported in other
cell systems (11).

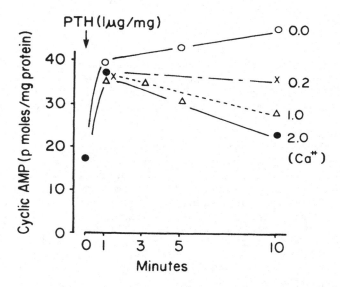

Fig. 2.   Effects of calcium concentration in the incubation
          medium on PTH-induced rises in renal tubular cyclic
          AMP. After 3 min preincubation in the medium with
          different calcium concentration (0, 0.2, 1.0 and
          2.0mM), PTH was added to the isolated renal cortical
          tubules. At 1,3,5 and 10 min after the hormone addi-
          tion the incubations were terminated and cyclic AMP
          contents (cell + medium) were measured.

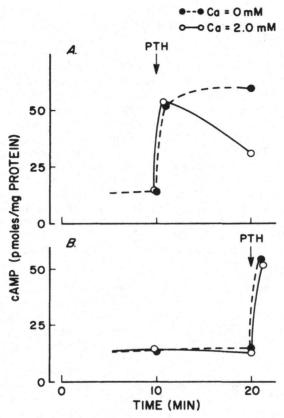

Fig. 3.   Changes in cell cyclic AMP in response to PTH after the
          longer preincubation of renal tubules in the presence
          and absence of 2.0 mM calcium in the incubation medium.
          See legend for Figure 2.

        Clues to the relative role of changes in cellular cAMP and Ca^{++}
as mediators of PTH actions may be obtained in several experimental
models. Firstly, it is of interest that both PTH and calcitonin,
physiologically antagonistic hormones, stimulate adenylate cyclase
activity and increase cyclic AMP levels of the kidney and bone (12-
14), and both increase urinary excretion of phosphorus which is pre-
ceded by a rise in renal tissue and urinary cyclic AMP (13).   However, these two hormones have opposite effects on some aspects of
renal cell metabolism. PTH stimulates and calcitonin inhibits the
conversion of $25(OH)D_3$ to $1,25(OH)_2D_3$ by the renal tubule cells (15).
Also, studies utilizing the in situ microfluorometric method to
evaluate the state of oxidation-reduction potential of the pyridine
nucleotide in the cortical tubules show a clear difference between

the effects of PTH and calcitonin (16); PTH or calcium infusion leads to the pyridine nucleotide potential to reduction, and the infusion of calcitonin or EGTA to oxidation. These results strongly suggest that PTH and calcitonin have opposing effects on Ca^{++} content of the renal tubule cells, with PTH increasing it while calcitonin decreasing it. It appears reasonable to speculate that the changes in cAMP in renal cells are responsible for the changes in renal transport mechanism induced by PTH and calcitonin, while the effects of PTH on some renal cell metabolism are mediated by the changes in the concentration of Ca^{++} within some subcellular compartments on which PTH and calcitonin may exert opposing effects (17).

Secondly, Kinne and his co-workers have demonstrated by separating the two different membranes of the tubular cells, i.e., the luminal and the anti-luminal membranes, that adenylate cyclase is localized almost exclusively in the anti-luminal or the basal-lateral membrane, and cAMP preferentially stimulates the phosphorylation of the luminal membrane (18,19). The demonstration of the direct effects of cAMP on luminal membrance strongly supports the important role of this nucleotide as a mediator of PTH-induced changes in renal transport mechanisms.

Thirdly, cholera toxin has been used extensively as a pharmacological tool to investigate the role of adenylate cyclase-cAMP system as a mediator of hormone action. This toxin has been shown to stimulate membrane-bound adenylate cyclase of almost all the tissues examined. The mode of stimulation of adenylate cyclase by this toxin seems quite different from that induced by other hormones in that a lag period of 15-60 minutes is necessary for the toxin to stimulate the enzyme. We have examined the effects of this toxin on the kidney (20,21). The toxin increases tubular cAMP levels in vitro after 30 minutes of latent period and this is due to an activation of adenylate cyclase. When the toxin is infused in one renal artery of thyroparathyroidectomized dogs there is an epilateral increase in urinary excretion of phosphorus, sodium, and other electrolytes 30-60 minutes after the initiation of the infusion. Furthermore, the assay of adenylate cyclase of cortex and outer medulla of the kidney at the height of renal effects of toxin revealed a marked enzyme activation in the infused side. These data again strongly support the notion that the stimulation of renal adenylate cyclase is accompanied by a change in urinary excretion of various electrolytes including phosphorus.

Finally, studies on patients with pseudohypoparathyroidism (PHP) provided us some valuable information on the mechanisms of PTH action on the kidney. Chase et al (22) have shown that, in contrast to the findings in normal and hypoparathyroid subjects, there is little rise in urinary cAMP and phosphorus excretion in PHP in response to intravenous PTH injection, suggesting a defective PTH-sensitive adenylate cyclase system. More recently, a subtype of PHP, Type II, has been proposed in which there is a normal rise in urinary cAMP with minimal phosphaturic response following PTH administration (23). In these patients some defects beyond the cAMP generation is speculated. A recent case of PHP, Type II, studied by Rodrigues et al (24) is of particular interest. They demonstrated that in a patient with PHP Type II the correction of hypocalcemia by rapid calcium infusion restored the full phosphaturic response to PTH, suggesting that normal plasma calcium concentration is crucial for the PTH-induced phosphaturia in this patient. It is not known how the rises in both cAMP and Ca^{++} were necessary for the full restoration of the phosphaturic response to PTH.

It is not known how cAMP and Ca^{++} regulate the cellular events responsible for the renal response to PTH. In this regard, of particular interest is the study by Heilmeyer et al (25). They have shown that, in the early sequence of events in muscle glycogenolysis, the activation of protein kinase stimulated by cAMP is followed by the activation of phosphorylase, the latter reaction being strikingly sensitive to Ca^{++} but minimally to cAMP. Thus, for the full cellular response to occur changes in both cAMP and Ca^{++} are of critical importance. It is probable that in the kidney similar metabolic sequence of events is also operative and the changes in both cAMP and Ca^{++} in a concerted manner are necessary for the PTH-induced renal cellular responses to occur.

ACKNOWLEDGEMENT

The author thanks Dr. Shaul G. Massry for his encouragement and critical reading of the manuscript.

REFERENCES

1. G.D. Aurbach and D.A. Heath: Parathyroid hormone and calci-
    tonin regulation of renal functions. Kidney Intl 6:331-345,
    1974.
2. S.G. Massry, J.W. Cobrun, R.M. Friedler, K. Kurokawa, and F.S.
    Singer: Relationship between the kidney and parathyroid
    hormone. Nephron 15:197-222, 1975.
3. L.R. Chase and G.D. Aurbach: Parathyroid function and the
    renal excretion of 3'5'-adenylic acid. Proc. Natl. Acad. Sci.
    USA 58:518-525, 1967.
4. L.R. Chase and G.D. Aurbach: Renal adenyl cyclase: Anatomi-
    cally separate sites for parathyroid hormone and vasopressin.
    Science 159:545-547, 1968.
5. H. Rasmussen, M. Pechet, and D. Fast: Effect of dibutyryl
    cyclic adenosine 3'5'-monophosphate, theophylline, and other
    nucleotide upon calcium and phosphate metabolism. J. Clin.
    Invest. 47:1843-1850, 1968.
6. A.B. Borle: Parathyroid hormone and cell calcium in Talmage
    and Munson, Calcium, Parathyroid Hormone, and the Calcitonin
    pp. 484-491, Excerpta Medica, Amsterdam, 1972.
7. N. Nagata and H. Rasmussen: Parathyroid hormone 3'5'-AMP,
    Ca^{++}, and renal gluconeogenesis. Proc. Natl. Acad. Sci. USA
    65:368-374, 1970.
8. H. Rasmussen and N. Nagata: Renal gluconeogenesis: Effects
    of parathyroid hormone and dibutyryl 3'5'-AMP. Biochem.
    Biophys. Acta 215:17-28, 1970.
9. K. Kurokawa and H. Rasmussen: Ionic control of renal gluco-
    neogenesis: IV. Effect of extracellular phosphate concentration.
    Biochem. Biophys. Acta 313:59-71, 1973.
10. H. Rasmussen and Ph. Bordier: The physiological and cellular
    basis of metabolic bone disease. Williams & Wilkins Co.,
    Baltimore, 1974.
11. J. Bockaert, M. Hunzicken-Dunn, I.L. Birnbaumer: Hormone-
    stimulated desentization of hormone dependent adenyl cyclase.
    J. Biol. Chem. 251:2653-2663, 1970.
12. F. Murad, H.B. Brewer, Jr., and M. Vaughan: Effect of thyro-
    calcitonin on adenosine 3',5'=cyclic phosphate formation by
    rat kidney and bone. Proc. Natl. Acad. Sci. USA 65:446-453,
    1970.
13. K. Kurokawa, N. Nagata, M. Sasaki, and K. Nakane: Effects of
    calcitonin on the concentration of cyclic adenosine 3',5'-
    monophosphate in rat kidney in vivo and in vitro. Endocrinology
    94:1514-1518, 1974.
14. N. Nagata, M. Sasaki, N. Kimura, and K. Nakane: Effects of
    porcine calcitonin on the metabolism of calcium and cyclic AMP
    in rat skeletal tissue in vivo. Endocrinology 97:527-535, 1975.

15. H. Rasmussen, M. Wong, D. Bickle, and D.B.P. Goodman: Hormonal control of the renal conversion of 25-hydroxycholecalciferol to 1,25-dihydroxycholecalciferol. J. Clin. Invest. 51:2502-2504, 1972.

16. S. Kimura, E. Ogata, S. Nishiki, S. Kobayashi, and Y. Yoshitoshi: Calcitonin, Ca^{++} and oxidation-reduction state of pyridine nucleotide in tubular cell. In Endocrinology 1973, eds. Taylor, Heineman, London 1974.

17. H. Rasmussen, P. Bordier, K. Kurokawa, N. Nagata, and E. Ogata: Hormonal control of skeletal and mineral homeostasis. Am. J. Med. 56:751-758, 1974.

18. L. Shlatz, I. Schwartz, E. Kinne-Saffran, and R. Kinne: Distribution of parathyroid hormone-stimulated adenylate cyclase in plasma membranes of the kidney cortex. J. Membrane Biol. 24:131-144, 1975.

19. R. Kinne, L. Shlatz, E. Kinne-Saffran, and I. Schwartz: Distribution of membrane-bound cyclic AMP-dependent protein kinase in plasma membranes of cells of the kidney cortex. J. Membrane Biol. 24:145-159, 1975.

20. R.M. Friedler, K. Kurokawa, J.W. Coburn, and S.G. Massry: Renal actions of cholera toxin. I. Effects on urinary excretion of electrolytes and cyclic AMP. Kidney Intl 7:77-85, 1975.

21. K. Kurokawa, R.M. Friedler, and S.G. Massry: Renal action of cholera toxin. V. Effects on adenylate cyclase-cyclic AMP system. Kidney Intl 7:137-144, 1975.

22. L.R. Chase, G.L. Nelson, and G.D. Aurbach: Pseudohypoparathyroidism: Efective excretion of 3',5'-AMP in response to parathyroid hormone. J. Clin. Invest. 48:1832-1844, 1969.

23. M. Drezner, F.A. Nelson, and H.E. Lebovitz: Pseudohypoparathyroidism Type V: A possible defect in the receptor of the cyclic AMP signal. N. Engl. J. Med. 289:1056-1060, 1973.

24. H.J. Rodrigues, H. Villarreal, Jr., S. Klahr, and E. Slatopolsky: Pseudohypoparathyroidism Type II: Restoration of normal renal responsiveness to parathyroid hormone by calcium administration. J. Clin. Endocrinol. Metab. 39:693-701, 1974.

25. L.M.G. Heilmeyer, Jr., F. Meyer, R.H. Haschke, and E.H. Fischer: Control of phosphorylase activity in a muscle glycogen particle. II. Activation by calcium. J. Biol. Chem. 245:6649-6656, 1970.

METABOLIC ACIDOSIS IN HYPERPARATHYROIDISM

ROLE OF PHOSPHATE DEPLETION AND OTHER FACTORS

Shaul G. Massry

University of Southern California School of Medicine

2025 Zonal Avenue, Los Angeles, California

Patients with primary or secondary hyperparathyroidism may display abnormalities in acid-base homeostasis and in renal handling of bicarbonate. Many investigators have observed mild acidosis, low levels of serum bicarbonate and impaired urinary acidification in patients with primary hyperparathyroidism (1-6) and in those with osteomalacia or malabsorption and secondary hyperparathyroidism (7-10). Successful treatment of the state of hyperparathyroidism is usually associated with reversal of these abnormalities. On the other hand, elevated levels of serum bicarbonate were noted in patients with hypercalcemia which was not due to excess parathyroid hormone and in patients with hypoparathyroidism (2,11-14). Also, Barzel reported that mild metabolic alkalosis may be present in patients with parathyroid hormone deficiency (13, 14).

The presence of hyperchloremic acidosis in patients with parathyroid adenoma is not an all or none phenomenon. We noticed this abnormality in 11 of 44 patients with parathyroid adenoma. In a recent study of 57 patients with primary hyperparathyroidism, Mallete et al (4) found that 24% had blood bicarbonate levels less than 24 mEq/l, and serum chloride level was above 107 mEq/l in 48% of the patients. In contrast, only one out of 13 patients with parathyroid adenoma reported by Coe had hyperchloremic acidosis (15). This patient has also very high blood levels of immunoreactive parathyroid hormone. Another patient had metabolic acidosis which could be attributed to reduced renal function. The reasons for these variations in the incidence of hyperchloremic acidosis in patients with hyperparathyroidism are not clear. The understanding of the mechanism(s) of the metabolic acidosis in such patients may provide an explanation for these variations.

It is theoretically possible that the abnormalities in acid-base homeostasis in patients with primary hyperparathyroidism are due to a direct effect of parathyroid hormone or are the results of some of the metabolic consequences of excess parathyroid hormone (hypercalcemia or hypophosphatemia and/or phosphate depletion), or both.

Muldowney et al, found that correction of the state of hyperparathyroidism abolished the renal bicarbonate wasting and ameliorated the metabolic acidosis (9,16). They postulated that parathyroid hormone directly inhibits the renal reabsorption of bicarbonate resulting in metabolic acidosis. Support for this hypothesis is found in the experimental observations that the acute administration of parathyroid extract produces a rise in urinary pH and an increase in urinary excretion of bicarbonate (17-20). Karlinsky et al (21), found that Tm bicarbonate is elevated in thyroparathyroidectomized dogs; the infusion of purified parathyroid hormone (60 units/hr) to these animals caused a fall in Tm bicarbonate from 30-32 to 24 mEq/l GFR but did not affect Tm bicarbonate in animals with intact parathyroid glands. These authors concluded that parathyroid hormone may have a major regulatory role over renal bicarbonate reabsorption, but excess hormone may not depress bicarbonate reabsorption to a level low enough to result in metabolic acidosis. In contrast, Crumb et al (22) were able to demonstrate a modest, but significant, fall in Tm bicarbonate during the infusion of a large amount of purified parathyroid hormone (300 units/hr) in dogs with intact parathyroid glands. These observations are consistent with the notion that very high blood levels of parathyroid hormone can suppress renal bicarbonate reabsorption. These authors also found that hypercalcemia, per se, can enhance tubular reabsorption of bicarbonate.

Since hypophosphatemia and phosphate depletion may occur in hyperparathyroidism, Gold, Massry, Arieff and Coburn postulated that phosphate depletion, per se, may be responsible for the abnormal renal handling of bicarbonate (23) in hyperparathyroidism. They found that phosphate depletion in dogs is associated with 1) a fall in blood levels of bicarbonate with a direct relationship between the levels of blood bicarbonate and phosphate, 2) a reduced renal threshold at which bicarbonate appeared in the urine and a reduced Tm for bicarbonate reabsorption (Figure 1), and 3) a rise in intracellular pH (Figure 2). These studies demonstrate that phosphate depleted dogs displayed abnormalities in both serum bicarbonate and in its renal handling which are similar to those seen in hyperparathyroidism. Since during phosphate depletion the parathyroid glands are hypoactive (24), any abnormality in bicarbonate reabsorption noted in the phosphate-depleted dogs could not be attributed to excess parathyroid hormone. These studies, therefore, support the concept that alterations in bicarbonate homeostasis in patients with hyperparathyroidism may be due, at least partly, to phosphate depletion. The latter could alter cell metabolism, resulting in reduced intracellular H^+ concentration, which may then impair H$^+$ secretion by the renal tubules and decrease their ability to reabsorb bicarbonate. Consequently, Tm bicarbonate and serum bicarbonate fall.

Micropuncture studies demonstrated an inverse linear relationship between serum levels of phosphate and the tubular fluid bicarbonate concentration both in intact and thyroparathyroidectomized dogs (25). These data support the results of Gold et al (23) and indicate that extracellular fluid phosphate concentration is an important modulator of proximal bicarbonate transport independent of the action of parathyroid hormone.

A possible explanation for the rise in the intracellular pH during phosphate depletion could be provided by considering the

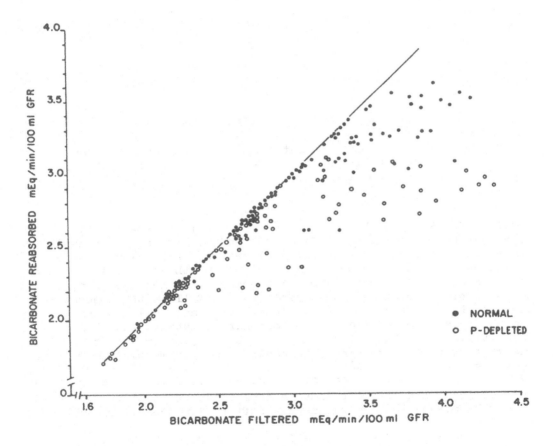

Fig 1. The relationship between the quantity of bicarbonate reabsorbed and that filtered for all clearance periods during bicarbonate infusion both before (●) and after (0) phosphate depletion.

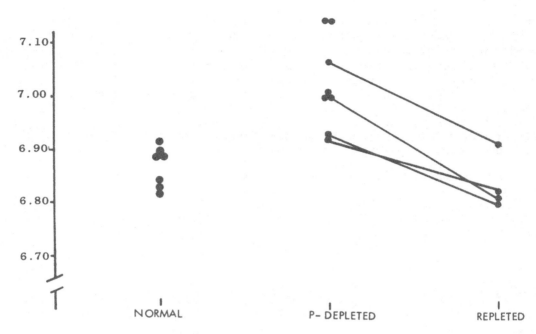

Fig 2. The effect of phosphate depletion and repletion on
        intracellular pH. The lines connect values obtained
        in the same animals.

model of Kurokawa and Rasmussen (26) for the interrelationship
between the concentration of Ca^{2+}, H^+, and HPO_4^{2-} in extracellular
space, cell cytosol and mitochondrial matrix. According to this
model, changes in the concentration of any of these ions in any one
compartment would be associated with changes in the other compartments. Thus, during phosphate depletion, a fall in the concentration of HPO_4^{2-} occurs in extracellular space and cell cytosol.
Phosphate is released from the mitochondrial matrix, and this pro-
cess utilizes H^+ (Ca_3 $(PO_4)_2$ + $2H^+$ → 3 Ca^{2+} + $2HPO_4^{2-}$). The H^+ is
supplied by the cytosol and mitochondrial compartments. In mild or
short-term phosphate depletion, the fall in cytosol H^+ may be adequately buffered with no change in intracellular pH. However, with
long standing and severe phosphate depletion, the fall in cytosol
H^+ may be marked and not adequately buffered; hence, intracellular
pH rises.

Figure 3 provides a scheme for the pathways through which
parathyroid hormone may affect renal bicarbonate handling and for
the possible interactions between parathyroid hormone, body stores
of phosphate, and hypercalcemia on renal tubular bicarbonate reabsorption in patients with primary hyperparathyroidism.

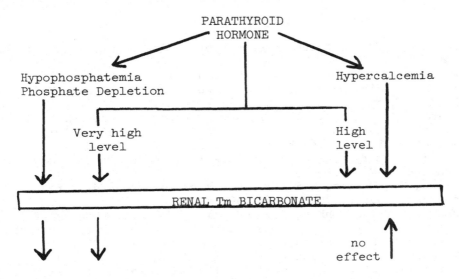

Fig 3. Pathways through which parathyroid hormone may affect
        renal handling of bicarbonate in patients with primary
        hyperparathyroidism.

It appears that a reduction in bicarbonate reabsorption in
patients with hyperparathyroidism may be due to a direct action of
parathyroid hormone on the renal tubule and/or to phosphate depletion which develops secondary to the sustained phosphaturic action
of excess parathyroid hormone. On the other hand, the hypercalcemia
in these patients may counteract the effect of parathyroid hormone
or phosphate depletion on bicarbonate reabsorption. The net effect
on the acid-base status of the patient will depend on the interaction
between these factors. Therefore, variations in the duration and
degree of elevated blood levels of parathyroid hormone, the magnitude of hypercalcemia, and the severity and duration of phosphate
depletion in patients with hyperparathyroidism may explain the
variations in the incidence of metabolic acidosis in these patients.
     Other factors may contribute to the metabolic acidosis in
patients with secondary hyperparathyroidism who are often hypocalcemic and may have vitamin D deficiency. Reports in this Workshop
(Peraino et al and Siegfried et al) indicated that Tm bicarbonate is
reduced by hypocalcemia, and vitamin D deficiency, per se, may be
associated with renal bicarbonate wasting. Thus, in patients
with secondary hyperparathyroidism, there may be four abnormalities
(excess parathyroid hormone, hypophosphatemia and/or phosphate
depletion, hypocalcemia, and vitamin D deficiency) responsible for
renal bicarbonate losses and, consequently, for the metabolic
acidosis.

REFERENCES

1. Lafferty, F.W.: Pseudohyperparathyroidism. Medicine, 45:247, 1965.
2. Wills, M.R., McGowan, G.K.: Plasma chloride levels in hyperparathyroidism and other hypercalcemia states. Brit. Med. J. 1:1153, 1964.
3. Dolman, M., Barzel, U.: Primary hyperparathyroidism: Diagnosis and treatment. New York State J. Med. 71:1201, 1971.
4. Mallette, L.E., Bilezikian, J.P., Heath, D.A., and Aurbach, G.D.: Primary hyperparathyroidism: Clinical and biochemical features. Medicine, 53:127, 1974.
5. Wrong, O., Davies, H.E.F.: The excretion of acid in renal disease. Quart. J. Med. 28:259, 1959.
6. Fourman, P., McConkey, B., and Smith, J.W.G.: Defects of water reabsorption and of hydrogen-ion excretion by the renal tubules in hyperparathyroidism. Lancet 1:619, 1960.
7. Muldowney, F.P., Freaney, R., and McGreeney, D.: Renal tubular acidosis and amino-aciduria in osteomalacia of dietary and intestinal origin. Quart. J. Med. 37:517, 1968.
8. York, S.E., and Yendt, E.R.: Osteomalacia associated with renal bicarbonate loss. Cand. Med. Assoc. J. 94:1329, 1966.
9. Muldowney, F.P., Freaney, R., and Brennan, F.: A case of osteomalacia in renal tubular acidosis associated with occult idiopathic steatorrhea: The effect of vitamin D on renal tubular hydrogen ion transport. Irish H. Med. Sci. 6:435, 1965.
10. Muldowney, F.P., Donohoe, J.F., Freaney, R., Kampff, C., and Swan, M.: Parathormone-induced renal bicarbonate wastage in intestinal malabsorption and in chronic renal failure. Irish J. Med. Sci. 3:221, 1970.
11. Thomas, W.C., Jr., Connor, T.B., and Morgan, G.: Some observations on patients with hypercalcemia examplifying problems in differential diagnosis, especially in hyperparathyroidism. J. Lab. Clin. Med. 52:11, 1958.
12. Heinemann, H.O.: Metabolic alkalosis in patients with hypercalcemia. Metabolism 14:1137, 1967.
13. Barzel, U.S.: Systemic alkalosis in hypoparathyroidism. J. Clin. Endocrinol. Metab. 29:17, 1969.
14. Barzel, U.S.: Parathyroid hormone, blood phosphorus, and acid-base metabolism. Lancet 1:1329, 1971.
15. Coe, F.L.: Magnitude of metabolic acidosis in primary hyperparathyroidism. Arch. Inter. Med. 134:262, 1974.
16. Muldowney, F.P., Carroll, D.V., Donohoe, J.F., and Freaney, R.: Correction of renal bicarbonate wasting by parathyroidectomy. Quart. J. Med. 40:487, 1971.
17. Ellsworth, R., Nicholson, W.M.: Further observations upon changes in the electrolytes of urine following the injection of parathyroid extract. J. Clin. Invest. 14:823, 1955.

18. Kleeman, C.R., and Cooke, R.R.E.: The acute effects of parathyroid hormone on the metabolism of endogenous phosphate. J. Lab. Clin. Med. 38:112, 1951.

19. Nordin, B.E.C.: The effect of intravenous parathyroid extract on urinary pH, bicarbonate and electrolyte excretion. Clin. Sci. 19:311, 1960.

20. Hellman, D.E., Au, W.Y.W., and Bartter, F.C.: Evidence for a direct effect of parathyroid hormone on urinary acidification. Amer. J. Physiol. 209:643, 1965.

21. Karlinsky, M.L., Sager, D.S., Kurtzman, N.A., and Pillay, V.K.: Effect of parathormone and cyclic adenosine monophosphate on renal bicarbonate reabsorption. Amer. J. Physiol. 227:1226, 1974.

22. Crumb, C.K., Martinez-Maldonado, M., Eknoyan, G., and Suki, W.N.: Effects of volume expansion, purified parathyroid extract, and calcium on renal bicarbonate absorption in the dog. J. Clin. Invest. 54:1287, 1974.

23. Gold, L.W., Massry, S.G., Arieff, A.I., and Coburn, J.W.: Renal bicarbonate wasting during phosphate depletion. A possible cause of altered acid-base homeostasis in hyperparathyroidism. J. Clin. Invest. 52:2556, 1973.

24. Stoerk, H.C., and Carnes, W.H.: The relation of the dietary Ca: P ratio to serum calcium and to parathyroid volume. J. Nutr. 29:43, 1945.

25. Puschett, J.B., and Fernandez, P.C.: Relationship between serum phosphate concentration and proximal tubular bicarbonate transport. Nephron, 1977 (in press).

26. Kurokawa, K., and Rasmussen, H.: Ionic control of renal gluconeogenesis: The interrelated effect of calcium and hydrogen ions. Biochem. Biophys. Acta. 313:17, 1973.

IDIOPATHIC HYPERCALCIURIA

Charles Y.C. Pak

The University of Texas Health Science Center at Dallas, Southwestern Medical School, Department of Internal Medicine, 5323 Harry Hines Blvd., Dallas, Texas, 75235

The term idiopathic hypercalciuria was originally used to describe the condition, characterized by hypercalciuria, normocalcemia and recurrent calcium (Ca) nephrolithiasis, for which no clear-cut etiology for the hypercalciuria could be found.[1] It is now recognized that this condition comprises a mixed group consisting of separate entities. Two subtypes,- renal hypercalciuria (RH) and absorptive hypercalciuria (AH), have now been well-characterized, depending on whether the hypercalciuria is the consequence of an impaired renal tubular reabsorption of Ca^2 or the intestinal hyperabsorption of Ca.[3,4] The objective of this discussion is to review diagnostic criteria, causes for the hypercalciuria and therapeutic considerations in renal and absorptive hypercalciurias.

DIAGNOSTIC CRITERIA

The RH and AH share common features of normocalcemia, hypercalciuria and passage of Ca-containing renal stones. However, the two conditions may be differentiated from each other from fasting urinary Ca and parathyroid function.

After an overnight fast, fasting urinary Ca is invariably increased (> 0.11 mg/mg urinary creatinine (Cr)) in RH, whereas, it is typically normal in AH (Fig. 1).[5] High values may sometimes be encountered in some patients with AH, if they were not prepared adequately on a low Ca diet prior to the test. Our preliminary studies indicate that "preparation" of patients by treatment with oral cellulose phosphate for 1-2 days prior to the collection of fasting urine sample provides improved discrimination between the two groups (Fig. 2). Whereas the "renal leak" of Ca persists in

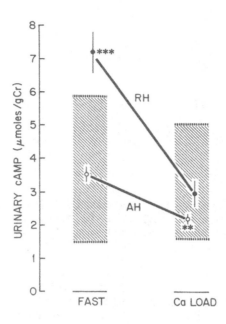

Figure 1. Fasting urinary Ca in renal hypercalciuria (RH) and absorptive hypercalciuria (AH). Shaded area indicates the range of values in control group. Significance from values in control groups is indicated by *** for p < 0.001. Results, following an oral load of 1 g Ca, are also shown.

RH during treatment, the high renal excretion of Ca resulting from inadequate dietary preparation in AH may be overcome. The results support the hypothesis that there is inadequate renal conservation of Ca in RH, not in AH.

Parathyroid function, as measured by circulating immunoreactive parathyroid hormone (PTH) or urinary cyclic AMP (cAMP), was stimulated in RH and normal or suppressed in AH.[5] During fasting state (after an overnight fast), the urinary cAMP was significantly elevated in RH, unlike in AH (Fig. 3). Following an oral load of 1 g Ca, urinary cAMP decreased to the normal range in RH. It was significantly below normal in AH. The findings suggest that parathyroid function is stimulated probably secondary to the "renal leak" of Ca in RH, whereas, it may be partially suppressed from the intestinal hyperabsorption of Ca in AH.

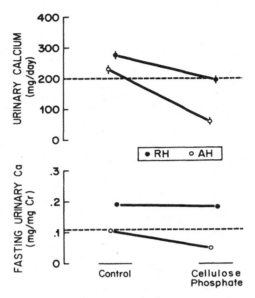

Figure 2. The effect of sodium cellulose phosphate on 24-hour urinary Ca and on fasting urinary Ca. A patient with RH and another
with AH were maintained for 5 days on a constant diet which contained 400 mg Ca/day; during last 2 days they were given sodium
cellulose phsophate, 5 gm three times each day with meals. In the
patient with RH, the inhibition of intestinal Ca absorption by
treatment did not lower 24-hour urinary Ca below 100 mg or the
fasting urinary Ca below 0.11 mg/mg Cr. In the patient with AH,
sodium cellulose phosphate lowered urinary Ca to less than 100 mg/
day and converted borderline fasting urinary Ca to normal. The
horizontal dashed lines indicate upper range of normal values.

MECHANISM OF INTESTINAL HYPERABSORPTION OF CA

The intestinal absorption of Ca is frequently increased in
RH and invariably so in AH.[4,6] Because of the well-known action
of vitamin D in stimulating intestinal Ca transport, vitamin D
metabolism was examined in hypercalciurias.

In states of hyperparathyroidism (RH and primary hyperparathyroidism), the circulating concentration of $1\alpha,25-(OH)_2$-vitamin
D was significantly increased and was positively correlated with
intestinal Ca absorption.[7] In RH, treatment with thiazide restored
intestinal Ca absorption towards normal, commensurate with the correction of renal leak of Ca and secondary hyperparathyroidism.[8]
Thus, the intestinal hyperabsorption of Ca in RH may be the consequence of PTH-mediated stimulation of $1\alpha,25-(OH)_2$-vitamin D synthesis.

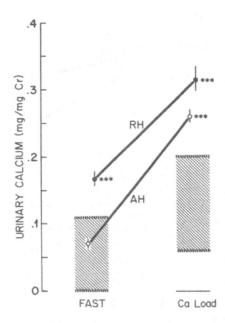

Figure 3. Urinary cyclic AMP during fast and following an oral load of 1 g Ca. The shaded area indicates the range of values in the control group. The significance from control group is given by ** for p < 0.01 and *** for p < 0.001.

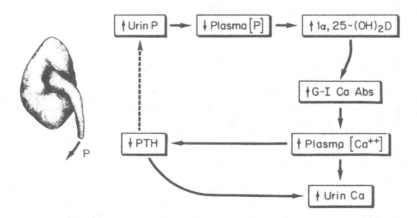

Figure 4. Scheme for hypophosphatemic absorptive hypercalciuria.

	Absorptive Hypercalciuria	Control Group
Serum P, mg %	3.73 ± .60	3.74 ± .70
Urin. P, mg/day	741 ± 159	698 ± 153
P Clearance, ml/min	13.8 ± 3.7	13.0 ± 5.7

Figure 5.   Serum P, urinary P and P clearance in AH and Control Group.   Studies were performed on a constant dietary regimen which contained daily 400 mg Ca and 800 mg P.   P clearance was obtained from 24-hour urinary P and the value for serum P obtained before breakfast during fasting state.   Values are presented as mean ± SD.

In contrast, the circulating concentration of the vitamin D metabolite was not correlated with intestinal Ca absorption in AH.[9] Although it was increased in 1/3 of patients, it was within the normal range in remaining two-thirds.   Thus, intestinal Ca absorption was inappropriately high in the majority of patients with AH.   Selected patients with AH were given Prednisone, 50 mg daily for 8 days.   The intestinal hyperabsorption of Ca persisted,[9] unlike in Sarcoidosis and vitamin D toxicity in which it was ameliorated.

Two other studies do not support an important role of vitamin D in the pathogenesis of AH.   Unlike in RH, thiazide did not significantly lower intestinal Ca absorption even though it corrected the hypercalciuria.[8]   Intestinal Ca perfusion by triple-lumen technique disclosed accelerated Ca transport in the jejunum, and normal absorption in the ileum.[10]   In contrast, 1α-OH-vitamin D has been shown to stimulate Ca absorption in both intestinal segments.[11]   The primary defect in AH may therefore be a selective jejunal hyperabsorption of Ca, which is mediated independently of vitamin D or PTH.

It has been postulated that the primary abnormality in AH is the impaired renal tubular reabsorption of P.[12]   The consequent hypophosphatemia stimulates the renal synthesis of $1\alpha,25-(OH)_2$-vitamin D and accounts for the intestinal hyperabsorption of Ca and hypercalciuria (Fig. 4).   Unfortunately, this hypothesis does not seem tenable in the majority of cases of AH.   In most cases of AH examined under a controlled regimen, serum P, urinary P and P clearance were normal (Fig. 5).   In one patient, persistently low serum P (< 2 mg/dl) and high P clearance (> 20 ml/min) were found in the setting of intestinal hyperabsorption of Ca and suppressed parathyroid function.   Treatment with orthophosphate (1.5 g P/day) increased serum P to 2.3 mg/dl.   However, in this patient as well

	Fractional Ca Absorption
Before	0.637 ± 0.016
Orthophosphate	0.640 ± 0.030

Figure 6. The effect of orthophosphate on fractional Ca absorption in AH. Orthophosphate was given orally at a dosage of 1.5 g P/day to four patients with AH. The fractional Ca absorption was measured before and after 1 month of treatment; it was obtained from the recovery of ^{47}Ca radioactivity in the feces following an oral administration of the isotope. After an overnight fast, the isotope was given in a 100 mg Ca load.

as in other patients with AH and normophosphatemia, the intestinal Ca absorption did not decline (Fig. 6). Thus, the postulated hypothesis for the hypophosphatemic AH, involving increased synthesis of $1\alpha,25$-$(OH)_2$-vitamin D, does not seem likely in this patient, although it is theoretically possible.

THERAPEUTIC CONSIDERATIONS

The delineation of causes for the hypercalciuria permits development of a rational mode of therapy, in which the treatment is directed at correcting the underlying cause for the hypercalciuria.[6] Thus, the optimum treatment for RH is the thiazide diuretic, which has been shown to restore the renal leak of Ca;[2] that for AH is sodium cellulose phosphate, which inhibits intestinal Ca absorption.[13] Furthermore, recent progress in the physical chemistry of stone formation permits quantitation of response to treatment.[14] These advances have allowed an appreciation of indications and mechanisms of action,-both physiological and physicochemical, for three drugs commonly used for RH and AH.

The thiazide diuretic possesses the unique property of augmenting renal tubular reabsorption of Ca.[15] In patients with RH, it has been shown to reduce urinary Ca and intestinal Ca absorption and to ameliorate secondary hyperparathyroidism.[2] During treatment, urine specimens usually become less saturated with respect to brushite $(CaHPO_4 \cdot 2H_2O)$[16] and Ca oxalate,[17] principally because of the fall in Ca content. Concurrently, the limit of metastability (formation product ratio) for both brushite[16] and Ca oxalate[17] often increases; thus, greater degree of supersaturation is required before spontaneous nucleation ensues. This action of the drug probably reflects increased renal excretion of certain inhibitors

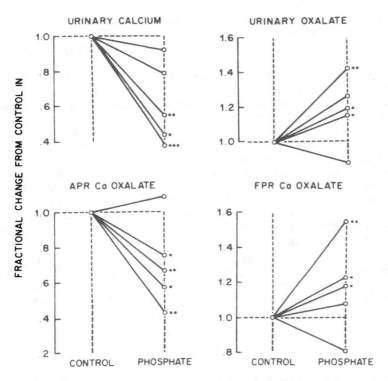

Figure 7. The effect of orthophosphate (1.5 g P/day orally) on urinary Ca, oxalate, activity product ratio (APR) and formation product
ratio (FPR) of Ca oxalate. For each patient, the effect of treatment
is expressed as the fractional change of values during treatment from
corresponding values during control period. The significance of
values are given by * for p < 0.05, ** for p < 0.01 and *** for p <
0.001.

of calcification, such as pyrophosphate[16] and zinc.[18]

Sodium cellulose phosphate is a non-absorbable ion-exchange
resin with a high affinity for Ca^{++}.[19] When appropriate amounts
of the drug are given to patients with AH (5 g two-3 times daily
on a Ca-restricted diet), excessive intestinal absorption and
renal excretion of Ca may be corrected, without adversely affecting parathyroid function and Ca metabolism.[13] Its principal
physicochemical effect is the reduction in the urinary state of
saturation with respect to brushite[19] and Ca oxalate,[20] which
occurs probably because of the fall in urinary Ca. The effect on
the state of saturation with respect to Ca oxalate is less pronounced because of the increased renal oxalate excretion.[20] Since

sodium cellulose phosphate probably does not alter renal excretion of inhibitors (pyrophosphate, citrate, zinc), it does not modify limit of metastability or the rate of crystal growth.

Orthophosphates (salts of sodium and/or potassium) are soluble and potentially absorbable following oral administration. When compared to sodium cellulose phosphate (of equivalent P content), orthophosphates cause a greater increase in urinary P and less pronounced decrease in urinary Ca.[21] Their effect on urinary oxalate is less consistent. As a result of these changes, urine specimens become more supersaturated with respect to brushite, and usually less saturated with respect to Ca oxalate (Fig. 7). Furthermore, orthophosphates promote renal excretion of pyrophosphate, an inhibitor of calcification.[22] Partly as a reflection of this response, the urinary formation product ratios of brushite and Ca oxalate are usually increased. Favorable clinical response may be accounted for by the decreased urinary state of saturation with respect to Ca oxalate and the requirement for increased supersaturation before spontaneous precipitation of brushite and Ca oxalate. However, the exact mechanism for the fall in urinary Ca is not clear, and the potential for soft-tissue calcification and parathyroid stimulation remains unresolved.

REFERENCES

1. Henneman, P.H., Benedict, P.H., Forbes, A.P., and Dudley, H.R.: Idiopathic hypercalciuria. New Engl. J. Med. 259:802, 1958.
2. Coe, F.L., Canterbury, J.M., Firpo, J.J., and Reiss, E.: Evidence for secondary hyperparathyroidism in idiopathic hypercalciuria. J. Clin. Invest. 52:134, 1973.
3. Nordin, B.E.C., Peacock, M., and Wilkinson, R.: Hypercalciuria and calcium stone disease. Clinics in Endocrinol. Metab. 1:169, 1972.
4. Pak, C.Y.C., Ohata, M., Lawrence, E.C., and Snyder, W.: The hypercalciurias: causes, parathyroid functions and diagnostic criteria. J. Clin. Invest. 52:387, 1974.
5. Pak, C.Y.C., Kaplan, R.A., Townsend, J., and Waters, O.: A simple test for the diagnosis of absorptive, resorptive, and renal hypercalciurias. New Engl. J. Med. 292:497, 1975.
6. Pak, C.Y.C., Barilla, D., Bone, H., and Northcutt, C.: Medical management of renal calculi. Presented at the symposium Advances in Endocrinology and Metabolism, Hahnemann Medical College and Hospital of Philadelphia, Philadelphia, Pennsylvania. February 24, 1976. In press.
7. Haussler, M.R., Bursac, K.M., Bone, H., and Pak, C.Y.C.: Increased circulating $1\alpha,25$-dihydroxyvitamin D_3 in patients with primary hyperparathyroidism. Clin. Res. 23:322A, 1975.

8. Barilla, D.E., Tolentino, R., Kaplan, R.A., and Pak, C.Y.C.: Selective effects of hydrochlorothiazide on the intestinal absorption of calcium in absorptive and renal hypercalciurias. Submitted for publication.

9. Kaplan, R.A., Haussler, M.R., and Pak, C.Y.C.: The role of 1α, 25-hydroxycholecalciferol in the mediation of intestinal hyperabsorption of calcium in primary hyperparathyroidism and hypercalciuria. Submitted for publication.

10. Fordtran, J.S., and Pak, C.Y.C.: Preliminary observations.

11. Vergne-Marini, P., Parker, T.F., Pak, C.Y.C., Hull, A.R., DeLuca, H.F., and Fordtran, J.S.: Jejunal and ileal calcium absorption in patients with chronic renal disease. Effect of 1α-hydroxycholecalciferol. J. Clin. Invest. 57:861, 1976.

12. Shen, F., Baylink, D., Nielson, R., Hughes, M., and Haussler, M.: Increased serum 1,25-dihydroxycholecalciferol (1,25-diOHD$_3$) in patients with idiopathic hypercalciuria (IH). Clin. Res. 23:423A, 1975.

13. Pak, C.Y.C., Delea, C.S., and Bartter, F.C.: Successful treatment of recurrent nephrolithiasis (calcium stones) with cellulose phosphate. New Engl. J. Med. 290:175, 1974.

14. Pak, C.Y.C.: Physicochemical and clinical aspects of nephrolithiasis. Symposium of International Colloquium on Renal Lithiasis. Univeristy of Florida, Gainesville, Fla. 1974. In press.

15. Brickman, A.S., Massry, S.G., and Coburn, J.W.: Changes in serum and urinary calcium during treatment with hydrochlorothiazide: studies on mechanisms. J. Clin. Invest. 51:945, 1972.

16. Pak, C.Y.C.: Hydrochlorothiazide therapy in nephrolithiasis: effect on urinary activity product and formation product of brushite. Clin. Pharm. Therap. 14:209, 1973.

17. Woelfel, A., and Pak, C.Y.C.: Effect of hydrochlorothiazide on the crystallization of calcium oxalate in urine. Submitted for publication.

18. Pak, C.Y.C., Ruskin, B., and Diller, E.: Enhancement of renal excretion of zinc by hydrochlorothiazide. Clin. Chim. Acta 39: 511, 1972.

19. Pak, C.Y.C.: Sodium cellulose phosphate: mechanism of action and effect on mineral metabolism. J. Clin. Pharm. New Drug 13:15, 1973.

20. Hayashi, Y., Kaplan, R.A., and Pak, C.Y.C.: Effect of sodium cellulose phosphate therapy on crystallization of calcium oxalate in urine. Metabolism 24:1273, 1975.

21. Pak, C.Y.C.: Effects of cellulose phosphate and of sodium phosphate on the formation product and activity product of brushite in urine. Metabolism 21:447, 1972.

22. Fleisch, H., and Bisaz, S.: Isolation from urine of pyrophosphate, a calcification inhibitor. Amer. J. Physiol. 203:671. 1962.

IS THERE A BONE-KIDNEY LINK IN THE HOMEOSTASIS OF INORGANIC PHOSPHATE (Pi)?

J.-P. Bonjour, U. Tröhler, R. Mühlbauer,
C. Preston and H. Fleisch
Department of Pathophysiology, University of
Berne, Murtenstrasse 35, 3010 Berne, Switzerland

The kidney responds to variations in the supply of inorganic phosphate (Pi) by changing its tubular capacity to transport Pi (1,2,3). This change represents very likely a homeostatic response which tends to adjust the rate of Pi excretion according to the needs of the organism. It would be logical to envisage that, according to this concept, variations in the needs of Pi should also lead to a homeostatic adjustment in the rate of tubular Pi transport. In the growing animals a large portion of the ingested Pi is taken up by the skeleton for mineralization. A decrease in the capacity of the bone to retain calcium and phosphate therefore should elicit a change in the renal handling of Pi similar to that promoted by an increment in the dietary Pi supply.

To test this hypothesis we have used as a tool the diphosphonate, disodium ethane-1-hydroxy-1,1-diphosphonate (EHDP). In vitro EHDP is a potent inhibitor of calcium phosphate precipitation (4,5). In vivo, in the growing rat, EHDP brings about a marked inhibition of bone mineralization when given at the dose of 10 mg P/kg per day (6,7). In the present experiments EHDP was given at this dose for 7 days to rats pair-fed either low (0.2 g %) or high (1.2 g %) Pi diet. In both diets the calcium content was 1.0 g %. After 5 days of treatment animals were thyroparathyroidectomized (TPTX). 2 days later the fractional excretion of Pi (FEPi) was measured over a wide range of plasma Pi ($[Pi]Pl.$).

The capacity of excretion as expressed by the function
relating [Pi]Pl to FEPi was enhanced by EHDP and dietary Pi. In fact, it appears that administering EHDP
in doses which block bone mineralization brings about
the same change in the renal handling of Pi than raising
the phosphorus content of the diet from 0.2 to 1.2 g %.
The increase in FEPi observed under EHDP was not associated with a change in cAMP excretion. It is probably
not due to inhibition of 1,25-dihydroxyvitamin D_3 (1,25-
$(OH)_2D_3$) production occurring at this dose of EHDP,
since it was not corrected by administration of 1,25-
$(OH)_2D_3$. Indeed 2 x 13 pmoles/day i.p. 1,25-$(OH)_2D_3$,
which is the dose which exerts a preventive effect on
the EHDP-induced reduction in intestinal calcium absorption (8), enhanced on the contrary significantly FEPi in
EHDP-treated rats fed a 0.2 g % Pi diet but not when the
animals are fed a 1.2 g % Pi diet. Interestingly this
dose of 1,25-$(OH)_2D_3$ also increased the FEPi of the non
EHDP-treated rats, bringing it back to that of non TPTX
animals. The metabolite furthermore restored the capability of the rats for adapting to variations of dietary
Pi to that of sham-operated animals. This would indicate
that 1,25-$(OH)_2D_3$ might play an important role in the
regulation of Pi excretion.

Free-flow micropunctures made at similar filtered load
of Pi in TPTX rats indicate that EHDP treatment affects
Pi transport mainly in the early proximal tubule and
apparently along the terminal nephron. This localization corresponds to that previously reported for the effect of dietary Pi (9). It differs from that described
for thyroparathyroidectomy which would affect the Pi
transport along the second portion of the proximal convoluted tubule (10). This difference in localization
along the proximal tubule could explain why we have observed that in TPTX rats, either increasing the dietary
Pi or treatment with EHDP enhanced the acute phosphaturic response to PTH even when measured at similar [Pi]Pl
and filtered load of Pi. By acting more proximally dietary Pi and EHDP could increase the delivery of Pi to
the site where PTH exerts its action.

In conclusion, blockage of bone mineralization by trea-
ting rats with large doses of EHDP (10 mg P/kg s.c. for
7 days) is associated with a change in the tubular capacity to transport Pi. This change could represent a
homeostatic response determined by the reduced capacity

of bone to retain Pi with respect to the dietary supply
of Pi. If so, it would imply the existence of a bone-
kidney link in the homeostasis of inorganic phosphate
similar to the bone-gut link postulated by Nicolaysen
(11) in the regulation of calcium metabolism.

Acknowledgements

This work has been supported by the Swiss National
Foundation for Scientific Research (3.121.73) and by
the Procter and Gamble Company, USA.

References

1. Tröhler, U., Bonjour, J.-P., and Fleisch, H.: In-
    organic phosphate homeostasis. Renal adaptation to
    the dietary intake in intact and thyroparathyroid-
    ectomized rats. J.Clin.Invest. 57: 264, 1976.

2. Steele, T.H., and DeLuca, H.F.: Influence of die-
    tary phosphorus on renal phosphate reabsorption in
    the parathyroidectomized rat. J.Clin.Invest. 57:
    867, 1976.

3. Tröhler, U., Bonjour, J.-P., and Fleisch, H.: Renal
    tubular adaptation to dietary phosphorus. Nature
    261: 145, 1976.

4. Francis, M.D., Russell, R.G.G., and Fleisch, H.:
    Diphosphonates inhibit formation of calcium phos-
    phate crystals in vitro and pathological calcifica-
    tion in vivo. Science 165: 1264, 1969.

5. Fleisch, H., Russell, R.G.G., Bisaz, S., Mühlbauer,
    R.C., and Williams, D.A.: The inhibitory effect of
    phosphonates on the formation of calcium phosphate
    crystals in vitro and on aortic and kidney calcifi-
    cation in vivo. Europ.J.Clin.Invest. 1: 12, 1970.

6. Schenk, R., Merz, W.A., Mühlbauer, R., Russell,
    R.G.G., and Fleisch, H.: Effect of ethane-1-hydroxy-
    1,1-diphosphonate (EHDP) and dichloromethylene di-
    phosphonate (Cl_2MDP) on the calcification and re-
    sorption of cartilage and bone in the tibial epi-
    physis and metaphysis of rats. Calc.Tiss.Res. 11:

196, 1973.

7.   Gasser, A.B., Morgan, D.B., Fleisch, H.A.,and Ri-
     chelle, L.J.: The influence of two diphosphonates
     on calcium metabolism in the rat. Clin.Sci. 43:
     31, 1972.

8.   Bonjour, J.-P., Trechsel, U., Fleisch, H., Schenk,
     R., DeLuca, H.F., and Baxter, L.A.: Action of 1,25-
     dihydroxyvitamin D_3 and a diphosphonate on calcium
     metabolism in rats. Am.J.Physiol. 229: 402, 1975.

9.   Tröhler, U., Mühlbauer, R., Bonjour, J.-P., and
     Fleisch, H.: Parathyroid hormone-independent regu-
     lation of the renal handling of inorganic phosphate
     (Pi) in the rat. Kidney Intern. 7: 367, 1975.

10. Amiel, C., Kuntziger, H., and Richet, G.: Micro-
     puncture study of handling of phosphate by proximal
     and distal nephron in normal and parathyroidecto-
     mized rat. Evidence for distal reabsorption.
     Pflügers Archiv: Europ.J.Physiol. 317: 93, 1970.

11. Nicolaysen, R.: The absorption of calcium as a func-
     tion of the body saturation of calcium. Acta Phy-
     siol.Scand. 5: 200, 1943.

EFFECT OF VITAMIN D$_3$ AND 1,25-DIHYDROXYVITAMIN D$_3$ ON INTESTINAL TRANSPORT OF PHOSPHATE

Meinrad Peterlik and Robert H. Wasserman

Department of Physical Biology, Cornell University

Ithaca, New York 14853, USA

Vitamin D plays an important role in the regulation of phosphate (P$_i$) metabolism. The fact that vitamin D exerts parallel effects on calcium and phosphate in its main target organs (intestine, bone and kidney) has created some difficulty in separating the effects of the vitamin on the cellular transport of these ions. There is now increasing evidence that vitamin D stimulates a phosphate transport mechanism in intestine quite independent of the calcium transport system (1,2). Two facts have eased the recognition of the unique effect of vitamin D on intestinal phosphate absorption. First, maximal stimulation of phosphate absorption occurs in the jejunum (3,4) while the duodenum is known as site of the maximal response of calcium absorption to vitamin D. Second, higher rates of transmural phosphate transport can be maintained in the virtual absence of extracellular calcium, i.e. phosphate does not require a simultaneous movement of calcium in order to be transported across the gut wall (1,2). In contrast to earlier reports that P$_i$ is transferred across the intestine along its electrochemical gradient (5) and that vitamin D enhances the passive permeability of P$_i$ (3), there is also evidence for the involvement of a vitamin D-sensitive active transport mechanism in the transintestinal movement of phosphate (1,2,4). However, at present no sufficient data are available on the kinetics of unidirectional phosphate fluxes across the luminal and serosal border of the intestine, and the site and nature of the vitamin D interaction with one or more of these reactions has not yet been established.

The everted gut sac technique seemed most suitable for the investigation of individual pathways of phosphate transfer in the intestine. Previous experiments had established that vitamin D

323

is capable of stimulating transmural phosphate transport in all
parts of the small intestine of the chick, but the jejunum showed
the highest increment in vitamin D-induced phosphate transport (2).
Therefore, this segment was exclusively used in the present study.
Everted gut sacs were derived from rachitic chicks which had been
raised on a vitamin D-deficient diet (-D) for 4 wk, or from vitamin
D-repleted animals (+D). Vitamin D repletion was achieved by intra-
muscular injection of 500 I.U. vitamin D_3 in 0.2 ml propylenglycol
48 hr before sacrifice. In some experiments the birds received
various doses of the active metabolite of vitamin D, 1,25-dihydroxy-
vitamin D_3, in 1.0 ml propylenglycol by gastric gavage. Incubation
of the everted sacs was in Krebs-Henseleit bicarbonate buffer at
32°C. $^{32}PO_4^{3-}$ was added either to the mucosal or to the serosal
incubation buffer for determination of P_i tracer fluxes.

CHARACTERIZATION OF THE PHOSPHATE TRANSPORT SYSTEM IN JEJUNUM

For the characterization of transmural phosphate transport in
everted sacs the initial concentration was 1.2 mM phosphate on both
sides of the gut and changes in luminal and serosal phosphate were
determined at various time intervals. The most obvious effect of
vitamin D repletion is the induction of phosphate net transfer
from the luminal side into the serosal compartment giving rise to
a pronounced asymmetrical distribution of P_i across the gut wall.
This concentrative transfer of phosphate in vitamin D-repleted
chicks is characterized by serosal/mucosal concentration ratios of
5.4 $\pm$ 0.7 (n = 20) vs. 1.5 $\pm$ 0.1 in the vitamin D-deficient group
(P <0.001). A detailed analysis of phosphate transfer across the
everted chick jejunum is shown in Fig. 1.

An almost constant net uptake of P_i from the mucosal solution
is observed in +D guts while -D segments show a slight secretion
of phosphate into the lumen. The difference in net movement can
be attributed to the approximately two-fold stimulation by vitamin
D of P_i entry into the tissue compartment. Phosphate influx rose
from an average of 0.21 $\pm$ 0.03 µmol/g per min in the vitamin D-
deficient group to 0.43 $\pm$ 0.02 µmol/g per min (n = 11, P <0.001)
after repletion with vitamin D_3. Vitamin D caused a reversal of
P_i net secretion into net uptake. Phosphate release (not shown)
was constant through 30 min and similar flux rates were calculated
for the -D (0.23 $\pm$ 0.02) and the +D group (0.18 $\pm$ 0.02 µmol/g
per min).

Net phosphate change in the serosal compartment could be
separated into two distinct phases. As indicated by the absence
of any radioactivity from the mucosal side, the first rapid increase of serosal P_i was caused by the efflux from the pool of
(stable) intracellular phosphate. This movement which is clearly

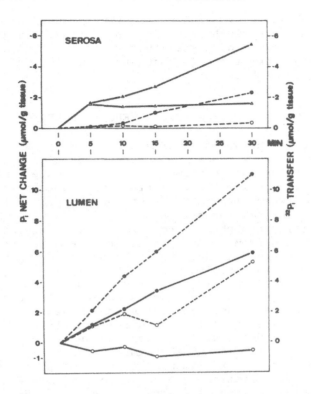

Fig. 1: Time course of mucosa-to-serosa phosphate transfer. Each point is an average from at least 6 determinations. Negative sign denotes out-of-tissue movement into serosal or mucosal volume. ●, ▲; +D chicks: o, △; -D. Solid lines: net P_i changes. Dashed lines: transfer of mucosal phosphate labelled with $^{32}P_i$.

insensitive to vitamin D was followed by a parallel increase of total and radiolabeled mucosal phosphate in the +D group. Only a slight rise in total P_i due to the migration of luminal P_i across the gut wall is observed in -D guts. There is an obvious lag time of about 7 to 10 min before phosphate originating from the lumen is released into the serosal space. Vitamin D stimulates this process by raising the rate from 0.015 ± 0.003 in the rachitic state to 0.103 ± 0.023 μmol/g per min (n = 13, P <0.001). Doubling the uptake of P_i from the lumen is certainly a reason for the higher accumulation of luminal phosphate in the serosal compartment observed in +D everted sacs, but cannot totally explain the above mentioned fivefold rate increase of phosphate discharge from intestinal tissue into the serosal extracellular space. It seems that in the vitamin D-deficient state, despite the relatively high rate of P_i entry at the luminal surface, only small amounts of mucosal phosphate are discharged into the serosal compartment. Therefore, it cannot be dismissed that vitamin D also influences the intracellular migration of phosphate to achieve an efficient lumen-to-serosa translocation.

PHOSPHATE FLUXES ACROSS SEROSAL BORDER

Also there is the question of whether the uptake process from the lumen in vitamin D-induced phosphate absorption or a stimulation of serosal P_i efflux is the primary event. In an effort to solve these questions, experimental conditions were sought which might differentiate between vitamin D effects on phosphate fluxes across the mucosal and serosal border of the gut. This was achieved by raising the initial phosphate concentration in the serosal buffer to 3.0 mM. Results from incubation under anaerobic conditions (not shown) had suggested that the early phase of the serosa directed vitamin D-insensitive efflux (Fig. 1) is by diffusion alone. Thus, it was expected that this net phosphate movement could be counteracted by raising the extracellular concentration and thereby reducing the outward concentration gradient. Fig. 2 shows that everted sacs when filled with buffer containing 3.0 mM P_i maintain this initial concentration in the serosal volume. No significant difference between +D and -D segments was detected. The mucosal buffer in these experiments was free of phosphate to minimize a possible contribution of mucosal to serosal P_i transfer to the serosal concentrations. Phosphate exchange under these "near equilibrium" conditions was measured from the disappearance of $^{32}P_i$ from the serosal solution. No influence of vitamin D became apparent on phosphate fluxes across the serosal border of the gut (Fig. 2). Identical rates of serosal P_i exchange were calculated for both the +D (0.046 $\pm$ 0.005) and the -D (0.047 $\pm$ 0.004 µmol/g per min) groups.

VITAMIN D EFFECT ON MUCOSAL PHOSPHATE FLUXES

Since luminal phosphate does not enter the serosal space within about 10 min and during this time any phosphate net transfer from intracellular sources into the serosal compartment can be counteracted by high extracellular phosphate, it seems possible to determine phosphate movements across the luminal surface without a major interference from out-of-tissue movements in the serosa direction. An incubation period of 10 min and an initial serosal concentration of 3.0 mM therefore were adopted as standard procedure for the determination of phosphate fluxes across the mucosal border and the vitamin D effect thereon.

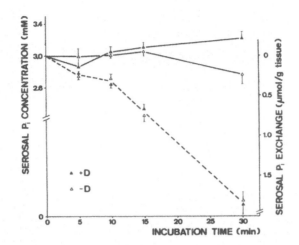

Fig. 2: Phosphate uptake across serosal border. Solid line: serosal P$_i$ concentration. Dashed line: 32-P$_i$ accumulation in tissue. Each point is an average from at least 6 determinations. S.E. is indicated by vertical bars. No significant differences between +D and -D values.

Phosphate influx into the epithelial cell layer determined from ^{32}P$_i$ tracer flux displayed a non-linear dependence on the initial P$_i$ concentration in the mucosal bathing solution in both the +D and the -D groups (Fig. 3). The nature of the vitamin D effect on this saturable entry of P$_i$ into the intestinal tissue became obvious when the kinetic constants were calculated from linearized plots (see insert in Fig. 3). Vitamin D exerts its effect on phosphate uptake by raising the maximal velocity (V$_{max}$) from 0.127 in the vitamin D-deficient state to 0.323 µmol/g tissue per min, but did not affect the affinity of the carrier for phosphate since K$_m$ is 0.2 mM with and without treatment with vitamin D.

Phosphate fluxes across the mucosal border were also measured under anaerobic conditions (Table 1). Incubation under nitrogen depressed the rate of P$_i$ entry significantly in both the vitamin D-deficient and the vitamin D-repleted state. On the other hand, phosphate release into the luminal solution was greatly enhanced during respiratory inhibition. This would force the conclusion that influx is by active transport while intracellular phosphate is transferred "downhill" into the lumen.

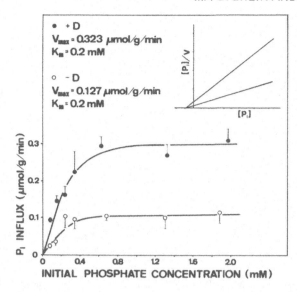

Fig. 3: Concentration dependence of mucosal P_i influx. Insert:
Linearized plot of uptake kinetics (initial P_i concentration).
Each point is an average from at least 6 determinations. S.E.
given by vertical bars.

CONCLUSIONS ON TRANSMURAL PHOSPHATE TRANSPORT

The experiments described in the preceding sections attempted
to separate basal and vitamin D-induced transmural phosphate transport into unidirectional fluxes across the mucosal and serosal
border of the everted jejunum. Notwithstanding a possible effect
of vitamin D on the intracellular compartmentalization of phosphate,
it is evident that the site of vitamin D interaction with intestinal
phosphate absorption is the mucosal surface. The primary event in
the stimulation of the absorptive process is an enhancement of P_i
entry into the epithelial cell layer. This pathway is carrier-
mediated and depends on respiratory energy and might therefore constitute an active transport mechanism. Movement of P_i in the
opposite direction is mainly diffusion controlled and not sensitive
to vitamin D. This excludes the possibility that vitamin D increases net absorption from the lumen by restricting phosphate
efflux. Diffusion of intracellular phosphate into the serosal
compartment is not controlled by vitamin D, neither is the re-
uptake from this extracellular space. Under standard experimental
conditions, the rate of P_i exchange across the serosal border is

Table 1:   Influence of respiratory inhibition on mucosal phosphate
fluxes.

Group	Influx[a]		Efflux[a]	
	O_2	N_2	O_2	N_2
+D	0.269 $\pm$0.030	0.183[b] $\pm$0.012	0.187 $\pm$0.019	0.418[c] $\pm$0.068
−D	0.109 $\pm$0.015	0.043[c] $\pm$0.007	0.251 $\pm$0.016	0.397[d] $\pm$0.030

[a]
   Flux rates are expressed as µmol P_i/g tissue per min.
   Means $\pm$ S.E. from 12 to 18 determinations.

[b-d]
   Significantly different from controls (O_2).
   b) P <0.025,   c) P <0.005, d) P <0.001.

considerably lower than the entry rates of phosphate at the mucosal
surface. Hence it is possible that the rate-limiting step in the
transintestinal movement of inorganic phosphate is located at the
serosal border of the gut.

REGULATION OF INTESTINAL PHOSPHATE ABSORPTION BY VITAMIN D

Prior to exertion of its biological function, vitamin D_3 is
metabolized in two subsequent hydroxylation steps to its active
metabolite, 1,25-dihydroxyvitamin D_3 (1,25-$(OH)_2D_3$) (6). Experiments were carried out to investigate a possible role of this
vitamin D metabolite in the regulation of intestinal phosphate
absorption. Mucosal P_i influx was measured under experimental
conditions which are known to modulate the metabolism of vitamin D.
The results are depicted in Fig. 4. Chicks on a normal diet with
an adequate intake of vitamin D_3 (20 I.U./day) showed a moderate
rate of P_i influx which was clearly above rachitic levels but, on
the other hand, also less than maximal stimulation. The latter is
exemplified by administration of a single dose of 500 I.U. vitamin
D_3 to rachitic chicks. Like intestinal calcium absorption, the
phosphate absorptive process undergoes adaptation to restriction
of dietary calcium or phosphorus. Chicks on a diet either low in
calcium or low in phosphorus but with otherwise adequate supply of
vitamin D_3 display elevated rates of phosphate influx (significantly

different from normal control values at P <0.001). There is evidence that both conditions influence the vitamin D-dependent regulation of calcium and phosphate metabolism by their stimulatory
effect on the kidney production of 1,25-(OH)$_2$D$_3$ (7). Further
support for the involvement of 1,25-(OH)$_2$D$_3$ in the regulation of
intestinal phosphate absorption comes from experiments where the
production of this sterol was blocked by high dietary strontium (8).
P$_i$ entry into everted guts derived from chicks on this experimental
diet was reduced when compared to normal controls (P <0.001) but
still significantly higher than in rachitic animals (P <0.025).
Strontium inhibition of phosphate influx is slightly but not significantly ameliorated by 500 I.U. vitamin D$_3$. A complete reversal
is achieved by administration of 1,25-(OH)$_2$D$_3$ to strontium-fed
chicks. Delivered in 6 single doses of 0.5 µg/chick at 12 hr intervals, 1,25-(OH)$_2$D$_3$ stimulates phosphate influx to maximal levels
(Fig. 4).

     The effect of 1,25-(OH)$_2$D$_3$ on intestinal phosphate absorption
was evaluated more directly by administration of the pure substance
to vitamin D-deficient chicks. After a single oral dose of 0.5 to
1.6 µg of 1,25-(OH)$_2$D$_3$, stimulation of phosphate influx was occasionally observed 4 hr later. More consistent responses were
achieved either with a high single dose (1.5 µg) after 9 hr, or
with multiple doses (three times 1.0 µg at 6 hr intervals) 18 hr
after administration of the first dose (Table 2). The induction of
phosphate transport by 1,25-(OH)$_2$D$_3$ was prevented, when doses of
50 µg/chick of cycloheximide were given at 6 hr intervals, starting

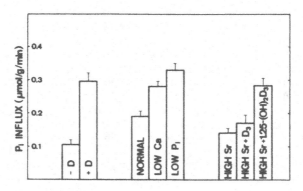

Fig. 4: Regulation of mucosal P$_i$ entry by dietary variations. For
experimental details see text. Data are given as means from 12 to
24 determinations ± S.E.

Table 2:   Enhancement of mucosal phosphate influx by 1,25-
           dihydroxyvitamin D_3 and effect of cycloheximide.

1,25-$(OH)_2D_3$	None		1 x 1.5 µg		3 x 1.0 µg	
Cycloheximide	0	+	0	+	0	+
P_i influx[a]	0.037 $\pm$0.011	0.045 $\pm$0.011	0.121[b] $\pm$0.011	0.044 $\pm$0.007	0.134[b] $\pm$0.019	0.071 $\pm$0.013

[a] Flux rates are expressed as µmol P_i/g tissue per min. Means from 12 determinations $\pm$ S.E.

[b] Significantly different from rachitic control (no 1,25-$(OH)_2D_3$) and from cycloheximide treated group, $P < 0.001$.

6 hr before the first dosage with 1,25-$(OH)_2D_3$. Cycloheximide had no influence on the non-stimulated phosphate influx (Table 2). These data indicate that a protein synthetic step is required for the full expression of the effect of 1,25-$(OH)_2D_3$ on intestinal phosphate absorption.

SUMMATION

Dietary variations (low calcium, low phosphorus, or high strontium) change phosphate transport by the jejunum according to their respective ability to increase or block the synthesis of 1,25-dihydroxyvitamin D_3, suggesting that the action of this active sterol underlies the response of intestinal phosphate absorption to vitamin D. 1,25-$(OH)_2D_3$ stimulates the active entry of P_i at the mucosal border by its action on protein synthesis. It is attractive to speculate that 1,25-$(OH)_2D_3$ might induce the synthesis of a "phosphate carrier" protein in the plasma membrane. The interpretation that the enhancement of the maximal velocity of the "phosphate pump" by vitamin D is due to the creation of new pump sites would be consistent with this hypothesis.

These investigations were supported by NIH grant AM-04652 and by Max Kade Fellowship (M.P.).

REFERENCES

1. Taylor, A. N.: In Vitro Phosphate Transport in Chick Ileum: Effect of Cholecalciferol, Sodium and Metabolic Inhibitors. J. Nutr. 104: 489, 1974.

2. Peterlik, M., and Wasserman, R. H.: Effect of Vitamin D on Transepithelial Phosphate Transport in Chick Intestine. Manuscript in preparation.

3. Hurwitz, S., and Bar, A.: Site of Vitamin D Action in Chick Intestine. Am. J. Physiol. 222: 761, 1972.

4. Wasserman, R. H., and Taylor, A. N.: Intestinal Absorption of Phosphate in the Chick: Effect of Vitamin D_3 and Other Parameters. J. Nutr. 103: 586, 1973.

5. MacHardy, G. J. R., and Parsons, D. S.: The absorption of inorganic phosphate from the small intestine of the rat. Quart. J. Exp. Physiol. 41: 398, 1956.

6. Fraser, D. R., and Kodicek, E.: Unique Biosynthesis by Kidney of a Biologically Active Vitamin D Metabolite. Nature 228: 764, 1970.

7. Hughes, M. R., Brumbaugh, P. F., Haussler, M. R., Wegedal, J. E., and Baylink, D. J.: Regulation of Serum 1α,25-Dihydroxyvitamin D_3 by Calcium and Phosphate in the Rat. Science 190: 578, 1975.

8. Omdahl, J. L., and DeLuca, H. F.: Rachitogenic Activity of Dietary Strontium. J. Biol. Chem. 247: 5520, 1972.

SODIUM-DEPENDENT TRANSPORT OF ORTHOPHOSPHATE IN NERVE FIBRES

R.W.Straub, J.Ferrero, P.Jirounek, M.Rouiller, A.Salamin

Département de Pharmacologie, Ecole de Médecine

CH - 1211 Genève 4 (Suisse)

The mechanism by which orthophosphate is concentrated in cells against an electrochemical concentration gradient has so far not been studied in detail. At first sight, such studies appear difficult and laborious, since transmembrane fluxes of phosphate are small (1) and since phosphate is involved in numerous metabolic reactions. An indication that a Na-dependent mechanism might be involved comes from experiments of Chambers (2) who observed that the uptake of labelled phosphate in sea urchin eggs is decreased when the Na of the seawater is replaced by other cations. Later, Harrison and Harrison (3) observed a similar effect of Na on phosphate transport in rat intestine. At that time, however, little was known on Na-dependent transport processes so that these authors did not study the effect of Na in more detail.

A few years ago, Anner, Ferrero, Jirounek and Straub (4) showed in mammalian nerve fibres that the uptake of radiophosphate is almost abolished when the extracellular Na is replaced by choline. A similar effect was found in fish nerve (5) and P.C. Caldwell (personal communication) found a Na dependence of phosphate influx in squid giant axons. Recently, Na-dependent phosphate fluxes have been described in the convoluted tubules of rat kidney (Baumann, de Rouffignac, Roinel, Rumrich and Ullrich, 6), in isolated brush border vesicles (Hoffmann, Thees and Kinne, 7), and Brown and Lamb (8) observed a Na-dependent influx and efflux of phosphate in cultured tumor cells. There is thus little doubt that Na-dependent phosphate transport is a fairly wide-spread phenomenon.

The present paper describes this transport system in more detail. For the experiments described here, small non-myelinated nerve fibres were used. These fibres have a mean diameter of about 0.7 μ (9) and therefore a large surface to volume ratio. They are thus particularly well suited for studying small transmembrane fluxes.

METHODS

The methods used have been described in detail (10,11,12). In brief, vagus nerves of rabbits were desheathed to allow easy access of ions to the nerve fibres. The preparations were then mounted in a polyethylene tube, where they were continuously perfused with either Locke or modified Locke. For measurements of the influx tracer amounts of ^{32}P were added to the perfusion fluid and the total radioactivity of the preparation and the surrounding fluid recorded. The rate of uptake of radiophosphate could easily be measured from these records.

For measurements of the efflux, the preparations were first loaded with radiophosphate as in the influx experiments. Afterwards, they were washed with tracer-free solutions and the effluent of the apparatus collected and counted. At the end of the experiment the preparations were removed, weighed, dissolved and their content in radiophosphate measured.

In addition, in both influx and efflux experiments, the labelling of several compounds of the nerve was studied at various times. Preparations were therefore removed after a brief wash with phosphate-free solution, weighed and then plunged in boiling triethanolamine buffer, rapidly cooled and homogenized. Chloroform was added, and after centrifugation, the phase containing the hydrosoluble compounds was separated from the chloroform fraction. The hydrosoluble compounds were further separated by chromatography; after elution, the amount of ATP, ADP, CrP and P_i and their radioactivity were measured. These compounds accounted for over 90% of the radioactivity of the hydrosoluble fraction. The radioactivity of the chloroform fraction, which contained several phosphoproteins and phospholipids, was also measured. In some experiments the efflux of ^{22}Na was studied, using the procedure described for the phosphate efflux. All experiments were done at 37°C; unless otherwise stated, the pH of the solutions was 7.40. Throughout this paper, the terms phosphate or P_i are used as synonyms for orthophosphate.

RESULTS

Influx

Fig. 1 shows the measurement of the phosphate influx. At the beginning of the experiment the preparation was perfused with Locke; radiophosphate labelled Locke was then applied. As shown, the recorded radioactivity then increased rapidly while the tube and the extracellular space were being filled by the labelled solution. Afterwards the increase in recorded radioactivity was slower. As discussed elsewhere (10), this phase corresponds to the influx of radiophosphate into the fibres. The slow increase in radioactivity was almost linear with time during the first 60 min. The initial rate of uptake could therefore be estimated. At 0.2 mM external phosphate, the uptake was around 3-4 μ-moles/kg wet nerve per min, which corresponds, with the dimensions of the axons given by Keynes and Ritchie (9) to an influx of 3 f-moles/cm^2 per sec (10). Phosphate fluxes are thus much smaller than the fluxes of K and Na. When the influx of P_i was measured at different extracellular phosphate concentrations, the upper curve of Fig. 2 was obtained. The curve shows a tendency to saturation with increasing phosphate concentrations.

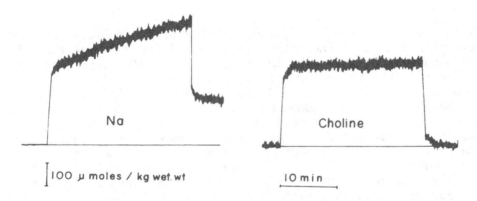

Fig. 1. Uptake of radiophosphate in Locke and choline-Locke. Radioactivity of preparation and surrounding fluid was recorded during perfusion with tracer-free solutions (base-line), after application of labelled solution (fast upstroke and slow increase in radioactivity) and finally again during perfusion in tracer-free solution (fast downstroke and slow loss of radioactivity). Fast changes were caused by filling or emptying of tube and extracellular space by the labelled solutions; slow increase in recorded radioactivity by influx of radiophosphate into the nerve fibres. External phosphate 0.2 mM.

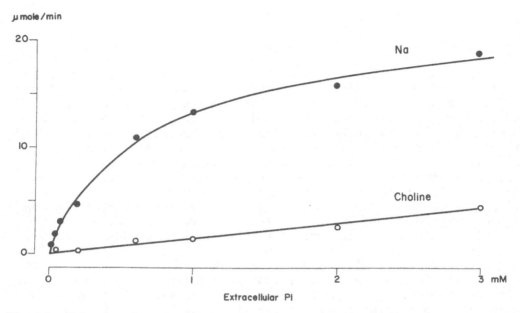

Fig. 2. Relation between extracellular phosphate concentration and phosphate influx in presence or absence of extracellular Na.

Measurements of the specific activities of the nucleotides, CrP and P_i extracted after incubation in labelled Locke showed that these compounds were slowly labelled (Fig. 3). The slow labelling seems to be due to slow influx and not to slow metabolism. Thus the rate constant of the influx, obtained from the measured influx and the total phosphate of these compounds is 0.001 min^{-1}. On the other hand, the rate constant of metabolic turnover of phosphate is about 0.2 min^{-1}, as calculated from the oxygen consumption of this preparation (13) and the total hydrosoluble phosphate. Compared to the rate constant of the influx, the turnover of phosphate of the hydrosoluble fraction is thus at least 100 times faster. After the first hour of incubation, little (about 10%) of the extracted radioactivity was found in the non-hydrosoluble fraction, which for these measurements can therefore be neglected.

When the influx experiments were repeated with Na-free Locke, the rate of uptake of radiophosphate was much slower (Fig. 1) than in Locke. The slowing was reversible; upon reintroduction of Na the rate of uptake recovered to the rate before the application of Na-free Locke, or even to a higher rate (12). If the rate of uptake

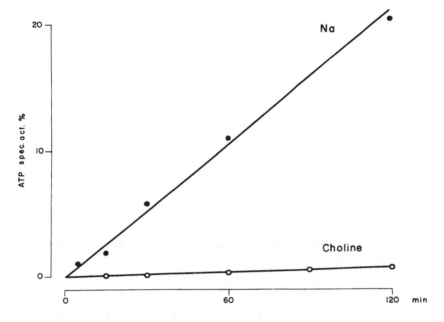

Fig. 3. Specific activity of ATP extracted during incubation in Lo-cke (Na) and choline-Locke (choline), given as percentage of spe-cific activity of extracellular phosphate. External phosphate 0.2 mM.

in Locke is taken as unity, the uptake was 0.1 when Na was replaced by choline or Tris, 0.2 in K-Locke and 0.5 in Li-Locke, at 0.2 mM external phosphate (12).

The influx in choline-Locke at different phosphate concentra-tions was always smaller than the influx in Locke (Fig. 2). Further-more, in choline-Locke the phosphate influx was approximately pro-portional to the phosphate concentration. The Na-dependent influx, given by the difference between uptake in Locke and uptake in cho-line-Locke, shows saturation kinetics with an apparent K_m of about 0.4 mM (12). In choline-Locke the labelling of extracted hydrosolu-ble compounds was also slowed (Fig. 3); the rate of labelling was decreased by about the same amount as the rate of uptake.

Fig. 4 shows the results of experiments in which the uptake was measured at different Na concentrations. The relation between Na-dependent phosphate uptake and the Na concentration of the solution shows a tendency to saturation with an apparent K_m of approximately 20 mM, at 0.2 mM external phosphate. The determination of the rela-tion between extracellular Na and phosphate influx is however rather

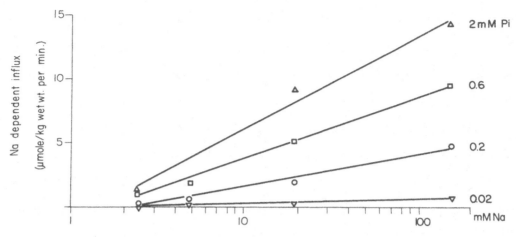

Fig. 4. Na-dependent phosphate influx at different extracellular Na concentrations. Note that Na concentrations are given on logarithmic scale. pH 8.4.

difficult, because the gradient between extracellular and intracellular Na changes rapidly. Thus in experiments, in which the efflux of ^{22}Na was measured, the rate constant of Na efflux was 0.047 min^{-1} in Locke and 0.03 min^{-1} in choline-Locke.

The phosphate influx does not seem directly to depend on the working of the Na-K-pump : inhibition of the pump by ouabain produced only a slow and small effect (14).

Efflux

When preparations that had been loaded with radiophosphate were washed with inactive Locke, it was found that the efflux of radiophosphate first decreased rapidly and then more slowly. The rate coefficient of the efflux calculated on the basis of the total counts in the preparation did not give a constant value (Fig. 5). This appears to be due to the fact that a fraction of the radiophosphate taken up by the preparation is slowly incorporated in phospholipids and phosphoproteins from where it is hardly released during the relatively short washout experiments (15). If the rate coefficient is calculated on the basis of the counts found in the hydrosoluble fraction alone, a coefficient is obtained that remains fairly constant during an experiment (Fig. 5). In the following,

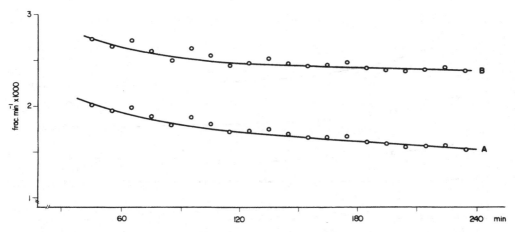

Fig. 5.Rate coefficient of phosphate efflux. For curve A, rate coefficient was calculated by dividing counts in effluent by total
radioactivity of preparation, curve B by dividing counts in effluent
by radioactivity of hydrosoluble extract of preparation.

this rate constant will be used. Moreover, the calculation of a rate constant on the basis of the hydrosoluble compounds is justified
by the fact that the rate of efflux is much smaller than the rate of
turnover.

The rate of efflux in Locke was found to depend on extracellular phosphate : an increase in phosphate caused an increase in efflux (Fig. 6). The rate constants of influx and efflux are about
equal at an extracellular phosphate concentration of 0.6 mM, which
is near the phosphate concentration of extracellular fluids in the
body, e.g. thoracic lymph contains about 1 mM phosphate and cerebro-
spinal fluid 0.6 mM (16).

The efflux measured 60 min after application of choline-Locke
was much slower than in Locke. A slow efflux was found for all phosphate concentrations tested. The slow efflux in Na-free solution
does not appear to be caused by the lack of Na in extracellular
medium; the immediate effect of application of choline-Locke was a
transient increase in efflux and a shorter transient increase was
also seen in Tris and Li-Locke. Comparison with the efflux of ^{22}Na
showed that the slowing of the efflux occured when the intracellular
Na was low.

The effect of external phosphate on phosphate efflux shown in

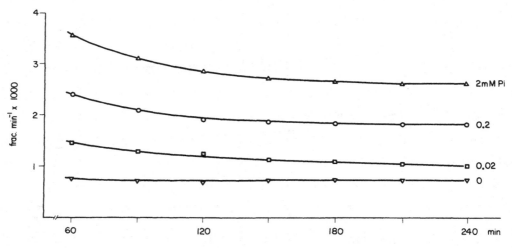

Fig. 6. Rate constant of phosphate efflux at different extracellular phosphate concentrations.

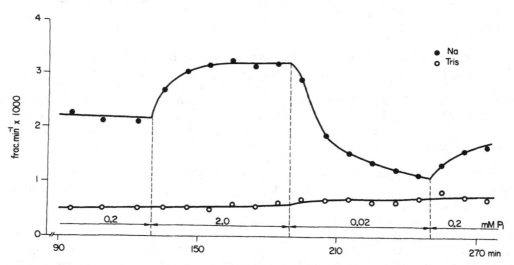

Fig. 7. Rate constant of phosphate efflux at different extracellular phosphate concentrations in presence of Na (full signs) and absence of Na (empty signs). Nerve was loaded for 2 hrs in presence of Na, time indicated refers to beginning of washing with Na or Na-free solutions.

Fig. 6 was also found when the extracellular phosphate was suddenly
changed (17). Fig. 7 (top) shows that this trans-effect was observed
in the presence of Na : a sudden increase in extracellular phosphate
then increased the efflux and a decrease in phosphate decreased it.
The bottom line of Fig. 7 shows that changes in extracellular phosphate had no effect when Na was absent. The loss of the trans-effect
appears to be caused by the lowering of intracellular Na. With solutions with intermediate Na concentrations, it was found that the
effect of extracellular phosphate disappeared when solutions with
less than 20 mM Na were used.

The trans-effect in Locke was found also when arsenate, a competitive inhibitor of phosphate influx (18) was added : on the other
hand, the addition of a dicarboxylic acid (malate) had no effect.

When the effect of external phosphate was abolished in Tris-
Locke, it could be partially restored by changing to Li-Locke or
KCl-Locke.

SUMMARY AND CONCLUSIONS

In order to discuss the possible mechanism involved in Na-dependent phosphate transport, it may be worth-while to summarize
briefly the main features of the system observed so far. Thus the
influx experiments showed that the Na-dependent phosphate influx
is saturable both with respect to extracellular phosphate and
Na, with an apparent K_m of 0.4 mM for phosphate and 20 mM for Na.
The efflux experiments showed that part of the efflux is also Na-
dependent; this part shows a trans-effect for phosphate which is
also saturable. Trans-effects are often described by a reaction
system in which the amount of transport system is limited and distributed between the two sides of the membrane. The following
scheme, a specific case of a more general system (19) can be
used as a basis for further discussion.

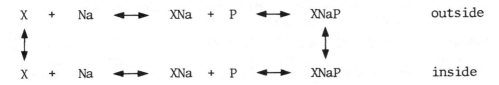

Fig . 8. Reaction scheme to explain trans-effect of external phosphate in presence of Na.

In this system, a trans-effect for phosphate is obtained only when Na reacts first. Using the same apparent K_m for both outside and inside reactions, and under the assumption that the reactions are much faster than the transfer which is taken to be the same for the Na-P_i charged and the uncharged carrier, the calculated rates are close to the observed ones.

As far as we know, phosphate can be replaced by arsenate with approximately the same affinity, and Na can be replaced by Li or by K with smaller affinities. The transport does not appear to involve a net charge transfer, so that the question of how the same system could work for divalent and monovalent phosphate remains to be further investigated (7). Preliminary studies (20) did not seem to indicate a pronounced difference in affinity between the mono- and divalent P_i, and it is therefore not clear whether we are dealing with one system or two. For the divalent P_i it might be necessary to assume that 2 Na could compensate for the charge. Simultaneous measurements of phosphate influx and Na gradient at different pH might allow to study this possibility further.

REFERENCES

1) Caldwell, P.C., and Lowe, A.G. : The influx of orthophosphate into squid giant axons. J. Physiol. 207:271, 1970.

2) Chambers, E.L. : Role of cations in phosphate transport by fertilized sea urchin eggs. Fed. Proc. 22:331, 1963.

3) Harrison, H.E., and Harrison, H.C. : Sodium, potassium, and intestinal transport of glucose, 1-tyrosine, phosphate, and calcium. Amer. J. Physiol. 205:107, 1963.

4) Anner, B., Ferrero, J., Jirounek, P., and Straub, R.W. : Inhibition of intracellular orthophosphate uptake in rabbit vagus nerve by Na withdrawal and low temperature. J. Physiol. 232:47 P, 1973.

5) Straub, R.W., Ferrero, J., Jirounek, P., Jones, G.J., and Salamin, A. : Na-dependent transport of orthophosphate in vertebrate non-myelinated nerves at different pH. Abstr. 6th int. Congr. Pharmacol., Helsinki, p. 367, 1975.

6) Baumann, K., de Rouffignac, C., Roinel, N., Rumrich, G., and Ullrich, K.J. : Renal phosphate transport : Inhomogeneity of local proximal transport rates and sodium dependence. Pflügers Arch. 356:287, 1975.

7) Hoffmann, N., Thees, M., and Kinne, R. : Phosphate transport by isolated renal brush border vesicles. Pflügers Arch. 362:147, 1976.

8) Brown, K.D., and Lamb, J.F. : Na-dependent phosphate transport in cultured cells. J. Physiol. 251:58 P, 1975.

9) Keynes, R.D., and Ritchie, J.M. : The movements of labelled ions in mammalian non-myelinated nerve fibres. J. Physiol. 179:333, 1965.

10) Anner, B., Ferrero, J., Jirounek, P., and Straub, R.W. : Uptake of orthophosphate by rabbit vagus nerve fibres. J. Physiol. 247: 759, 1975.

11) Anner, B., and Moosmayer, M. : Rapid determination of inorganic phosphate in biological systems by a highly sensitive photometric method. Anal. Biochem. 65:305, 1975.

12) Anner, B., Ferrero, J., Jirounek, P., Jones, G.J., Salamin, A., and Straub, R.W. : Sodium-dependent influx of orthophosphate in mammalian non-myelinated nerve. J. Physiol., in the Press.

13) Ritchie, J.M. : The oxygen consumption of mammalian non-myelinated nerve fibres at rest and during activity. J. Physiol. 188:309, 1967.

14) Straub, R.W., Anner, B., Ferrero, J., and Jirounek, P. : Transport of inorganic phosphates across nerve membranes. In : Comparative Physiology", ed. Bolis, L., Maddrell, H.P., and Schmidt-Nielsen, K., pp 249-257, Amsterdam : North-Holland, 1975.

15) Ferrero, J., Jirounek, P., Rouiller, M., Salamin, A., and Straub, R.W. : Efflux of inorganic phosphate and intracellular phosphate turnover in nerve. Experientia 32:755, 1976.

16) Straub, R.W., Ferrero, J., Jirounek, P., Jones, G.J., and Salamin, A. : Transmembranal transport of inorganic phosphate and its implication in some diseases. In : "Membrane and Diseases", ed. Bolis, L., Hoffman, J.F., and Leaf, A., New York : Raven Press, 1976.

17) Ferrero J., Jirounek, P., Rouiller, M., Salamin, A., and Straub, R.W. : Efflux of inorganic phosphate from rabbit vagus in Locke and Na-free Locke. Proc. Physiol. Soc., Cambridge, 2-3 July 1976.

18) Anner, B., Ferrero, J., Jirounek, P., and Straub, R.W. : Na-dependent phosphate-influx into mammalian nerve fibres. Experientia, 29:740, 1973.

19) Berger, E., Long, E., and Semenza, G. : The sodium activation of biotin absorption in hamster small intestine in vitro. Biochem. Biophys. Acta 255:873, 1972.

20) Ferrero, J., Jirounek, P., Jones, G.J., Salamin, A., and Straub, R.W. : Monovalent and divalent orthophosphate uptake in desheathed rabbit vagus nerve. Experientia 31:709, 1975.

OCCURRENCE OF HYPERPARATHYROIDISM IN CHILDREN WITH X-LINKED HYPOPHOSPHATEMIA UNDER TREATMENT WITH VITAMIN D AND PHOSPHATE

Krohn,H.P., Offermann,G., Brandis,M.,

Brodehl,J., Hanke,K., Offner,G.

Kinderklinik,Med.Hochschule Hannover,

Medizinische Klinik, FU Berlin, Germany

X-linked familial hypophosphatemia (XLH) is a hereditary disorder of phosphate metabolism. The marked reduction of renal tubular phosphate reabsorption is followed by chronic hypophosphatemia with rickets and growth retardation. The rickets are resistant to a normal dosage of vitamin D, but they can be healed or prevented by pharmacological doses of vitamin D. An additional oral phosphate substitution was shown by West (1) and Glorieux (2) to induce growth acceleration.

Prior to treatment there was no hyperparathyroidism in this disease, but hyperparathyroidism occured under oral phosphate therapy, as shown by Arnaud and Scriver (3). Other investigators as Lewy (4) and Reitz (6) however observed elevated values of iPTH before treatment. Fanconi (5) could not find hyperparathyroidism following phosphate loading. Since these data are controversial our investigations were performed in order to look for hyperparathyroidism in this disease before and under phosphate therapy.

15 patients with XLH could be investigated, 5 of them before starting of treatment, 5 after treatment with vitamin D alone and 10 after treatment with vitamin D and phosphate for at least 12 months. The therapeutic approach is shown in the first figure. Each patient

received an individual dose of vitamin D between 10 000
and 100 000 units per day, sufficient to treat the
rickets. In addition, inorganic phosphate was administered orally in 5 divided doses, beginning in the morning
and ending late in the evening in order to elevate the
serum phosphate concentration continuously. The total
amount of phosphate was 1 to 4 g per day.

Tubular reabsorption of phosphate was measured during
standard inulin clearance (10). The data of fractional
reabsorption of phosphate are expressed as T_p/C_{in} in
umol/ml. iPTH was measured by radioimmunoassay with the
antibody chicken M 12 according to Arnaud (7) and
Fischer. 25 Hydroxycalciferol (25 HCC) was measured
simultaneously by a protein binding assay (8).

In the following slide the values of iPTH are depicted
in patients with XLH under different treatment situations.

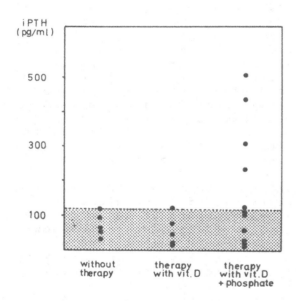

Figure 1
iPTH values in
patients with
XLH under different
treatment situation

In the first column the values of 5 patients without any
treatment are shown. They are within a normal range or
close to normal, as earlier reported by Arnaud (3) and
by Fanconi (5). In the second column the iPTH values are
shown in 5 patients, who were treated with vitamin D
alone. There is no change in iPTH values, as you can see.

In 5 out of 10 patients however an oral treatment with
phosphate induces hyperparathyroidism as it is shown in
the third column.

In 5 patients we were able to measure the iPTH values
and 25 HCC values under treatment with vitamin D alone
as well as under combined treatment (represented by
the triangels). Under vitamin D alone (circle) the
25 HCC levels were elevated, as expected. The iPTH
values were within a normal range. Following an additi-
onaloral phosphate therapy an increase in iPTH values
was seen in 4 out of 5 patients. There was no systema-
tical change in 25 HCC.

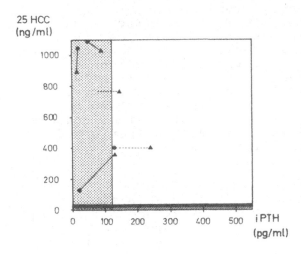

Figure 2
25 HCC values and
iPTH values in
5 patients with XLH
under treatment
with vitamin D
alone (●) and in
combination with
oral phosphate (▲)

It is concluded therefore, that this disease is not
associated with hyperparathyroidism prior to treatment, but that oral phosphate substitution can induce
hyperparathyroidism as it was shown by Arnaud and Scriver

The pathogenic mechanism for the development of hyperparathyroidism under oral phosphate substitution may be
initiated by changes of the Ca concentration in extracellular fluid.
To test this theory, Ca concentration was measured over
24 hours correlated to the oral phosphate intake. The
measurements were performed directly before and one
hour after oral phosphate load.

Serum phosphate concentration is diminished before
phosphate loading. The levels rise following each single
load nearly to normal values and decrease in the following hours. Serum Ca concentration is in the lower range
of normal before treatment, but tends to decrease
following the single phosphate intake within one hour.
There is another increase in the following hours.

Following an oral phosphate substitution a slight short
time decrease in total Ca concentration can be recognized. Hypocalcemia is able to elevate iPTH levels, as
it is shown by Reiss and Canterbury (9).

In 4 out of 5 patients with phosphate induced hyperparathyroidism the dosage of vitamin D was further
elevated individually. The effect of this therapeutic
regimen is demonstrated in the next figure. As expected
25 HCC values are further increased. This is accompanied
by a decrease in the former elevated iPTH values in
all patients. Serum Ca concentration rose slightly,
but remained within a normal range in all patients.
The development of hyperparathyroidism therefore may be
reversed by elevation of vitamin D, but control measurements of Ca concentration in serum must be performed
exactly to prevent vitamin D intoxication.

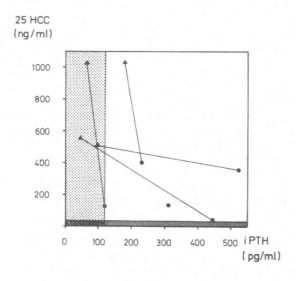

Figure 3
25 HCC values and
iPTH values in 5
patients with XLH
with phosphate
induced hyperpara-
thyroidism before
(•) and after(▲)
elevation of
vitamin D

A physiological effect of PTH is the reduction of renal
tubular reabsorption of phosphate. In XLH Glorieux and
Scriver (2) postulated a loss of PTH-sensitive phosphate transport mechanism in the kidney, which is complete in males and can be incomplete in females.

To test this hypothesis we investigated renal tubular
phosphate reabsorption prior and after oral phosphate
therapy. Prior to   therapy T_P/C_{In} is markedly reduced
as compared to controls, as shown in the shadowed area.
Following phosphate therapy fractional tubular reabsorption of phosphate is even further decreased in all
patients.

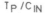

T_P/C_{IN}

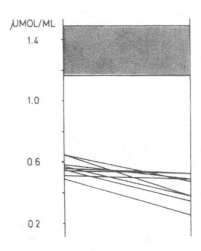

Figure 4
Tubular reabsorption
of phosphate in patients
with XLH before and
after treatment with
vitamin D and oral
phosphate substitu-
tion

In the following figure this reduction in fractional
phosphate reabsorption is depicted in those patients,
who developed hyperparathyroidism by phosphate therapy
compared to those patients, who had normal iPTH values
under treatment. T_P/C_{In} decreased significantly in
patients with hyperparathyroidism from an average of
0.58 to an average of 0.37 umol/ml, while there was
only a minimal decrease in the other group, which was
not significant.
This is in contrast to observations of Arnaud, Glorieux
and Scriver (3), who could not find a decrease of
phosphate reabsorption in XLH in association with hyperparathyroidism.
Further it seems to be worthwhile that the reduction of
phosphate reabsorption, observed in our patients, could

be found in both sexes, in 4 girls and in 1 boy, who is
supposed to have a total absence of PTH sensitive
phosphate transport.

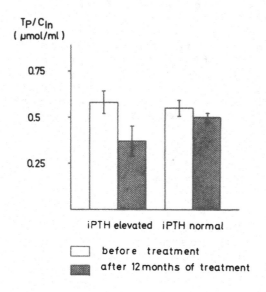

Figure 5
Tubular reabsorption
of phosphate in pat.
with XLH, who developed
hyperparathyroidism
under phosphate treat-
ment compared to pat.
who had no hyperpara-
thyroidism under treat-
ment

Finally it can be concluded:
1. Some patients with XLH develop hyperparathyroidism
under treatment with vitamin D and phosphate.
2. Hyperparathyroidism is accompanied by a further
decrease in tubular reabsorption of phosphate in boys
and girls.
3. The development of hyperparathyroidism is assumed
to be related to a short time decrease of serum Ca
concentration.
4. Hyperparathyroidism is lowered in these patients by
an elevation of vitamin D therapy.

Reference

1. West,C.D., Blanton,J.C., Silverman,F.N., Holland,N.
   Use of phosphate salts as an adjunct to vitamin D
   in the treatment of hypophosphatemic vitamin D refractory rickets.   J.Pediat. 64, 469-477 (1964)

2. Glorieux,F., Scriver,C.R.
   Loss of a parathyroid hormone sensitive component
   of phosphate transport in x-linked hypophosphatemia
   Science 175, 997 (1972)

3. Arnaud,C., Glorieux,F., Scriver,C.R.
   Serum parathyroid hormone in x-linked hypophosphatemia. Science 173, 845-847 (1971)

4. Lewy,J.E., Cabana,E.C., Repetto,H.A., Canterbury,J.
   Reiss,E.
   Serum parathyroid hormone in hypophosphatemic
   vitamin D resistant rickets
   J.Pediat. 81, 294-300 (1972)

5. Fanconi,A., Fischer,J.A., Prader,A.
   Serum parathyroid hormone concentrations in hypo-
   phosphatemic vitamin D resistant rickets.
   Helv.paediat.Acta 29, 187-194 (1974)

6. Reitz,R.E., Weinstein,R.L.
   Parathyroid hormone secretion in familial vitamin D
   resistant rickets
   N.Engl.J.Med. 289, 941-945 (1973)

7. Arnaud,C., Tsao,H.S., Littledike,E.T.
   Radioimmunoassay of human parathyroid hormone in
   serum.
   J.clin.Invest. 50,21 (1971)

8. Offermann,G., Dittmar,F.
   A direct protein-binding assay for 25 Hydroxy-
   calciferol.
   Horm.Metab.Res. 6, 534 (1974)

9. Reiss,E., Canterbury,J.M., Bercovitz,M.A., Kaplan,E.
   The role of phosphate in the secretion of para-
   thyroid hormone in man.
   J.clin.Invest. 49, 2146-2149 (1970)

10. Krohn,H.P., Brandis,M., Brodehl,J., Offner,G.
    Vitamin D resistente Rachtis: Ergebnis einer zwölf-
    monatigen Behandlung mit Vitamin D und Phosphat
    Mschr.Kinderheilk. 124, 417-419 (1976)

A POSSIBLE RELATIONSHIP BETWEEN HIGH-EXTRACTION CEREAL AND RICKETS AND OSTEOMALACIA

J.A. Ford, W.B. McIntosh and M.G. Dunnigan

Departments of Medicine and Paediatrics

Stobhill General Hospital, Glasgow, Scotland

Rickets and osteomalacia are common among the Asian population of the United Kingdom.[1,2] Rickets occurs in the neo-natal period, infancy and adolescence and osteomalacia in adult life, particularly in pregnancy. The condition is due to vitamin-D deficiency as shown by the demonstration of low levels of serum 25-hydroxychole-calciferol (25-H.C.C.) in affected patients and by their prompt theraputic response to low doses of vitamin-D.[3] The reasons for the Asian population's proneness to vitamin-D deficiency remain unclear. Low dietary intakes of vitamin-D, ultra-violet deprivation associated with the "purdah" way of life,[4] skin pigmentation and mode of dress, a high dietary phytate intake,[5] and possible genetic differences in vitamin-D metabolism have all been incriminated.

Significant vitamin-D deficiency is not found outside infancy and old age in the white and West Indian populations although northern latitude, atmospheric pollution and limited food forti-fication place severe constraints on the availability of vitamin-D in Britain. It seems possible that discriminants between the white, Asian and West Indian populations with respect to possible rachitogenic factors may provide clues to the aetiology of Asian rickets. The present study measured the daylight outdoor exposure of Asian and white schoolchildren in mid-summer and mid-winter and by inference their relative capacity to synthesize cholecalciferol in response to ultra-violet radiation. A weighed diet survey of Asian and white schoolchildren was re-analyzed to provide a measure of the two groups' relative intakes of high-extraction cereal (chupatty flour), phytate, phosphorus, calcium and vitamin-D and of the relationship of these components to the severity of biochemical rickets in individual Asian children. The findings were assessed

353

with epidemiological data linking high-extraction cereal diets to
rickets and osteomalacia.

SUBJECTS AND METHODS

Measurement of Outdoor Activity

Forty Asian and white children took part in the survey.
Twenty Asian children (mean age 12.9 years) had been examined in
a prior survey and 10 had been found to have clinical, radiological
or biochemical evidence of rickets.   The remaining 10 children
showed no evidence of rickets.   Twenty white children (mean age
13.3 years) formed a control group.   The white children were not
venesected and it was assumed that they were non-rachitic.
Previous surveys of white schoolchildren in Glasgow have shown no
evidence of vitamin-D deficiency and no case of "nutritional"
rickets in this age group is known to us.   The Asian and white
schoolchildren recorded and timed their daylight outdoor activities
over a 7-day period in July 1974.   Ten of the Asian children
(5 rachitic) and 10 of the white children subsequently recorded
their daylight outdoor activities over a 7-day period in January
1975.   The childrens' records were checked at home daily by a
medical social worker.

Weighed Diet Survey

Forty Asian and white children participated in a weighed diet
survey[6]   The Asian group contained 11 children with clinical,
radiological or biochemical evidence of rickets (mean age 12 years)
and 14 children with no evidence of rickets (mean age 8.7 years).
The white control group comprised 15 children (mean age 10.4 years)
with no biochemical evidence of rickets.

The dietary survey was an individual one, each item of food
being weighed and recorded separately for a period of seven days.
The results were calculated from the food tables of McCance and
Widdowson[7]

In the present study the original data were reviewed and
additional calculations were made of individual intakes of chupatty
flour and phosphorus.   The data were also examined for significant
correlations between intakes of chupatty flour, carbohydrate,
calories, phytate, phosphorus, calcium and vitamin-D and the
presence of rickets as judged by individual levels of serum calcium,
phosphate and alkaline phosphatase.

TABLE 1 - Mean Daylight Outdoor Exposures of White and Asian
Schoolchildren in July and January (7-Day Survey).

| Group | No. | Exposure (h/day) (mean ± S.E.M.) | |
		Summer	Winter
White	20	3.13 ± 0.34	1.34 ± 0.12
Asian	20	2.62 ± 0.63	1.08 ± 0.09
	10	3.03 ± 0.50	1.01 ± 0.17

RESULTS

Measurement of outdoor exposure

The mean daylight outdoor exposure of the white children did
not differ significantly from those of the Asian children either in
summer or winter (Table 1). The mean outdoor exposure of rachitic
Asian children did not differ significantly from the groups as a
whole. Some Asian and white children spent many hours a day outdoors in summer but a number of both groups went out comparatively
little even in fine weather. The medical social workers conducting
the survey concluded that the time spent outdoors by each child
during the survey was reasonably typical of his normal pattern of
activity, reflecting leisure interests, sociability and age.

TABLE 2 - Chupatty flour, phosphorus and "phosphorus excess"
(P-Ca) intakes in Asian and white children
(7-Day weighed dietary inventory).

	Chupatty flour g per day Mean ± S.E.M.	Phosphorus mg per day Mean ± S.E.M.	P-Ca mg per day Mean ± S.E.M.
Rachitic Asian children (n=11) (1)*	213 ± 25 <0.01	1590 ± 117 <0.02	643 ± 64 <0.001
Non-rachitic Asian children (n=14) (2)*	104 ± 20	1189 ± 83 <0.01	358 ± 64 <0.05
White children (n=15) (3)*	-	1264 ± 67 n.s.	249 ± 37 <0.05

*Students 't' tests.

1. Rachitic Asian children - white children
2. Rachitic Asian children - non-rachitic Asian children.
3. Non-rachitic Asian children - white children.

Weighed Diet Survey

The Asian and white diets were similar in calorie, protein, carbohydrate, calcium and vitamin-D content.[6] The most significant discriminant between the diets of Asian and white children and of rachitic and non-rachitic Asian children was their consumption of high-extraction cereal as chupatty flour (Table 2). An age-matched sub-group of seven rachitic Asian children (mean age 11.4 years) and seven non-rachitic children (mean age 11.3 years) consumed 242 ± 30 (S.E.M.) g per day and 119 ± 28 g per day respectively ($p<0.02$), confirming that the differences were not simply age-related. Because of its much higher content of high-extraction cereal, the Asian diet also contained significantly more phytate and total phosphorus than the white diet. Discrimination between Asian and white diets and between the diets of rachitic and non-rachitic Asian children with regard to phosphorus was improved if the excess of dietary phosphorus over dietary calcium (P-Ca; "phosphorus excess") was compared. The significant difference between rachitic Asian children and white children with respect to "phosphorus excess" intakes was retained when smaller age-matched sub-groups were compared but that between rachitic and non-rachitic Asian children was lost.

In a vitamin-D deficient population levels of serum alkaline phosphatase show an inverse correlation with levels of serum 25-hydroxycholecalciferol[3] and therefore provide a measure of the severity of vitamin-D deficiency in individual subjects. A highly significant correlation was found between individual intakes of chupatty flour and serum alkaline phosphatase levels (Table 3). The further significant correlations found with dietary phytate, "phosphorus excess", phosphorus, carbohydrate and caloric intakes reflect intakes of chupatty flour. Levels of serum calcium and phosphate showed no significant correlations with any dietary component.

TABLE 3 – Significant Correlations Between Components of the Diet of 25 Asian Children and their Levels of Serum-Alkaline-Phosphatase (7-Day Weighed Survey).

Dietary component	r	P
Chupatty flour (g/day)	+ 0.63	< 0.001
Phytate phosphorus (mg/day)	+ 0.63	< 0.001
Total phosphorus (mg/day)	+ 0.53	< 0.01
Carbohydrate (g/day)	+ 0.55	< 0.01
Energy (K cal/day)	+ 0.46	< 0.02

DISCUSSION

Vitamin-D Intakes of Asian and White Children

Vitamin-D in man is derived from a limited number of dietary sources and from the endogenous synthesis of cholecalciferol in skin from 7-dehydrocholesterol in response to ultra-violet radiation. Current evidence suggests that even in the northern latitude of the United Kingdom endogenous cholecalciferol is the major source of vitamin-D in subjects not receiving vitamin-D supplements.[8,9] Thus, in theory, adequate ultra-violet exposure should prevent rickets or osteomalacia.

The observations on the daylight outdoor exposures of Asian and white children confirm earlier impressions that Asian children in Glasgow are in this respect culturally assimilated and play out as much as white children; they dress similarly except that Asian girls more usually wear trousers. The findings do not support earlier suggestions that ultra-violet deprivation may explain Asian rickets[4] as several white children in our survey went out relatively little.

Skin pigmentation does not appear to impair cholecalciferol synthesis following ultra-violet radiation;[4] the absence of significant vitamin-D deficiency in the more deeply pigmented West Indian population supports this view. Our own and subsequent diet surveys have shown no good evidence of a relative lack of dietary vitamin-D in the Asian compared with the white diet.[6,10] It therefore seems likely that the average amount of vitamin-D derived from diet and endogenous synthesis is similar in both Asian and white populations. As a corollary, the presence of Asian vitamin-D deficiency implies that the vitamin-D requirement of the Asian population exceeds that of the white population, particularly at times of increased demand.

A Possible Relationship Between High-Extraction Cereal and Rickets and Osteomalacia

The reasons for the Asian population's increased vitamin-D requirement are at present unclear. The sequential hydroxylations of cholecalciferol in liver and kidney to 25-hydroxycholecalciferol (25-H.C.C.) and 1,25-hydroxycholecalciferol (1,25-D.H.C.C.) are determined enzymically. The quantitive rates of these reactions may be genetically influenced although they are not at present known with precision. In the absence of this information, it is possible that slight differences in the intermediary metabolism of vitamin-D may be significant in a situation of borderline vitamin-D self-sufficiency.

Chupatty flour is a high-extraction wheat flour to which a quantity of millings (bran) is added according to the type of flour required; the extraction rate is thus effectively over 90%. The dough is cooked without the addition of yeast to produce a form of unleavened bread or chupatty. The present study has established that the consumption of chupatty flour discriminates well between white children, and rachitic and non-rachitic Asian children. The study also established a highly significant correlation between individual intakes of chupatty flour and the severity of biochemical rickets. Whether these correlations are causal remains to be established.

It now seems unlikely that the high phytate content of high-extraction cereal can produce vitamin-D deficiency leading to rickets and osteomalacia.[11] Low calcium intakes are not _per se_ likely to produce vitamin-D deficiency and the intestinal enzyme phytase probably inactivates much phytate allowing adaptation to high phytate diets.

Phytate-derived inositol polyphosphate esters have been shown to be potent inhibitors of the calcification of rachitic rat cartilage _in vitro_ and of aortic calcification in rats with vitamin-D intoxication when injected parenterally.[12] Synthetic diphosphonates will similarly inhibit calcification in the living animal and have been reported to produce radiological changes of rickets in children treated with ethane-1-hydroxy, 1-diphosphonate (E.D.H.P.) for recurrent renal stone formation.[13] It may therefore be necessary to reconsider the biological role of phytate and to explore possible interactions between polyphosphate esters and cholecalciferol and its metabolites.

In the present study, the "phosphorus excess" (P-Ca) intakes which proved a better discriminant than total phosphorus intakes between rachitic Asian, non-rachitic Asian and white diets may be assumed to be a measure of phosphorus absorption; this has been shown to depend in part on the ratio of phosphorus to calcium in the diet.[14] A number of links are already established between dietary phosphorus, vitamin-D metabolism and metabolic bone disease. A pulsed dose of dietary phosphorus will produce a rapid rise in serum parathormone levels with a peak about one hour after administration; this is achieved by means of a corresponding slight fall in serum calcium.[15] Parathormone has a regulatory role in the conversion of 25-H.C.C. to 1,25-D.H.C.C. in the kidney[16] and in man can increase the formation of 1,25-D.H.C.C. three- or four-fold.[17] In several animals high phosphorus intakes produce the condition of nutritional secondary hyperparathyroidism in the presence of a presumably adequate vitamin-D intake.[18]

The possibility may therefore be considered that a high phosphorus intake is rachitogenic where vitamin-D status is borderline by inducing a relative increase in parathyroid secretion with accelerated conversion of 25-H.C.C. to 1,25-D.H.C.C. If the 25-H.C.C. is derived from a limited substrate (ultra-violet irradiated 7-dehydrocholesterol or cholecalciferol), depletion of 25-H.C.C. and eventually of 1,25-D.H.C.C. may be envisaged, particularly at times of increased demand during puberty or in pregnancy. This intermittent relative increase in parathyroid secretion would, of course, antedate the sustained secondary hyperparathyroidism associated with the establishment of rickets.

Phosphorus has also been shown to inhibit the synthesis of 1,25-D.H.C. in the kidney by direct inhibition of 1α-hydroxylase[19] but this mechanism seems less likely _in vivo_ in the absence of a high serum phosphorus level and would not explain the low levels of 25-H.C.C. found in Asian rickets.

Epidemiological Relationships between High-extraction Cereal and Rickets and Osteomalacia

The paradox of rural rickets. The possible causal association between high-extraction cereal diets and rickets and osteomalacia may be more fully examined in situations where co-existing severe ultra-violet deprivation can be excluded and endogenous cholecalciferol synthesis is not severely limited. These conditions are fulfilled by certain examples of rural rickets, a condition met with in several parts of Asia. Wilson[20] found severe rickets and osteomalacia in the Kangra district of Kashmir among field workers leading an open air life with plentiful sunshine at an altitude of over 4,000 feet. The diets of those most affected consisted exclusively of cereals with no milk and little ghi or cooked vegetables. From Wilson's dietary data it can be estimated that the subjects of his survey who were most affected had a calcium intake of about 250 mg daily and a phosphorus intake of 2,000 mg daily. More recently Rheinhold[21] has described the occurrence of rural rickets in Iran in subjects who derive a major portion of their calorie intakes from wholemeal unleavened bread (tanok). The paradox of rickets and osteomalacia occurring in the presence of adequate sunshine may be resolved by postulating a rachitogenic role for the high-extraction cereal in the diet. In the presence of adequate endogenous cholecalciferol synthesis the low dietary vitamin-D content of the diet seems unlikely to be responsible. The parallel with rickets in Asian children in Britain who do not suffer from gross ultra-violet deprivation, as shown above, is apparent.

Rickets in Ireland 1941-48. The Irish National Nutrition Survey between 1943 and 1948 provided detailed evidence relating a rise in the extraction rate of flour to a marked increase in the incidence of rickets.[22] Between 1940 and 1942 the extraction rate of flour in Ireland was raised from 70% to 100% and in 1942 clinicians in Dublin

noticed a two-fold rise in the incidence of rickets.   No obvious
change in the vitamin-D intake of Irish children between 1939 and
1942 was found to explain the rise and it was thought possible that
the increased extraction rate of the national flour might be
responsible.   Between 1943 and 1948 the extraction rate of flour
was progressively reduced and the flour was fortified with calcium
carbonate in 1947 and 1948.   In those years the annual incidence
of rickets in children from one to four years (whose staple diet
was bread and butter) fell progressively without any measurable
change in their vitamin-D intake.   The incidence of rickets in
children under one year (whose intake of bread was small) did not
significantly alter.

    Correlations between the extraction rate of flour and the
annual incidence of rickets in children under one year and from one
to four years were not significant.   When the extraction rate of
the national flour was examined in terms of its "phosphorus excess"
(P-Ca) content, a similarity was apparent between the reduction in
the annual incidence of rickets in older children and the "phosphorus
excess" content of the flour in that year.   The "phosphorus excess"
content of flour between 1943 and 1948 showed a highly significant
correlation with the annual incidence of rickets in older children
(r= +0.86; p < 0.02) and an insignificant correlation with children
under one year (r= +0.09; n.s).   Correlations between the incidence
of rickets in older and younger children and their estimated dietary
vitamin-D intakes were not significant.

    The incidence of rickets in Dublin between 1943 and 1948 shows
the same lack of correlation with vitamin-D intake (assuming constant
ultra-violet exposure) as is shown by Asian rickets in Glasgow in
the present study and a similar correlation with high-extraction
flour and a measure of phosphorus absorption ("phosphorus excess"
intake).   Moreover, the findings indicate that the association of
rickets with high-extraction flour is not confined to Asians and
that genetic mechanisms are therefore less likely to be responsible
for rickets in the latter.

CONCLUSION

    The evidence of the present study suggests a strong and
possibly causal relationship between high-extraction cereal and
rickets and osteomalacia.   It seems likely that this occurs when
vitamin-D status is border-line.   The rachitogenic component of
high-extraction cereal remains to be identified; dietary phytate
now seems unlikely and phytate-derived polyphosphate esters or
dietary phosphorus may be incriminated.   The present study strongly
indicates that Mellanby's original suggestion of an "anti-calcifying
substance" in high-extraction cereal remains valid.[23]

REFERENCES

1. Dunnigan, M.G., Paton, J.P.J., Haase, S., McNicol, G.W., Gardner, M.D., and Smith, C.M.: Late rickets and osteomalacia in the Pakistani community in Glasgow. Scott.med.J. 7 : 159, 1962.

2. Ford, J.A. Colhoun, E.M., McIntosh, W.B., and Dunnigan, M.G.: Rickets and osteomalacia in the Glasgow Pakistani community 1961-71. Brit. med. J. ii : 677, 1972.

3. Preece, M.A., McIntosh, W.B., Tomlinson, S., Ford, J.A., Dunnigan, M.G., and O'Riordan, J.L.H. : Vitamin-D deficiency among Asian immigrants to Britain. Lancet, i : 907, 1973.

4. Gupta, M.M., Round, J.M., and Stamp, T.C.B. : Spontaneous cure of vitamin-D deficiency in Asians during summer in Britain. Lancet, i : 586, 1974.

5. Wills, M.R., Day, R.C. , Phillips. J.B., and Bateman, E.C. : Phytic acid and nutritional rickets in immigrants. Lancet, ii : 771, 1972.

6. Dunnigan, M.G., and Smith, C.M.: The aetiology of late rickets in Pakistani children in Glasgow. Report of a diet survey. Scott. med. J. 10 : 1, 1965.

7. McCance, R.A., and Widdowson, E.M. : The composition of foods. Spec. Rep. Ser. Med. Res. Counc. Lond., No. 235. London. H.M. Stationery Office, 1960.

8. Preece, M.A., Tomlinson, S., Pietrek, J., Robot, C.A., Ford, J.A., Dunnigan, M.G., and O'Riordan, J.L.H. : Serum 25-hydroxyvitamin-D concentration in man. Proceedings of the Fifth Parathyroid Conference, Oxford. Excerpta Medica International Congress Series No. 346 : 448, 1974.

9. Preece, M.A. Tomlinson, S., Ribot, C.A., Pietrek, J., Korn, H.T., Davies, D.M., Ford, J.A., Dunnigan, M.G., and O'Riordan, J.L.H. : Studies of vitamin-D deficiency in man. Quart. J. Med. 44 : 575, 1975.

10. Cooke, W.T., Asquith, P., Ruck, N., Melikian, V., and Swan, C.H.J. : Rickets, growth and alkaline phosphatase in urban adolescents. Brit. med. J. ii : 293, 1974.

11. Walker, A.R.P., Fox, F.W., and Irving, J.T. : Studies in human mineral metabolism : effect of bread rich in phytate phosphorus on metabolism of certain mineral salts with special reference to calcium. Biochem. J. 42 : 452, 1948.

12. Van den Berg, C.J., Hill. L.F., and Stanbury, S.W. :
    Inositol polyphosphates and phytic acid as inhibitors of
    biological calcification in the rat.   Clin.Sci. 43 : 377, 1972.

13. McCredie, D.A., Powell, H.R., and Rotenberg, E. : Diphosphonate
    therapy in nephrocalcinosis.   Brit. J. Urol. 48 : 93, 1976.

14. Clark, I. : Importance of dietary calcium : phosphate ratios
    in skeletal calcium, magnesium and phosphate metabolism.
    Am. J. Physiol. 217 : 865, 1969.

15. Reiss, E., Canterbury, J.M., Bercovitz, M.A., and Kaplan,E.L. :
    The role of phosphate in the secretion of parathyroid hormone
    in man.   J. clin. Invest. 49 : 2146, 1970.

16. Kodicek, E. : The story of vitamin-D from vitamin to hormone.
    Lancet, i : 325, 1974.

17. Mawer, E.B., Backhouse, J., Hill, L.F., Lumb, G.A., De Silva,P.,
    Taylor, C.M., and Stanbury, S.W. : Vitamin-D metabolism and
    parathyroid function in man.   Clin. Sci. 48 : 348, 1975.

18. Laflamme, G.H., and Jowsey, J. : Bone and soft tissue changes
    with oral phosphate supplements.   J. clin. Invest. 51 :
    2834, 1972.

19. Tanaka, Y., and De Luca, H.F. :   The control of 25-hydroxy-
    vitamin-D metabolism by inorganic phosphorus.   Arch. Biochem.
    Biophys. 154 : 566, 1973.

20. Wilson, D.C. : Incidence of osteomalacia and late rickets in
    Northern India.   Lancet, ii : 10, 1931.

21. Reinhold, J.G. : High phytate content of rural Iranian bread :
    a possible cause of human zinc deficiency.   Am. J. clin.
    Nutr. 24 : 1204, 1971.

22. Jessop, W.J.E. : Results of rickets surveys in Dublin.
    Brit. J. Nutr. 4 : 289, 1950.

23. Mellanby, E. : Rickets-producing and anti-calcifying action
    of phytate.   J. Physiol. 109 : 488, 1949.

INHIBITION OF PARATHYROID HORMONE SECRETION BY ISOPROTERENOL

Christensen, M.S., Brandsborg, O. and Christensen, N.J.

Institute of Pharmacology, University of Aarhus, Second
Clinic of Internal Medicine and Surgical Department of
Gastroenterology, Kommunehospitalet, Aarhus, Denmark

The beta-receptor agonists stimulate the secretion of
many hormones, for example insulin, gastrin, glucagon and renin.
The serum parathyroid hormone concentration has also been reported
to rise in response to intradermal injection of epinephrine and
isoproterenol in patients with allergic diseases (1) and to intravenous infusion of the two catecholamines in cows (2).

During an investigation of the effect of isoproterenol on
gastrin secretion in man (3) we observed, contrary to the expectation, a fall in the serum concentration of parathyroid hormone in
response to intravenous isoproterenol. We have therefore reexamined
the effect of isoproterenol on the serum parathyroid hormone concentration in man. The effect of an oral glucose load on the serum
parathyroid hormone concentration was also studied in order to mimic
the plasma phosphate lowering effect of isoproterenol and the rise
in serum insulin and blood glucose.

SUBJECTS AND PROCEDURE

The following groups of subjects were investigated:
1) 14 subjects (mean age 33 years, range 22-44 years, 9 normal male
subjects and 3 male and 2 female patients with duodenal ulcer) were
studied in the basal state and during i.v. infusion of isoproterenol
in a dose of 2 μg/min for 2o min.
2) 4 subjects were studied during beta-adrenergic receptor blockade
employing propranolol. Propranolol was given orally in a dose of
10 + 10 + 20 mg the day before the experiment and 20 mg 2 hours before the experiment. Isoproterenol was given as described above.
3) 8 normal male subjects (age range 21-24 years) were examined
before and 30, 60 and 90 min after an oral glucose load (70 g). The
glucose was dissolved in calcium free water.

The experiments were performed while the subjects rested in the supine position. All subjects had rested for at least 30 min before the first blood sample was withdrawn. Venous blood was collected through a catheter in the antecubital space.

METHODS

Blood glucose concentration was determined by a glucose oxidase method (4). Serum calcium, serum phosphate and serum protein concentrations were determined on an autoanalyser (SMA). Serum insulin concentration was determined by radioimmunoassay (5).

The serum concentration of parathyroid hormone (s-PTH) was measured by radioimmunoassay after extraction of the hormone from serum by adsorption to and acid elution from Quso G 32, a microfine silicate. The extraction procedure provides a hormone concentration 3.2 times greater in extract than in serum (6). The antibody used was AS 211/32. Bovine PTH was used for ^{125}I-labelling. The sensitivity of the assay was 10 pg bPTH present in the incubation mixture. The coefficient of variation in % was 16 for measurements within normal range (30-105 pg/ml bovine equivalents,MRC bPTH standard 71/324). The normal range of s-PTH in this assay is in accordance with a recent report (7). With this PTH assay we can measure the concentration of PTH in serum from 95% of normal subjects. S-PTH was found elevated in 96% of primary hyperparathyroid patients and undetectable in patients with non-parathyroid hypercalcemia and in hypoparathyroid sera (6). It has been shown that about 75% of the PTH measured by this assay in sera from primary hyperparathyroid patients has a half life of approximately 5 min or less (6). S-PTH is suppressed to undetectable values 10 min after intravenous calcium infusion. Most likely the assay mainly measures the secreted PTH(1-84) (6).

Isoproterenol added to control sera in a concentration of 2 ng/ml had no influence on the results of the immunoassay.

The paired t-test was used in the statistical analysis.

RESULTS

Table I shows the mean s-PTH in the 14 subjects studied before and at the end of intravenous infusion of isoproterenol (2 µg/min). In the basal state s-PTH averaged 71 and 72 pg/ml, which corresponds to the mean value previously found in a group of 76 normal subjects (6). At the end of the infusion of isoproterenol s-PTH had decreased in all subjects to a mean value of 40 pg/ml (p<0.001). There was no difference between the normal subjects and the patients with duodenal ulcer.

During isoproterenol infusion the serum calcium concentration was unchanged when corrected for individual variations in serum

Table I. The mean serum concentration of parathyroid hormone ($\pm$ SEM) before and after an i.v. infusion of isoproterenol (2 µg/min, 20 min) in 14 subjects.

	Basal		Isoproterenol
	-15 min.	0 min.	20 min.
Serum PTH, pg/ml mean (SEM) n = 14	71 (6)	72 (6)	40 (4)

basal versus isoproterenol: $p<0.001$

protein (8) (9.60 mg/100 ml both before and after isoproterenol). The serum phosphate concentration decreased on average 0.44 mg/100 ml ($p<0.001$) during the isoproterenol infusion.

The blood glucose concentration rose from a mean value of 70 mg/100 ml in the basal state to 76 mg/100 ml at the end of the isoproterenol infusion ($p<0.002$). Mean basal insulin concentration was 4 µU/ml and increased to 17 µU/ml at 20 min ($p<0.05$). The mean pulse rate was 69 beats/min in the basal state and rose to 97 beats/min at the end of the infusion period ($p<0.002$).

In 4 subjects the isoproterenol infusion was performed during beta-adrenergic blockade with propranolol. The serum PTH concentration remained unchanged in one subject, increased in one, and decreased slightly in two subjects. The mean serum PTH value before (71 pg/ml) and after infusion (64 pg/ml) were not significantly different.

DISCUSSION

The present study showed that i.v. infusion of isoproterenol decreased serum PTH concentration in all subjects examined. This effect was blocked by propranolol and therefore induced by an increased beta-adrenergic receptor activity.

The decrease in serum PTH concentration during the infusion of isoproterenol was probably due to inhibition of PTH secretion although an effect of isoproterenol on the degradation of circulating PTH cannot be excluded. It is unclear, however, if the inhibition of PTH secretion was due to a direct effect of isoproterenol

on the PTH producing cells or secondary to the effects of isoproterenol on other parts of the endocrine system or the cardiovascular
system. Isoproterenol increased blood glucose concentration, serum
insulin and the pulse rate, while serum phosphate decreased. The
oral glucose loads produced the same lowering of phosphate in serum,
but did not affect the serum concentration of PTH significantly.

The response of the parathyroid gland in man to isoproterenol
is unique in the sense that the secretion of other endocrine glands
is increased by isoproterenol, e.g. insulin and glucagon (9), gastrin
(3) and renin (10). The parathyroid gland also responds anomalously

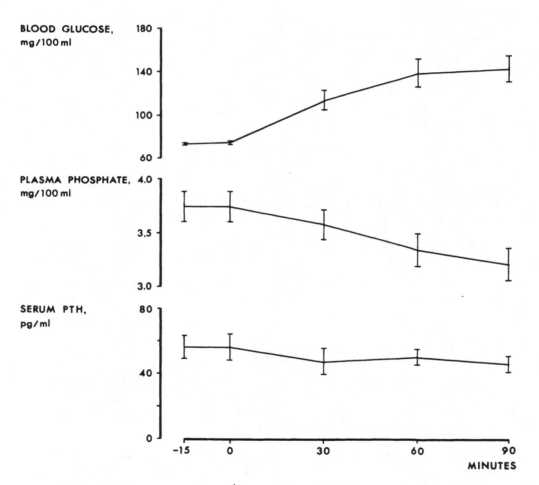

Fig.1 Concentrations (mean $\pm$ SEM) of glucose in blood, phosphate in
plasma and parathyroid hormone in serum following an oral glucose
load of 70 g to 8 normal subjects.

to a rise in the extracellular calcium concentration, which inhibits PTH secretion but stimulates the secretion of other glands (10).

It has to be emphasized that our findings of a decrease in the serum PTH concentration in response to isoproterenol is inconsistent with the report by Kukreja et al. (1). These authors studied the serum PTH concentration in patients with allergic disorders before and after intradermal injection of isoproterenol. We are not able to explain the reason for this discrepancy. The specificity of the authors PTH assay was, however, barely discussed. The fact that their lowest normal range is reported to be 7 times the detection limit of the assay indicates that the assay to a high degree measures PTH fragments reported to be the dominant form of PTH in the circulating blood and biologically inactive (11,12).

SUMMARY

Intravenous infusion of the beta-adrenergic agonist isoproterenol produced a fall in the serum concentration of parathyroid hormone. It also produced a pronounced fall in the serum phosphate concentration, and significant increases in blood glucose and serum insulin concentration and in pulse rate.

The fall in serum parathyroid hormone was abolished by beta-adrenergic blockade with propranolol.

Oral glucose loads produced a pronounced fall in serum phosphate concentration, comparable to the fall after isoproterenol infusion, but no significant changes in serum parathyroid hormone.

It is concluded that the fall in serum parathyroid hormone after isoproterenol is due to a beta-adrenergic effect. It is unknown, if isoproterenol acts directly on the parathyroid hormone secreting cell, or the fall in serum parathyroid hormone is secondary to the effect of isoproterenol on other endocrine glands or the cardiovascular system.

REFERENCES

1. Kukreja S.C., Hargis G.K., Bowser E.N., Henderson W.J., Fisherman E.W. & Williams G.A.: Role of adrenergic stimuli in parathyroid hormone secretion in man. J.Endocr.Clin.Metab. 40:478 (1975)

2. Fischer J.A., Blum J.W. & Binswanger U.: Acute parathyroid hormone response to epinephrine in vivo. J.Clin.Invest. 52:2434 (1973)

3. Brandsborg O., Brandsborg M. & Christensen N.J.: The role of the betaadrenergic receptor in the secretion of gastrin: Studies in normal subjects and in patients with duodenal ulcer. Europ.J. clin.Invest. In press (1976).

4. Christensen N.J.: Notes on the glucose oxidase method. Scand.J. clin.Lab.Invest. 19:379 (1967).

5. Ørskov H.: Wick-chromatography for the immunoassay of insulin. Scand. J. clin. Lab. Invest. 20:297 (1967)

6. Christensen M.S.: A sensitive radioimmunoassay of parathyroid hormone in human serum using a specific extraction procedure. Scand. J. clin. Lab. Invest. 36 pp (1976).

7. Hannsjoerg, W. S., Segre, G. V., Morgan, J. L., Sweetman, B. J., Potts, J. T., Jr. & Oates, J. A.:Prostaglandins as mediators of hypercalcemia associated with cancer. New Engl.J.Med. 293: 1278 (1975).

8. Pedersen K.O.: Protein-bound calcium in human serum. Quantitative examination of binding and its variables by a molecular binding model and clinical chemical implications for measurement of ionized calcium. J. Clin. Lab. Invest. 30:321 (1972).

9. Iversen, J.: Adrenergic receptors and the secretion of glucagon and insulin from the isolated, perfused canine pancreas. J. Clin. Invest. 52:2102 (1973).

10. Rubin R.P.: Calcium and the secretory process. Plenum Press. New York 1974.

11. Silverman R & Yalow, R. S.: Heterogeneity of parathyroid hormone. Clinical and physiological implications. J.Clin.Invest. 52:1958 (1973).

12. Reiss E. & Canterbury, J. M.: Emerging concepts of the nature of circulating parathyroid hormones: implications for clinical research. Recent Progr.Hormone Res. 30:391 (1974).

EFFECT OF PARATHYROID HORMONE AND VOLUME EXPANSION ON JEJUNAL CALCIUM, SODIUM, AND WATER TRANSPORT IN THE RAT

T. Drüeke, J. Chanard, E. Pujade-Lauraine, B. Lacour

and J.L. Funck-Brentano

Université de Paris V, INSERM U.90, Hôpital NECKER

It seems well established that parathyroid hormone (PTH) increases intestinal calcium absorption and that this effect is indirect, possibly via enhanced production of 1,25 dihydroxy-cholecalciferol $(1,25-(OH)_2D_3)$ by the kidney (1,2). The time-lag between PTH administration and $1,25-(OH)_2D_3$ synthesis is likely to be several hours (2). A possible direct PTH effect on the intestine in the absence of $1,25-(OH)_2D_3$ mediation remains questionable.

In the proximal renal tubule, the acute administration of PTH results in a parallel inhibition of sodium and calcium reabsorption (7), and the acute stimulation of endogenous PTH secretion by plasma volume expansion with calcium-poor albumin has a similar effect on proximal tubular reabsorption of sodium (8).

The purpose of the present study was to investigate possible direct effects of acute PTH administration or secretion on jejunal calcium, sodium, and water transport.

METHODS

Five groups of experiments were performed in rats. In group I, calcium-poor albumin infusion experiments were done in which PTH secretion was stimulated ; in group II, calcium-rich albumin infusions were done in which PTH secretion were not stimulated ; in group III, purified bovine PTH was infused, while in group IV, only the PTH vehicle was infused ; in group V, bovine PTH was infused to thyro-parathyroidectomized rats (TPTx).

Male Wistar AF rats weighing 200-300 g were fed a commercial diet containing 1.5% calcium, 0.2% magnesium, 0.95% phosphorus,

and 200 I.U. % vitamin D. The rats were fasted for 18 hours prior
to the experiment with free access to distilled water.

   Rats were anesthetized with intraperitoneal pentobarbital.
The surgical procedure was conducted according to Humphreys et
al. (9). In short, 10-12 cm loop of proximal jejunum was perfused
in situ using a modified Tyrode's solution containing NaCl 137,
NaHCO$_3$ 11.9, NaH$_2$ PO$_4$ 0.4, KCl 3.4, CaCl$_2$ 3.0, MgCl$_2$ 0.1, and
glucose 5.0 mM, respectively. 45 Ca was added to measure lumen-
to-blood flux, pH was maintained constant (7.0) by previous
bubbling of the solution with CO$_2$ (5%) and air (95%). The perfusion rate was 200 µl/min. Phenolsulfonphtalein was added as an
index of volume change.

   In each group, the experimental protocol consisted in 1)three
control collection periods of jejunal fluid starting 60 min after
completion of surgery and 2) four   experimental collection
periods. Each period was 15 min in length. The experimental collection periods started 15 min after completion of the infusion
of albumin solution or after starting PTH infusion. In groups
I and II, 0.6 ml per 100 g body wt of a 25% human albumin solution were infused. The albumin solution of group I contained
1.75 mM and that of group II 6.0 mM calcium.

   In groups III and V, 2 I.U. of bovine (b) PTH (Wilson Lab.)
per 100 g body wt were diluted in ice-cold isotonic saline and
infused for 2 hours ; 20% of the solution was given as priming
dose and the remaining dose was infused at the rate of 0.32 ml/h.
In group IV, no PTH was added to the saline.

   Isotonic saline was infused in all rats after completion of
surgery (0.32 ml/h) until the experimental period. In groups III,
IV and V, the saline of control periods contained additionally
the acidic PTH vehicle in the same v/v ratio as during the experimental period.

   TPTx was performed 2 to 5 days prior to the experiments.
Calcium was measured by atomic absorption spectrometry and
plasma iPTH as previously described (10).

   Net and unidirectional movement of solute and water was
calculated according to Wensel et al (5).

                              RESULTS

            1 - Plasma volume expansion

   Figure 1 shows net calcium, sodium, and water flux before
and after expansion with calcium-poor (group I) and calcium-rich
(group II) albumin. In group I, net calcium flux was significantly decreased in the volume expanded state when compared to control
(p < 0.01). No such change was found in group II. Net sodium and
water fluxes were found significantly decreased after plasma

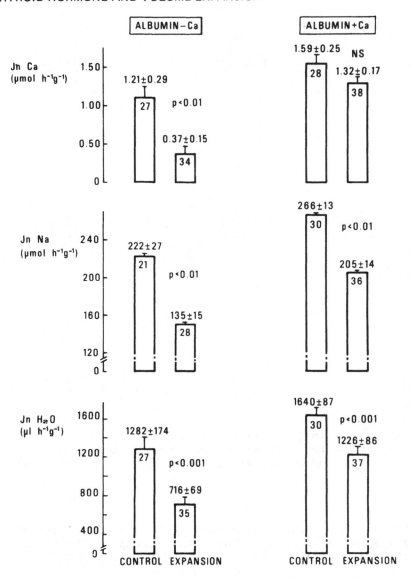

Figure 1 : Effects of plasma volume expansion with hyperoncotic albumin on jejunal net fluxes of Ca, Na, and water. Calcium-poor albumin contained 1.75 mM Ca and calcium-rich albumin 6.0 mM Ca.

volume expansion in both groups when compared to control.

Total plasma calcium increased significantly from 2.26 ± 0.05 to 2.59 ± 0.03 in group I (p<0.001) and from 2.37 ± 0.04 to 2.67 ± 0.03 in group II (p<0.001).

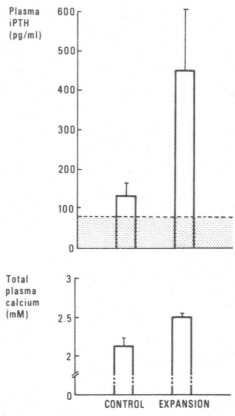

Figure 2 : Effects of plasma volume expansion with Ca-poor
hyperoncotic albumin on total plasma calcium concentration and
plasma iPTH level expressed as pg equivalent of b-PTH per ml.

After albumin expansion, plasma iPTH level increased significantly ($p < 0.05$) in group I but not in group II when compared
to control (figure 2).

2 - Effects of b-PTH infusion

Figure 3 shows the decrease of net calcium, sodium, and
water flux in normal rats induced by b-PTH infusion during 60 min
when compared to control (group III). No such changes were observed
during the experimental period when perfusing the PTH vehicle
only (group IV).
The effects induced by b-PTH infusion in normal rats were
also observed in TPTx rats (group V).

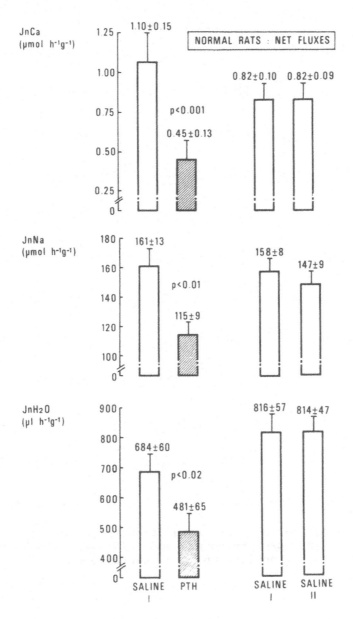

Figure 3 : Effects of b–PTH infusion on jejunal net fluxes of Ca, Na, and water in normal rats. During the control period, saline (I) was infused. During the experimental period, either PTH (dashed column) or saline (II) was infused.

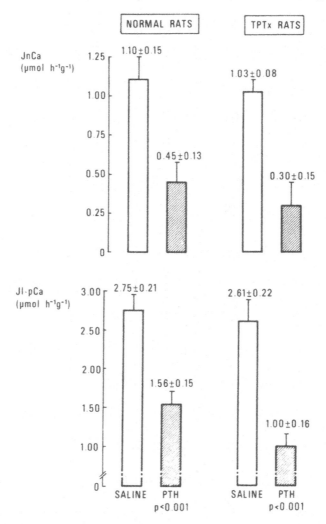

Figure 4 : Effects of b-PTH infusion on jejunal net and lumen-to-blood Ca fluxes in normal and TPTx rats. The open columns indicate the control periods and the dashed columns the experimental periods.

Figure 4 demonstrates a similar decrease of net calcium flux in both groups. Moreover, lumen-to-plasma flux decreased significantly in groups III and V.

During the experiments, total plasma calcium changed from

2.22 + 0.03 to 2.30 + 0.04 mM and from 1.24 + 0.06 to 1.33 + 0.07 mM in groups III and V respectively. These changes were not significant.

DISCUSSION

All recent reports demonstrate an increased intestinal calcium absorption after PTH admnistration (1). The effect of PTH is not immediate and depends on the effects of calcium and phosphate in the diet (1,3,11). When PTH was acutely administered, no immediate effect on the intestinal transport of calcium was documented in man (5,6). However, one in vitro study in isolated vascularly perfused rat small intestine (3) indicated an increase in calcium absorption brought about by an acute PTH infusion. Moreover, Birge et al. (4,12) suggested a direct influence of PTH on calcium release from intestinal mucosal cell and identified an intestinal sodium and calcium-dependent phosphatase stimulated by PTH.

The present results are at variance with those of Olson et al. (3) : they document a decrease in net and lumen-to-blood calcium transfer within 60 minutes following intravenously administered PTH. The present data were obtained with an in vivo model using b-PTH, the activity of which had been previously checked by measurement of cAMP formation in renal tubule membrane. Total plasma calcium did not change significantly 60 min after PTH injection. However, we have seen a significant increase in plasma calcium 2 h after PTH injection under similar conditions.

In addition to the effect of exogenous PTH on jejunal calcium movement, acute infusion of calcium-poor hyperoncotic albumin was a potent stimulus for endogenous PTH secretion (Fig. 2) and induced a similar decrease in net calcium transfer. Such an effect was blunted when calcium-rich hyperoncotic albumin was used.

Under the present experimental conditions, jejunal net sodium and water transport paralleled that of calcium following exogenous and endogenous increase in plasma PTH. However, a dissociation of jejunal calcium and sodium absorption following plasma volume expansion with hyperoncotic calcium-rich albumin was observed : net sodium flux was decreased as during plasma volume expansion with calcium-poor albumin, but net calcium flux was not different from control.

Effects of PTH similar to those observed on the jejunum were documented on the renal proximal tubule, where Agus et al. (7) have shown a parallel decrease in calcium and sodium reabsorption. In addition, plasma volume expansion with calcium-poor hyperoncotic albumin as a potent stimulus of endogenous PTH secretion was used by Knox et al. (8) to study changes in sodium reabsorption by the proximal renal tubule in the dog : sodium reabsorption decreased only when animals were not parathyroidectomized.

It appears that PTH acutely decreases jejunal net calcium, sodium, and water flux and lumen-to-blood calcium flux. These effects do not require calcitonin because they were documented in TPTx animals. They seem also unrelated to the hypercalcemic effect of PTH as total plasma calcium did not change during the first hour following PTH injection. However, plasma ionized calcium which was not measured could increase without change in total plasma calcium. Increase in plasma ionized calcium could lead to an increased passive plasma-to-lumen flux of calcium but not a decrease in lumen-to-blood flux. The mechanism of the direct effect of PTH on transjejunal calcium, sodium, and water transport is not clear. The present results do not indicate whether the observed PTH effect is primarily involving calcium or sodium transport.

SUMMARY

The effects of PTH on jejunal calcium, sodium, and water transport were studied in the rat in situ. In TPTx rats, as well as in normal rats, bovine PTH induced a decrease in net calcium, sodium, and water absorption. Additionally, lumen-to-plasma calcium flux was found decreased in both groups.

Stimulation of endogenous PTH secretion by calcium-poor hyperoncotic albumin resulted in a similar decrease in net calcium, sodium, and water absorption.

It is suggested that PTH has a direct inhibitory effect on jejunal calcium, sodium, and water absorption.

REFERENCES

1 - Borle, A.B. : Calcium and Phosphate Metabolism. Ann. Rev. Physiol. , 36 : 361, 1974.

2 - De Luca, J.F. : Recent advances in our understanding of the vitamin D endocrine system. J. Lab. Clin. Med. 87 : 7, 1976.

3 - Olson, B.E., Jr. , De Luca, H.F. , Potts, J.T., Jr. : The effect of calcitonin and parathyroid hormone on calcium transport of isolated intestine, in : Calcium, Parathyroid Hormone and the Calcitonins, R.V. Talmage and P.L. Munson ed. 1972, Excerpta Medica, Amsterdam, p. 240-246.

4 - Birge, S.J. , Switzer, S.C. , Leonard, D.R. : Influence of sodium and parathyroid hormone on calcium release from intestinal mucosal cells. J. Clin. Invest. 54 : 702, 1974.

5 - Wensel, R.H. , Rich, C. , Brown, A.C. , Volwiler, W. : Absorption of calcium measured by intubation and perfusion of the intact human small intestine. J. Clin. Invest. 48 : 1768, 1969.

6 - Walton, J. , Williams, M.E. , Shea, T.L. , Gray, T.K. : Effects of parathyroid extract on jejunal absorption of phosphate and calcium. Clin. Res. 24 : 30 A, 1976.

7 - Agus, Z.S. , Gardner, L.B. , Beck, L.H. , Goldberg, M. : Effects of parathyroid hormone on renal tubular reabsorption of calcium, sodium and phosphate. Amer. J. Physiol. 224 : 1143, 1973.

8 - Knox, F.G. , Schneider, E.G. , Willis, L.R. , Strandhoy, J.W., Ott, C.E. , Cuche, J.L. , Goldsmith, R.S. , Arnaud, C.D. : Proximal tubule reabsorption after hyperoncotic albumin infusion. J. Clin. Invest. 53 : 501, 1974.

9 - Humphreys, M.H. , Earley, L.E. : The mechanism of decreased intestinal sodium and water absorption after acute volume expansion in the rat. J. Clin. Invest. 50 : 2355, 1971.

10 - Chanard, J. , Klahr, S. , Slatopolsky, E. : Microtubule disrupters and secretion of parathyroid hormone in vivo. J. Urol. Nephrol. 82 : 355, 1976.

11 - Winter, M. , Morava, E. , Simon, G. , Sos, J. : The role of parathyroid glands in the absorption of calcium from the small intestine. J. Endocrinol. 47 : 65, 1970.

12 - Birge, S.J. , Gilbert, H.R. : Identification of an intestinal sodium and calcium-dependent phosphatase stimulated by parathyroid hormone. J. Clin. Invest. 54 : 710, 1974.

AKNOWLEDGMENTS

We thank Mrs. D. Coraboeuf for technical assistance.

CHOLECALCIFEROL METABOLITES BINDING IN PORCINE PARATHYROID GLANDS

A. ULMANN, J.F. CLOIX and J.L. FUNCK-BRENTANO

I.N.S.E.R.M. U.90 - Hôpital Necker

161, rue de Sèvres - 75015 - PARIS - FRANCE

Among vitamin D_3 metabolites, 1α,25-dihydroxycholecalciferol [1,25-$(OH)_2D_3$] appears to have marked effects on calcium or phosphate intestinal absorption (1, 2) and can be considered a hormone. 1,25-$(OH)_2D_3$ renal production from 25-hydroxycholecalciferol [25-$(OH)D_3$] is in part regulated by phosphate (3) and by parathyroid hormone (PTH) (4). On the other hand, some in vivo and in vitro experiments (5, 6, 7) suggest that 1,25-$(OH)_2D_3$ might control PTH production via a direct mechanism.

At the cellular level, 1,25-$(OH)_2D_3$ may act in a similar way than steroid hormone do, i.e. binding of the hormone to a cytoplasmic protein or receptor and migration of the hormone-receptor complex to the nucleus. The complex then associates to the chromatin, thus resulting in enhanced synthesis of a hormone-specific protein. Such events have been demonstrated in chick intestinal mucosa (8), and, more recently, in chick parathyroid glands (7).

We report here our findings on 25-$(OH)D_3$ or 1,25-$(OH)_2D_3$ binding to cytoplasm or nuclei from porcine parathyroid glands.

MATERIALS AND METHODS

Sterols

Tritiated 25-$(OH)D_3$ [^{3}H-25-$(OH)D_3$] (9.7 Ci/mmole) was obtained from Amersham. Crystalline 25-$(OH)D_3$ was the gift of Roussel Laboratories. High specific activity (9.7 Ci/mmole) or low specific activity (0.8 mCi/mmole) tritiated 1,25-$(OH)_2D_3$ [^{3}H-1,25-$(OH)_2D_3$] was prepared in vitro as previously described (9). Low specific activity ^{3}H-1,25-$(OH)_2D_3$ was used as "unlabelled" 1,25-$(OH)_2D_3$.

Preparation of Cytosol

Immediately after slaughter, porcine parathyroid glands (100 mg approximately) were defatted and homogenized at 4° in 2 ml of buffer A (10 mM Tris, 25 mM KCl, 5 mM $MgCl_2$, pH 7.4). Homogenates were centrifuged at 800 x g for 10 min at 4°. The resulting supernatant, centrifuged at 105,000 x g for 1 hour at 4°, yielded a final supernatant which was considered the cytosol.

Preparation of Nuclei

Porcine parathyroid glands (20 to 30 mg) were cut into 200 um slices and incubated with sterols for 18 h at 4° and 30 min at 37° in 0.5 ml of buffer B (10 mM Tris, 250 mM sucrose, 1 mM $MgCl_2$, pH 7.4). After incubation, slices were extensively washed with sterol-free buffer B, and homogenized in the same buffer. The homogenates were then centrifuged three times at 800 x g for 10 min at 4° and the resulting crude nuclear pellets were mixed with 8 ml of a 2 M sucrose solution and centrifuged at 50,000 x g for 45 min at 4°. The purified nuclear pellets were then resuspended in buffer B, and were assayed for radioactivity and DNA content. In some experiments, the purified nuclear pellets were resuspended in buffer B containing 1.2 % Triton X-100 (Sigma). After 10 min at 4°, nuclei were centrifuged and washed twice with Triton-free buffer B.

Additional Procedures

Protein was measured according to Lowry (10) with bovine serum albumin as standard. DNA was measured according to Burton (11) with calf thymus DNA as standard.

RESULTS

25-(OH)D_3 and 1,25-(OH)$_2D_3$ Cytosol Binding

Aliquots of cytosol from porcine parathyroid glands were incubated with 10^{-8} M of either ^{3}H-25-(OH)D_3 or ^{3}H-1,25-(OH)$_2D_3$ for 8 hours at 4° and centrifuged on 5 to 20 % sucrose gradients. The upper panel of Fig. 1 shows that ^{3}H-25-(OH)D_3 binds to 6 S cytosolic macromolecules. Binding is saturable since a 100-fold excess unlabelled 25-(OH)D_3 displaces ^{3}H-25-(OH)D_3 by 60 %. In addition, incubation in the presence of a 100-fold excess unlabelled 1,25-(OH)$_2D_3$ results in a 30 % ^{3}H-25-(OH)D_3 binding decrease. It appears on the lower panel of Fig. 1 that ^{3}H-1,25-(OH)$_2D_3$ interacts with a macromolecular component (sedimentation rate : 5 S).

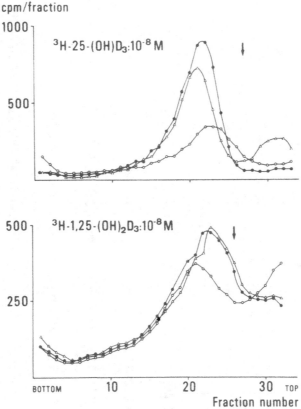

Fig. 1 : Sucrose gradient sedimentation of porcine parathyroid cytosol incubated with ^3H-1,25-(OH)$_2$D$_3$ or ^3H-25-(OH)D$_3$. Upper panel : incubation with ^3H-25-(OH)D$_3$ alone (●), or in the presence of a 100-fold cold 25-(OH)D$_3$ (o) or 1,25-(OH)$_2$D$_3$ (△). Lower panel : incubation with ^3H-1,25-(OH)$_2$D$_3$ alone (●), or in the presence of a 100-fold cold 1,25-(OH)$_2$D$_3$ (o) or 25-(OH)D$_3$ (△). Arrows indicate bovine serum albumine (4.6 S).

Binding is saturable since abolished when incubation are performed in the presence of a 100-fold excess unlabelled 1,25-(OH)$_2$D$_3$. No displacement is observed in the presence of a 100-fold excess unlabelled 25-(OH)D$_3$.

25-(OH)D$_3$ and 1,25-(OH)$_2$D$_3$ Nuclear Uptake

Parathyroid slices were incubated with increasing amounts of radioactive sterols for 18 h at 4° and 30 min at 37°. Nuclei were then prepared as described above. At each concentration of either ^3H-1,25-(OH)$_2$D$_3$ or ^3H-25-(OH)D$_3$ non-specific binding was determined

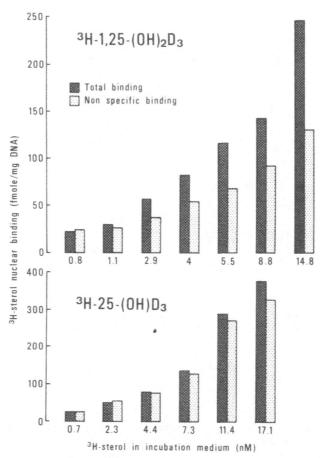

Fig. 2: Nuclear binding of either ^{3}H-1,25(OH)$_2$D3 or ^{3}H-25-(OH)D3
in parathyroid slices incubated with increasing amounts of these
sterols. ▨ : total binding (indubations with tritiated sterol
alone). ▩ : non specific binding (incubations with tritiated
plus a 100-fold excess unlabelled sterol).

by parallel incubations in the presence of a 100-fold excess of unlabelled 1,25-(OH)$_2$D3 or 25-(OH)D3 respectively. Figure 2 gives the
evidence of a 1,25-(OH)$_2$D3 nuclear specific uptake (total minus non
specific uptake) for 1,25-(OH)$_2$D3 medium concentrations as low as
10-9 M. No saturation is evident while increasing 1,25-(OH)$_2$D3
concentration. A 25-(OH)D3 specific nuclear uptake is demonstrated
only for 25-(OH)D3 medium concentrations above 4.4 x 10-9 M. In
some experiments, nuclei were washed with Triton X-100 (see "Materials and Methods"): that lowered nuclear specific uptake of both

sterols, but 1,25-(OH)2D3 specific nuclear uptake was still 4 times that of 25-(OH)D3.

In some experiments incubations were performed with either ^{3}H-1,25-(OH)2D3 or [3]H-25-(OH)D3 alone or in the presence of a 100-fold excess unlabelled progesterone. Progesterone completely abolished 25-(OH)$_2$D$_3$ uptake by Triton-washed nuclei, whereas it had almost no effect on 1,25-(OH)$_2$D$_3$ nuclear uptake.

DISCUSSION

Cytosolic macromolecules exist in porcine parathyroid glands that bind both 25-(OH)D$_3$ and 1,25-(OH)$_2$D$_3$. Incubations in the presence of unlabelled sterols indicate that 25-(OH)D$_3$ has no affinity for [3]H-25-(OH)D$_3$ binder. Preliminary experiments have shown that these binders differ from 25-(OH)D$_3$ and 1,25-(OH)$_2$D$_3$ porcine plasma binding proteins. Recently, Brumbaugh et al. (7) have demonstrated the existence inside the cytoplasm from rachitic chick parathyroid glands of binders for 1,25-(OH)D$_3$ and 25-(OH)D$_3$. 1,25-(OH)$_2$D$_3$ was found to bind to a 3.1 S binder, whereas 25-(OH)D$_3$ binds to 6 S component having a low affinity for 1,25-(OH)$_2$D$_3$. Species differences may explain different sedimentation rates observed for 1,25-(OH)$_2$D3 cytosolic binders in chick or porcine parathyroid glands.

It appears from our data that 25-(OH)D$_3$ and 1,25-(OH)$_2$D$_3$ can be found in association with porcine parathyroid glands nuclei. Washing of the nuclei with Triton X-100 does not abolish nuclear binding of either 1,25-(OH)$_2$D$_3$ or 25-(OH)D$_3$. When parathyroid slices are incubated with equal amounts of either [3]H-25-(OH)D$_3$ or ^{3}H-1,25-(OH)$_2$D$_3$, this latter sterol nuclear uptake is 3 or 4 times greater than that of 25-(OH)D$_3$ whether nuclei are Triton-washed or not. However competitions experiments with progesterone suggest that 25-(OH)D$_3$ nuclear binding may not be specific in contrast with that of 1,25-(OH)$_2$D$_3$.

PTH production has been shown to be impaired in the presence of 1,25-(OH)$_2$D$_3$ both in the rat, in vivo or by bovine parathyroid glands, in vitro (5). A possible direct action of 1,25-(OH)$_2$D$_3$ on parathyroid cells was suggested by Henry and Norman (6) : after injection of radioactive 1,25-(OH)$_2$D$_3$ in rachitic chicks they found that this sterol was concentrated by parathyroid glands. In addition, Brumbaugh et al. (7) have shown that 1,25-(OH)$_2$D$_3$ but not 25-(OH)D$_3$ binds to chromatin from chick parathyroid glands. Similarly, our results suggest that porcine parathyroid glands, which contain a calcium binding protein (12) could be a target organ for 1,25-(OH)$_2$D$_3$.

REFERENCES

1 – Fraser, D.R. and Kodicek, E. : Unique biosynthesis by kidney
    of a biological active vitamine D metabolite. Nature 228 :
    764, 1970.

2 – Gray, R., Boyle, I. and DeLuca, H.F. : Vitamin D metabolism :
    the role of kidney tissue. Science, 172 : 1232, 1971.

3 – Tanaka, Y. and DeLuca, H.F. : The control of 25-hydroxyvitamin
    D metabolism by inorganic phosphorus. Arch. Biochem. Biophys.
    154 : 566, 1973.

4 – Garabedian, M., Holick, M.F., DeLuca, H.F. and Boyle, I.T. :
    Control of 25-hydroxycholecalciferol metabolism by parathy-
    roid glands. Proc. Nat. Acad. Sci. USA 69 : 1673, 1972.

5 – Chertow, B.S., Baylink, D.J., Wergedal, J.E., Su, M.H.H. and
    Norman, A.W. : Decrease in serum immunoreactive parathyroid
    hormone in rats and in parathyroid hormone secretion in vitro
    by 1,25-dihydroxycholecalciferol. J. Clin. Invest. 56 : 668,
    1975.

6 – Henry, H.L. and Norman, A.W. : Studies on the mechanism of
    action of calciferol. VII. Localization of 1,25-dihydroxy-
    vitamin D_3 in chick parathyroid glands. Biochem. Biophys.
    Res. Commun. 62 : 781, 1975.

7 – Brumbaugh, P.F., Hughes, M.R. and Haussler, M.R. : Cytoplas-
    mic and nuclear binding components for 1α-25-dihydroxyvitamin
    D in chick parathyroid glands. Proc. Nat. Acad. Sci. USA, 72 :
    4871, 1975.

8 – Brumbaugh, P.F. and Haussler, M.R. : 1α,25-dihydroxycholecal-
    ciferol receptors in intestine. J. Biol. Chem. 249, 1251,
    1974.

9 – Omdahl, H.L., Gray, R.N., Boyle, I.T., Knutson, J. and DeLuca,
    H.F. : Regulation of metabolism of 25-hydroxycholecalciferol
    by kidney tissue in vitro by dieterary calcium. Nature New.
    Biol. 237 : 63, 1972.

10 – Lowry, O.H., Rosebrough, N.J., Farr, A.L. and Randall, R.J.
    Protein measurement with the folin phenol reageant. J. Biol.
    Chem.. 193 : 265, 1951.

11 – Burton, K : A study of the condition and mechanism of the
    diphenylamine reaction for the colorimetric estimation of
    deoxyribonucleic acid. Biochem. J. 62 : 315, 1956.

12 – Oldham, S.B., Fischer, J.A. and Arnaud, C.D. : Isolation and
    properties of a calcium binding protein (CaBP) from normal
    porcine parathyroid glands (pPTGs). Excerpta Med. Int. Congr.
    Ser. 256 : 95, 1972.

ACKNOWLEDGMENTS

This work was supported by a grant of the Centre National de
la Recherche Scientifique.

Effect of a Ca^{2+} dependent protein kinase and a protein phosphatase on the Ca^{2+}-phosphate transport ATPase

W.H. Hörl and L.M.G. Heilmeyer, jr.
Institut für Physiologische Chemie, Ruhr-
Universität, 4630 Bochum, West Germany

Phosphorylase kinase, a large oligomer of the composi-
tion $\alpha_4\ \beta_4\ \gamma_4$, is the key enzyme for the regulation of
glycogen degradation. It catalyzes, activated by low
concentration of Ca^{2+} ions, the conversion of phosphorylase b to a, i.e. the phosphorylation of one
specific serine residue of each of the two subunits of
phosphorylase b (1). In addition this kinase in-
corporates phosphate into its own subunit α (2,3,4)
and into troponin (5). Fluoresceineisothiocyanate
labelled antibodies against phosphorylase kinase stain
the sarcolemma and the sarcoplasmic reticulum of
striated muscle cells (4,6,7,8). These immunological
results indicate the presence of this enzyme in
membraneous structures. This paper will further demonstrate that this kinase in combination with a phosphatase influences the Ca^{2+} transport ATPase.

In order to study the role of phosphorylase kinase and
-phosphatase for the function of the sarcoplasmic
reticulum these membranes were isolated according to
De Meis and Hasselbach (9). The distribution of glycogen metabolizing enzymes during preparation of these
vesicles is shown in Table 1. About 5% of the total
protein is attributable to the presence of glycogen
metabolizing enzymes of which phosphorylase b consti-
tutes the main component. These enzymes may be associated with a protein-glycogen complex which is
probably copurified with this vesicular fraction (9).
Phosphorylase b can be completly separated from the

DISTRIBUTION OF GLYCOGEN METABOLIZING ENZYMES IN PREPARATION OF
SARCOPLASMIC RETICULUM

Fraction	Volume ml	Protein mg/ml	ATPase Units	%	Phosphorylase Kinase Units	%	Phosphorylase Phosphatase Units	%
1. crude extract	900	14.2	1751	100	709239	100	981	100
2. 44000 x g sediment	190	13.2	697	39.8	50942	7.2	251	25.6
3. ATP wash	410	5.7	961	54.9	51220	7.2	291	29.7
4. KCl wash	260	3.4	498	28.4	11304	1.6	362	36.9
5. KCl wash	215	2.9	420	24.0	4300	0.6	286	29.2
6. crude vesicles	38	16.1	497	28.4	2621	0.4	155	15.8

Fraction	Phosphorylase Units	%	Protein Kinase Units	%	Glycogen Synthetase Units	%	Glycogen mg	%
1. crude extract	116100	100	1.476	100	137.70	100	68.4	100
2. 44000 x g sediment	20330	17.5	0.263	17.8	41.04	29.8	57.0	83.3
3. ATP wash	20910	18.0	0.262	17.8	41.82	30.4	53.3	77.9
4. KCl wash	6000	5.1	0.120	8.1	14.75	10.7	14.0	20.5
5. KCl wash	4515	3.9	0.095	6.4	8.39	6.1	7.3	10.7
6. crude vesicles	3002	2.6	0.011	0.8	3.95	2.9	1.4	2.1

Table 1 : Enzymes were assayed as described (14), glycogen as modified according to Montgomery (15) and Protein according to Lowry (16).

membranes by sucrose gradient centrifugation. Fig. 1
shows that phosphorylase kinase and phosphorylase phosphatase cosediment with these membranes which are
characterized by the Ca²⁺ transport ATPase. Phosphorylase b does not sediment under these conditions. It
was tested that soluble phosphorylase kinase and -phos-
phatase do also not sediment into the gradient.

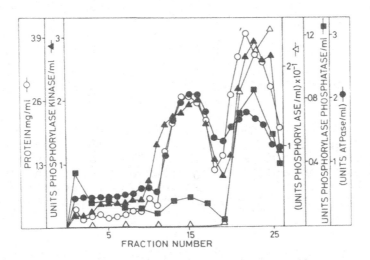

Fig. 1
Sucrose gradient centrifugation of vesicles of sarcoplasmic reticulum. 45 mg vesicles were layered on top
of a linear gradient between 0.3 and 0.9 M sucrose and
centrifuged for 1 hr at 8000 x g in a swing out rotor
at 4°. Fractions (1.3 ml) were collected and assayed
for enzyme activity as described (14).

Upon recentrifugation of the vesicular proteins (Fig 2)
phosphorylase kinase and -phosphatase again cosediment
with the Ca²⁺ transport ATPase. These results are in
agreement with the immunological localization of phosphorylase kinase and phosphorylase b. The latter protein is only found in the sarcoplasm, whereas the
kinase is also present in these membranes. Consequently
the weight ratio of phosphorylase kinase to phosphorylase b which is 1 : 5 in the crude extract reverses
during this purification to 10 : 1. Furthermore the
pH 6.8/8.2 activity ratio of this kinase increases from
0.07 to 0.45. Such an activity ratio is characteristic
for the phosphorylated or the partially proteolytic degraded kinase (2,3).

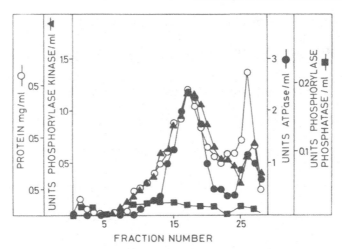

FRACTION NUMBER

Fig. 2
Membrane fractions of gradient 1 (10-18) were pooled
and dialyzed against 0.1 M NaCl. Thereafter the
solution was concentrated by ultra filtration over an
Amicon filter XM 100. The material was recentrifuged
on a sucrose gradient and analyzed as described above.

Polypeptides corresponding in molecular weight to the
α and β subunits but not the γ subunit of phosphorylase kinase are detectible by SDS gel electrophoresis
in the purified vesicles of the sarcoplasmic reticuhm
(4,7,8).
An indication of the function of this membraneous
kinase can be deduced from studies of the Ca^{2+} transport ATPase. Fig. 3 shows the time dependency of the
phosphate liberation from ATP catalyzed by the transport ATPase (11). As can be seen addition of anti-
phosphorylase kinase inhibits the oxalate stimulation
only. Similarely this oxalate effect can be suppressed
by phosphorylase b. Concomitantly with the splitting
of ATP a Ca^{2+} dependent conversion of phosphorylase b
to a can be demonstrated. Therefore the suppression
of the oxalate effect can be correlated with an inhibition of this kinase either by antibodies or by
competition with phosphorylase b. Both proteins reduce
the Ca^{2+} accumulation in the vesicles by 20 to 30 %
(see Fig. 4) which indicates that they do not act by
closing channels for the anions. It seems therefore
that oxalate influences the Ca^{2+} transport ATPase
mediated through this kinase or phosphatase. Fig. 5

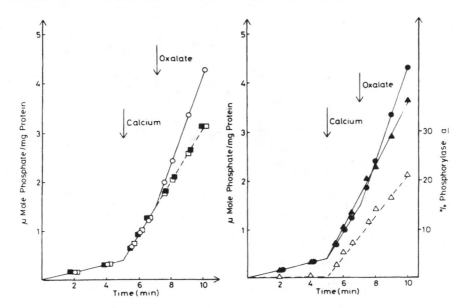

Fig. 3
Effect of anti-phosphorylase kinase and phosphorylase
b on the Ca²⁺ transport ATPase. Antibodies (3.0 mg/ml
purified γ-globulin fraction) were added in the
presence of oxalate (■ — ■) to the control mixture
with (o — o) and without (□ — □) oxalate, (▲ — ▲) represents the presence of phosphorylase b (4.5 mg/ml)
and oxalate, (● — ●) represents the control with BSA
(3.0 mg/ml) and oxalate, (△ — △) shows % conversion
of phosphorylase b into a in the Ca²⁺ ATPase test
mixture according to Hasselbach (11).

shows the effects of oxalate and fluoride anions on
the purified phosphorylase kinase and -phosphatase. As
can be seen both anions are potent inhibitors of the
phosphatase. Phosphate is also known to be a phosphorylase phosphatase inhibitor (12).

Up to a concentration of 20 mM these anions do not affect phosphorylase kinase activity. Therefore the
stimulation of the Ca²⁺ transport ATPase by all these
anions may be mediated through the phosphatase inhibition and not only by precipitation of calciumoxalate
(13). In agreement with this interpretation the Ca²⁺
transport ATPase can be stimulated with fluoride like
with oxalate (Table 2). More directly the Ca²⁺transport
ATPase activity can be inhibited by addition of phos-

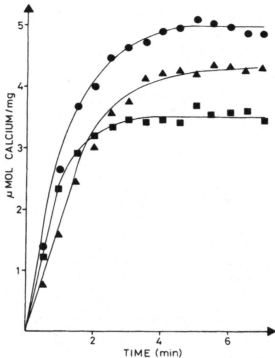

Fig.4
Caclium transport into vesicles of the sarcoplasmic
reticulum. Calcium transport was determined in aliquots filtered through Millipore filter (450 n)
Anti-phosphorylase kinase (■ — ■) was added in a
concentration of 3 mg/ml and phosphorylase b (▲—▲)
in a concentration of 4.5 mg/ml, vesicular protein
was 0.5 mg/ml (●—●) represents the control without
addition.

phorylase phosphatase in absence of these anions. This
effect of the phosphatase can be suppressed by low
molecular weight phosphatase inhibitors, fluoride or
oxalate, which results in an augmentation of the
stimulatory effect of these anions (see Table 2).
Similarly, the antagonistic enzyme phosphorylase
kinase reverses the Ca^{2+} transport ATPase inhibition
by the phosphatase and lowers the activity ratio of
the ATPase in absence and presence of oxalate. These
results indicate that the Ca^{2+} transport ATPase
activity is influenced by two enzymes: a Ca^{2+}dependent
protein kinase and a protein phosphatase.

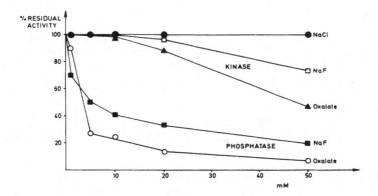

Fig. 5
Influence of oxalate, NaF and NaCl on the activity of
purified phosphorylase kinase and phosphorylase phosphatase. These enzymes were prepared as described in
Table 2. 100 % activity of phosphorylase kinase represents 1.6 Units/ml (7960 nMol x min^{-1} x mg^{-1}).
100 % activity of phosphorylase phosphatase represents
0.45 Units in a total test volume of 200 μl (45 nMol
x min^{-1} x mg^{-1}). NaCl has no effect on phosphorylase
kinase and phosphorylase phosphatase activity($\bullet$——$\bullet$).

Table 2
Influence of oxalate, fluoride, phosphorylase kinase
and -phosphatase on the Ca^{2+} transport ATPase. Phosphorylase phosphatase was prepared according to
Djovkar (17) and phosphorylase b kinase according to
Jennissen and Heilmeyer (14). Ca^{2+} ATPase was determined according to Hasselbach (11).

	Intact Vesicles	Intact Vesicles + 0.055 mg/ml Phosphorylase Phosphatase	Intact Vesicles + 0.03 mg/ml Phosphorylase Phosphatase + 0.02 mg/ml Phosphorylase Kinase
+ ATP μ Mole x min^{-1} x mg^{-1}	0.10	0.11	0.10
+ Calcium μ Mole x min^{-1} x mg^{-1}	0.69	0.35	0.68
+ Oxalate (4 mM) μ Mole x min^{-1} x mg^{-1}	1.83	1.71	1.55
Oxalate Stimulation n – Fold	2.65	4.89	2.28
+ Na F (20 mM) μ Mole x min^{-1} x mg^{-1}	1.95	1.95	
Fluoride Stimulation n – Fold	2.83	5.57	

References

1.) Fischer, E.H., Heilmeyer, jr., L.M.G., and
    Haschke, R.H.: Phosphorylase and the Control of
    Glycogen Degradation; in: Current Topics in Cel-
    lular Regulation, 4 : 211, 1971.

2.) Hayakawa, T., Perkins, J.P., Walsh, D.A., and
    Krebs, E.G.: Physicochemical Properties of Rabbit
    Skeletal Muscle Phosphorylase Kinase: Biochemistry
    12 : 567, 1973.

3.) Cohen, P.: The Subunit Structure of Rabbit Skeletal
    Muscle Phosphorylase Kinase and the Molecular Basis
    of Its Activation Reactions; Eur. J. Biochem.
    34 : 1, 1973

4.) Hörl, W.H., Jennissen, H.P., Gröschel-Stewart, U.,
    and Heilmeyer, jr., L.M.G.: Calcium and Cyclic
    AMP Dependent Phosphorylation of Enzymes and
    Contractile Proteins; in: Calcium Transport in
    Contraction and Secretion (Carafoli, E. et al. eds)
    North Holland Publishing Company 535, 1975.

5.) England, P.J., Stull, J.T., Huang, T.S., and Krebs,
    E.G.:Phosphorylation and Dephosphorylation of
    Skeletal Muscle Troponin; in: Metabolic Inter-
    conversion of Enzymes (Fischer, E.H., et al. eds.)
    Springer-Verlag Berlin, Heidelberg, New York 175,
    1974.

6.) Hörl, W.H., Jennissen, H.P., Gröschel-Stewart, U.,
    and Heilmeyer, jr., L.M.G.: Evidence for the
    Presence of a Ca^{2+} Dependent Protein Kinase (Phos-
    phorylase Kinase) in Sarcoplasmic Reticulum Mem-
    branes; Hoppe-Seyler's Z. Physiol. Chem. 356 : 239,
    1975.

7.) Jennissen, H.P., Hörl, W.H., Gröschel-Stewart,U.,
    Velick, S.V., and Heilmeyer, jr., L.M.G.;
    Localization and Turnover of Phosphorylase Kinase
    in Rabbit Skeletal Muscle; in: Metabolic Inter-
    conversion of Enzymes (Shaltiel, S., ed.), Springer-
    Verlag Berlin, Heidelberg, New York, in press,
    1975.

8.) Jennissen, H.P., Hörl, W.H., Gröschel-Stewart, U., and Heilmeyer, jr., L.M.G.: Localization of a Calcium Dependent Protein Kinase in Rabbit Muscle Cell Membranes by Immunofluorescence and Activity Distribution Studies; Eur. J. Biochem., in preparation

9.) De Meis, L., and Hasselbach, W.: Acetyl Phosphate as Substrate for Ca²⁺ Uptake in Skeletal Muscle Microsomes; J. Biol. Chem. 246 : 4759, 1971.

10.) Meyer, F., Heilmeyer, jr., L.M.G., Haschke, R.H., and Fischer, E.H.: Control of Phosphorylase Activity in a Muscle Glycogen Particle: I. Isolation and Characterization of the Protein-Glycogen Complex. J. Biol. Chem 245 : 6649, 1970.

11.) Hasselbach, W. :Structural and Enzymatic Properties of the Calcium Transporting Membranes of the Sarcoplasmic Reticulum. Ann. New York Acad. Sci. 137 : 1041, 1966.

12.) Martensen, T.M., Brotherton, l.E., and Graves,D.J., Kinetic Studies of the Inhibition of Muscle Phosphorylase Phosphatase. J. Biol. Chem. 248 : 8323, 1973.

13.) Hasselbach, W., and Makinose, M.: Über den Mechanismus des Calciumtransportes durch die Membranen des sarkoplasmatischen Retikulums. Biochem. Z. 339 : 94, 1963.

14.) Jennissen, H.P., and Heilmeyer, jr., L.M.G.,: General Aspects of Hydrophobic Chromatography. Adsorption and Elution Characteristics of Some Skeletal Muscle Enzymes. Biochemistry, 14 : 754, 1975.

15.) Lowry, O.H., Rosebrough, H.J., Farr, A.L., Randall, R.L.: Protein Measurements with the Folin Phenol Reagent. J. Biol. Chem. 193 : 265, 1951.

16.) Montgomery, R.,: Determination of Glycogen. Arch. Biochem. Biophys. 67 : 378, 1957.

17.) Djovkar, A.,: Diplomarbeit, Partielle Charakteri-
     sierung verschiedener Enzyme des Glycogen-Stoff-
     wechsels nach Anreicherung durch hydrophobe
     Chromatographie, Universität Würzburg, 1974.

Acknowledgments

The authors are much indebted to Dr. H.P. Jennissen
for a gift of anti-phosphorylase kinase.
For excellent technical help we wish to thank Miss
R. Wittal.

INFLUENCE OF VITAMIN D ON BICARBONATE REABSORPTION

David Siegfried, Rajiv Kumar, Jose Arruda and
Neil Kurtzman
Section of Nephrology, University of Illinois
Abraham Lincoln School of Medicine
Chicago, Illinois 60612

INTRODUCTION

It seems well established that acute administration of
vitamin D enhances renal reabsorption of sodium, phosphate and
calcium in the dog and in the rat (1-5). These effects are
thought to be the result of vitamin D action on the proximal
tubule (1,2). Vitamin D deficiency secondary either to
inadequate dietary intake or to intestinal malabsorption may
be associated with the development of metabolic acidosis.
This metabolic acidosis has been attributed to the secondary
hyperparathyroidism of vitamin D deficiency (6,7). Pharmacological doses of parathyroid hormone depress renal bicarbonate
reabsorption but not to a level low enough to result in
metabolic acidosis (8,9). These studies have cast doubt on
the role of parathyroid hormone per se in the generation of
metabolic acidosis of hyperparathyroidism. The occurrance of
metabolic acidosis in vitamin D deficiency (10) suggests that
vitamin D may play a role in renal hydrogen ion secretion.
Accordingly, we measured bicarbonate reabsorption before and
after administration of 25 hydroxycholecalciferol (25 OHD) to
dogs.

METHODS

Twenty experiments were performed on twenty female mongrel
dogs. The dogs were anesthetized with sodium pentobarbital
(30 mg/kg intravenously); subsequent small doses were given
to maintain light anesthesia. An endotracheal tube was

inserted and connected to a Bird respirator; arterial CO_2 tension was kept between 35 and 45 mm Hg by appropriate manipulation of the respirator. An arterial catheter was used to sample arterial blood and monitor blood pressure. A femoral vein catheter was used for infusions. Saline (0.9%) containing I^{125} iothalamate (115 μC/l) was infused at 0.5 ml/min throughout the experiments as a marker of glomerular filtration rate (GFR). 0.9 M $NaHCO_3$ was infused at varying rates to maintain plasma HCO_3 between 30 and 35 mEq/l. An equilibration period of at least 40 minutes was allowed before collection was started. Collections were of ten minutes duration. Urine was collected separately from both kidneys through ureteral catheters. The right renal artery was isolated and cannulated with a 25 guage needle for infusion of 25 OHD or the vehicle. The following groups of animals were studied.

Group I - Intact Dogs

Group IA - 25 OHD Infusion. Six intact dogs were included in this group. After three control clearances 25 OHD was infused into the right renal artery at a rate of 0.2 μg/kg/h for one hour. 25 OHD was dissolved in propylene glycol.
Group IB - Propylene Glycol (PG) Infusion. Six intact dogs were studied exactly the same way as those in group IA except they were infused with propylene glycol.

Group II - Thyroparathyroidectomized (TPTX) Dogs

TPTX was performed 24 hours prior to the study. TPTX was considered successful if serum Ca dropped at least 2 mg%.
Group IIA - 25 OHD Infusion. Four dogs were studied in this group. After three control clearance collections 25 OHD was infused into the renal artery at a dose of 0.2 μg/kg/h for one hour.
Group IIB - Propylene Glycol. Four dogs were studied in an identical manner to those in Group IIA except they were infused with propylene glycol.
Fluid losses were carefully replaced every ten minutes with 0.9% saline. Specimen collection, GFR, blood and urinary electrolyte determinations and statistical analysis were performed as previously described (11).

RESULTS

Table I and II show the results obtained in intact and TPTX dogs infused with PG and 25OHD. As can be seen intact and TPTX dogs infused with PG showed no significant change in

TABLE I

Effect of 25 hydroxycholecalciferol on renal HCO_3 reabsorption in intact dogs.

		GFR	Tm/GFR	Plasma HCO_3	FE Cl	FE PO_4	Filt PO_4*	Plasma PO_4
		ml/min	mEq/l GFR	mEq/l	%	%	µg/min	mg/100 ml
Intact Propylene Glycol (n = 6)								
*Right	C	17.7±2.22	23.8±0.86	32.7±0.36	3.0±0.86	23.4±5.02	6360±117.55	3.5±0.33
		NS	NS	NS	NS	NS	NS	NS
	E	16.1±1.85	24.1±0.87	32.3±0.46	3.3±0.81	24.3±5.30	549±103.02	3.7±0.36
*Left	C	18.7±2.48	23.2±0.76		3.8±1.22	27.0±5.70	6760±132.80	
		NS	NS		NS	NS	NS	
	E	17.4±2.21	23.5±0.94		3.5±1.37	28.4±6.44	618±130.20	
Intact 25 OHD (n = 6)								
Right	C	15.4±1.89	24.4±1.11	31.4±0.58	3.4±1.12	20.7±7.62	562±107.92	3.7±0.51
		$p<0.01$	$p<0.05$	NS	NS	NS	$p<0.05$	NS
	E	13.2±1.76	26.0±1.15	31.9±0.43	2.1±0.08	22.7±7.20	457± 91.96	3.5±0.60
Left	C	17.2±2.82	24.0±1.39		4.2±1.16	20.6±6.92	602±121.31	
		$p<0.05$	$p<0.05$		NS	NS	$p<0.05$	
	E	14.7±2.92	26.0±1.15		1.9±0.68	21.1±6.54	478±108.04	

*Filt PO_4 = filtered phosphate. Right and left stand for right and left kidneys.

TABLE II

Effect of 25 hydroxycholecalciferol on renal HCO_3 reabsorption in TPTX dogs.

		GFR	Tm/GFR	Plasma HCO_3	FE Cl	FE PO_4	Filt PO_4	Plasma PO_4
		ml/min	mEq/l GFR	mEq/l	%	%	µg/min	mg/100 ml
TPTX Propylene Glycol (n = 4)								
Right	C	22.0±1.71	27.6±1.83	31.6±0.72	1.1±0.61	3.2±1.93	1007±140.18	4.5±0.29
		NS	NS	NS	NS	NS	NS	NS
	E	19.2±1.33	27.8±1.85	33.0±0.51	1.4±0.75	9.9±6.78	927± 92.30	4.8±0.32
Left	C	29.9±4.05	26.8±1.64		1.6±0.55	5.6±2.70	1365±321.00	
		NS	NS		NS	NS	NS	
	E	24.1±4.50	27.1±1.72		1.9±1.05	13.5±7.52	1151±205.90	
TPTX 25 OHD (n = 4)								
Right	C	29.1±1.92	28.6±0.69	32.5±0.48	1.0±0.29	6.6±3.31	1353±166.97	4.6±0.40
		NS	NS	p<0.02	NS	NS	NS	NS
	E	29.1±2.73	29.3±0.59	34.4±0.29	1.2±0.39	11.6±5.81	1378±193.61	4.7±0.34
Left	C	33.1±0.94	28.1±0.56		1.0±0.28	9.6±7.50	1532±144.14	
		NS	NS		NS	NS	NS	
	E	30.7±2.63	29.0±0.50		1.4±0.41	9.6±6.50	1447±184.95	

GFR, HCO_3 reabsorption, Cl and PO_4 excretion. Intact dogs
infused with 25 OHD showed a significant increase in HCO_3
reabsorption in both the infused and in the contralateral
kidney (figure 1).   Plasma HCO_3 and fractional Cl excretion
were unchanged before and after 25 OHD infusion. Fractional
PO_4 excretion was high in the control period due to HCO_3 infusion; it remained unchanged after 25 OHD administration
(figure 2).
     In TPTX dogs 25 OHD administration did not result in any
change in HCO_3 reabsorption (figure 3), GFR, fractional Cl
excretion, or fractional PO_4 excretion.

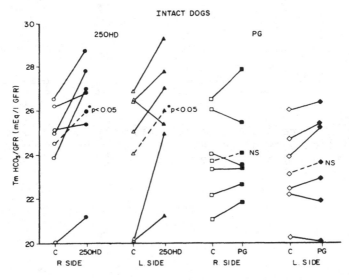

Fig. 1. The left panel shows HCO_3 reabsorption (Tm/GFR)
in intact dogs before (C) and during 25 OHD administration. The right panel shows HCO_3 reabsorption before
and during propylene glycol infusion. The dashes
indicate the mean for all dogs.

DISCUSSION

     Our results clearly demonstrate that acute infusion of 25
OHD increases renal bicarbonate reabsorption in the dog. The
increase in bicarbonate reabsorption was observed only in the
presence of parathyroid glands which suggests that the presence of parathyroid hormone is essential for this effect of
vitamin D. This observation agrees with the data of Popovtzer
et al who demonstrated an effect of vitamin D on phosphate
reabsorption only in the presence of parathyroid hormone (5).
     Vitamin D administration did not decrease the phospha-

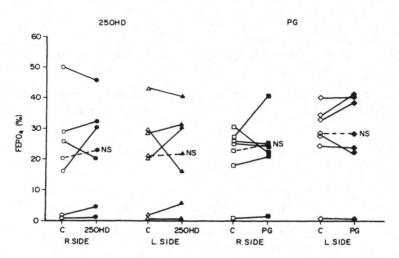

Fig. 2.   Fractional PO$_4$ excretion (FEPO$_4$) is presented in intact dogs before and during 25 OHD administration (left panel) and before and during PG administration (right panel).

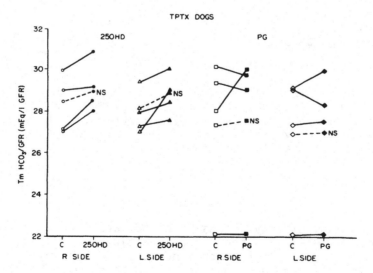

Fig. 3.   HCO$_3$ reabsorption in TPTX dogs treat with 25 OHD (left panel) and PG (right panel).

turia of bicarbonate loading. This is somewhat suprising
since it has been recently demonstrated that increased levels
of parathyroid hormone is the main factor responsible for the
phosphaturia of bicarbonate administration (12). We have no
clear cut explanation for this finding but it is possible that
the tendency for vitamin D to enhance phosphate reabsorption
under these circumstances was overridden by increased levels
of parathyroid hormone and volume expansion caused by sodium
bicarbonate administration.

The mechanism whereby vitamin D enhances bicarbonate
reabsorption is not clear. It is possible that enhanced
bicarbonate reabsorption is secondary to a generalized action
of vitamin D in the proximal tubule but a specific effect of
vitamin D in the distal nephron cannot be excluded.

The finding that vitamin D enhances renal bicarbonate
reabsorption may be relevant to the problem of hyperchloremic
acidosis of hyperparathyroidism. Muldowney et al described the
occurrance of hyperchloremic acidosis in patients with primary
hyperparathyroidism and in secondary hyperparathyroidism due
to malabsorption (6,7,13). They demonstrated that the maximal
rate of bicarbonate reabsorption was depressed in these
patients and that with successful treatment of the hyperparathyroidism metabolic acidosis was corrected. They suggested
that parathyroid hormone inhibits renal bicarbonate reabsorption and that increased levels of parathyroid hormone can
cause metabolic acidosis. More recently, the effect of
parathyroid hormone on renal bicarbonate reabsorption was
studied. Karlinsky et al (8) demonstrated that pharmacologic
doses of parathyroid hormone had a small effect on bicarbonate
reabsorption in intact dogs. In thyroparathyroidectomized
dogs bicarbonate reabsorption was increased; administration of
parathyroid hormone to these animals depressed bicarbonate
reabsorption to control levels. Crumb et al (9) demonstrated
that pharmacologic doses of parathyroid hormone depresses
whereas hypercalcemia enhances bicarbonate reabsorption in
intact and thyroparathyroidectomized dogs. These studies
demonstrate that parathyroid hormone plays an important role
in renal bicarbonate reabsorption; however, in order to
demonstrate that parathyroid hormone causes renal tubular
acidosis one must show that parathyroid hormone administration
lowers bicarbonate reabsorption below the normal plasma
bicarbonate concentration (8). The failure to demonstrate
this with pharmacologic doses of parathyroid hormone has cast
doubt that parathyroid hormone per se can cause metabolic
acidosis (8). Coe studied thirteen patients with hyperparathyroidism and found only two patients with metabolic acidosis.
He concluded that parathyroid hormone was not an important
regulator of acid excretion (14).

Gold et al demonstrated that chronic phosphate depletion in dogs leads to a decrease in bicarbonate reabsorption (15). Since phosphate depletion occurs in hyperparathyroidism they suggested that phosphate depletion, rather than increased levels of parathyroid hormone, is responsible for the metabolic acidosis of hyperparathyroidism (15,16). The depression of bicarbonate reabsorption was of small magnitude and could hardly account for the metabolic acidosis in hyperparathyroidism. It is possible that the presence of more than one factor is necessary for the development of metabolic acidosis with hyperparathyroidism. The ideal situation for the generation of metabolic acidosis in hyperparathyroid patients without renal failure would be the simultaneous presence of high parathyroid hormone levels, phosphate depletion, hypocalcemia and vitamin D deficiency. All these factors are present in malabsorption and this could explain the more frequent occurrance of metabolic acidosis in secondary hyperparathyroidism than in primary hyperparathyroidism.

SUMMARY

The effects of acute administration of 25 hydroxycholecalciferol on bicarbonate reabsorption was studied in dogs. 25 hydroxycholecalciferol infused into the renal artery at a dose of 0.2 μg/kg/hour led to a small but significant bilateral increase in bicarbonate reabsorption in intact dogs. 25 hydroxycholecalciferol had no effect on bicarbonate reabsorption in thyroparathyroidectomized dogs. The phosphaturia of bicarbonate administration was not altered by 25 hydroxycholecalciferol administration.

REFERENCES

1. Cekle, D., Stroder, J., and Rostock, D.: The effect of vitamin D on renal inorganic phosphate reabsorption of normal rats, parathyroidectomiaed rats and rats with rickets. Pediat. Res. 5:40, 1971.

2. Puschett, J.B., Moranz, J., and Kurnick W.S.: Evidence for a direct action of cholecalciferol and 25-hydroxycholecalciferol on the renal transport of phosphate, sodium, and calcium. J. Clin. Invest. 51:373, 1972.

3. Puschett, J.B., Fernandez, P.C., Boyle, I.T., Gray, R.W., Omdahl, J.L., and DeLuca H.F.: The acute renal tubular effects of 1,25-dihydroxycholecalciferol. Proc. Soc. Exp. Biol. Med. 141:379, 1972.

4. Puschett, J.B., Beck. W.S.Jr., Jelonek, A., and Fernandez, P.C.: Study of the renal tubular interactions of thyro-calcitonin cyclic adenosine 3',5'-monophosphate, 25-hydroxycholecalciferol, and calcium ion. J. Clin. Invest. 53:756, 1974.

5. Popovtzer, M.M., Robinette, J.B., Deluca, H.F., and Holick, M.F.: The acute effect of 25-hydroxycholecal-ciferol on renal handling of phosphorus. J. Clin. Invest. 53:913, 1974.

6. Muldowney, F.P., Donohoe, J.F., Freaney, R, Kampff, C., and Swan, M.: Parathormone induced renal bicarbonate wastage in intestinal malabsorption and in chronic renal failure. Irish J. Med. Sci. 3:221, 1970.

7. Muldowney, F.P., Freaney R., and McGeeney, D.: Renal tubular acidosis and amino-aciduria in osteomalacia of dietary or intestinal origin. Quart. J. Med. 37:517, 1968.

8. Karlinsky, M.L., Sager, D.S., Kurtzman, N.A., and Pillay, V.K.G.: Effect of parathormone and cyclic adenosine monophosphate on renal bicarbonate reabsorption. Am. J. Physiol. 227:1226, 1974.

9. Crumb, C.K., Martinez-Maldonado, M., Eknoyan, G., and Suki, W.: Effects of volume expansion, purified para-thyroid extract and calcium on renal bicarbonate absorp-tion in the dog. J. Clin. Invest. 54:1287, 1974.

10. Booth, B.E., Tsai, H.C., and Curtis-Morris, R. Jr.: Metabolic acidosis in the vitamin D deficient chick. Proc. VIII Ann. Cong. Neph. page 10, 1975.

11. Kurtzman, N.A.: Regulation of renal bicarbonate reab-sorption by extracellular volume. J. Clin. Invest. 49:586, 1970.

12. Mercado, A., Slatopolsky, E., and Klahr, S.: On the mechanisms responsible for the phosphaturia of bicar-bonate administration. J. Clin. Invest. 56:1386, 1975.

13. Muldowney, F.P., Carroll, D.V., Donohoe, J.F., and Freaney, R.F.: Correction of renal bicarbonate wastage by parathyroidectomy. Quart. J. Med. 40:487, 1971.

14. Coe, F.L.: Magnitude of metabolic acidosis in primary hyperparathyroidism. Arch. Int. Med. 134:262, 1974.

15. Gold, L.W., Massry, S.G., Arieff, A.I. and Coburn, J.W.:
     Renal bicarbonate wasting during phosphate depletion - A
     possible cause of altered acid-base homeostasis in
     hyperparathyroidism. J. Clin. Invest. 52:2556, 1973.

16. Massry, S.G., Kurokawa, K., Arieff, A.I., and Ben-Isaac,
     C.: Metabolic acidosis of hyperparathyroidism. Arch.
     Int. Med. 134:385, 1974.

ACKNOWLEDGEMENT

We would like to thank Dr. Hector DeLuca who kindly
provided the 25 hydroxycholecalciferol used in this study.

PARTIAL BODY PHOSPHORUS BY NEUTRON ACTIVATION ANALYSIS AND ITS

CLINICAL APPLICATION

J.T. DABEK, B.H.B. ROBINSON, B.J. THOMAS, K. AL-HITI,
P.W. DYKES, J.H. FREMLIN, D.A. HEATH
UNIVERSITY OF BIRMINGHAM, ENGLAND

INTRODUCTION

About 780g of phosphorus is present in the average 70Kg man
(1), 85% of this is associated with calcium in bone and 15% is
present in soft tissue (2). Thus only $\frac{1}{2}$% of total body phosphorus
is present as phosphate in blood plasma and extracellular fluid.
Serum inorganic phosphorus is not strictly controlled, like serum
Ca but may vary in the individual up to 2 mg/100 ml or so, i.e.
about 30-40% (2). Obviously the PO4 content of a particular bone
will vary in diseases such as osteomalacia, osteoporosis and hyperparathyroidism both during development of the disease and during
treatment. Likewise the phosphorus content of soft tissue may vary
in these diseases. Because so little of the total body phosphorus
is present in the blood plasma and because its concentration is
variable (2), the plasma phosphate concentration does not reflect
soft tissue or bone phosphorus accurately. The present paper reports
on a non-invasive method for measuring tissue phosphorus changes
in a section of the thoraco-lumbar region of the trunk, using in-
vivo neutron activation analysis.

METHOD

(a) Outline

A collimated beam of fast neutrons produced by the reaction of
10.2 MeV cyclotron protons with a thick lithium target is directed
at a 20 x 10 cm area of the lumbo-thoracic trunk. ^{28}Al($T\frac{1}{2}$ = 2.31
mins: γ = 1.78 MeV) is produced from ^{31}P by an n, α fast neutron reaction in the irradiated bone and soft tissue with a dose of 3 Rem
(quality factor = 10) to the skin over 150 seconds. Counting is

commenced 150 seconds from the end of radiation, using a 15cm x 12 cm
NaI (Tl) detector. The ^{28}Al counts recorded in the first 5 minutes
of counting divided by the neutron dose, measured by a cadmium-coated
BF$_3$ counter, gives a measure of the phosphorus content of the irradiated tissue. Serial changes in this index reflect changes in soft-
tissue or bone phosphorus content.

(b) Production of Neutrons

The 152 cm fixed energy cyclotron of the University of
Birmingham is used to produce 10.2 MeV protons. These impinge on a
Lithium target to produce neutrons by the reaction ^{7}Li (p,n)^{7}Be.
The energy of these neutrons varies from 0 to 8 MeV with mean 3.5 MeV.

(c) Collimation of Neutrons (Fig. 1)

The lithium target is surrounded by neutron-absorbing boron-
doped paraffin wax except in the forward direction, where the beam
passes into a tapering rectangular-section steel collimator which
gives a spot 20 cm high x 10 cm wide, 1 metre from the target. This
collimator is surrounded by boron-doped paraffin wax. The neutron
flux in the umbra of the collimator is 3% of that in beam.

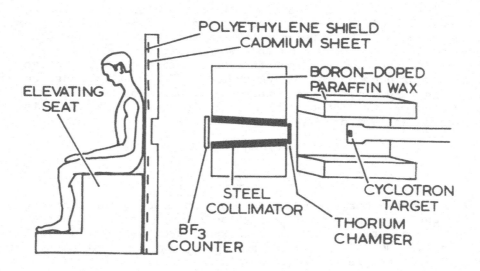

Fig. 1 Irradiation Geometry

(d) Positioning of the Patient for Irradiation (Fig. 1)

The lower limit of irradiation is defined by the line joining
the iliac crests and the midline is positioned in the midplane of the
collimator. Thus, a 20 cm high x 10 cm wide volume of tissue symmetrical about the midline, is irradiated. Repositioning is according to these bony landmarks.

(e) Counting the Induced Activity (Fig. 2)

A single 15 cm diameter x 12 cm NaI (Tl) detector is used. The
patient sits in a chair with a perspex back support. The midline is
positioned along a vertical mark on the perspex. The crystal is positioned up to the perspex support and its height adjusted so that the
lowest point of its lead shielding is at the point of intersection of
the midline and the line of iliac crests. Counting begins 150 seconds
after the end of irradiation and continues for twenty minutes in consecutive 5 minute periods. Correction for patient movement is by a
small ^{137}Cs source ($\gamma = \cdot 662$ MeV, $T\frac{1}{2} = 30$ yrs) taped to the skin at the

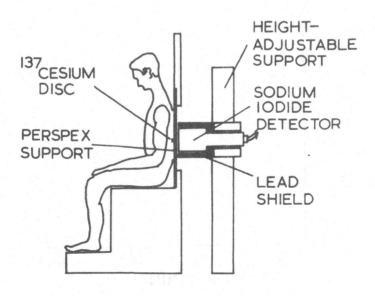

Fig. 2 Counting Geometry

midpoint of the irradiated area. The change in Cs counts with distance from the crystal has been correlated with changes in ^{28}Al
counts from the spine of a human skeleton so that correction to a
'zero position' is possible (Fig. 3). Standard electronics and
multi-channel analysis is employed.

(f) Dosimetry

The total skin dose is measured using fast neutron badges and
γ/β badges both processed by the National Radiation Protection Board.
The incident fast neutron flux is monitored by both a Thorium Fission
counter and a Boron Trifloride counter. The latter is placed in a
thin cadmium sheath. The total dose to the area irradiated is 3 Rem.
The BF$_3$ counter, which is correct to ± 1% is used to normalize the
^{28}Al counts.

(g) Calculation of the Results

The partial body phosphorus content is expressed in arbitrary
units and represents ^{28}Al counts divided by BF$_3$ neutron monitor

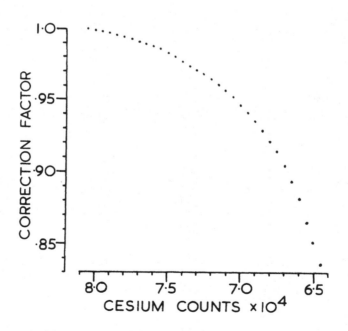

Fig. 3 Position Correction Factor

dose readings. The ^{28}Al count is obtained by subtracting the sum of counts under the ^{28}Al peak in the five-minute counting period beginning 17½ minutes after the end of radiation, from the sum for the period beginning 2½' after irradiation. (Fig. 4). Typically about 1500 counts would be subtracted from 3500 counts. The statistical error is thus about 3%. The overall reproducibility in phantom studies is about 5%.

THE PATIENTS

The patients were attending the local Birmingham hospitals for treatment of chronic renal failure, hypercalcaemia without apparent cause after investigation, hyperparathyroidism or osteomalacia. Details of these patients are shown in Table 1.

Eight patients had chronic renal failure and 3 of these were under treatment with 1 alpha hydroxycholecalciferol (1∝ -OHD$_3$) and none received regular aludrox therapy. Four patients had parathyroidectomy for primary hyperparathyroidism, 5 patients had mild hypercalcaemia and 3 had small doses of vitamin D$_2$ and calcium as treatment for osteomalacia. All the patients gave their consent to be studied after a brief explanation of the aims.

In all cases the measurements were made at intervals of several months.

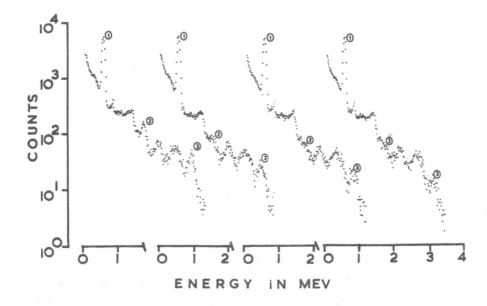

Fig. 4 Typical Spectra : 1 = ^{137}Cs ; 2 = ^{28}AL ; 3 = ^{49}Ca

TABLE 1

Details of Patients Studied

Initials	Diagnosis		Age	Sex	Treatment	Bone Disease
C.B.	C.R.F.	Alports Synd.	36	M	Diet	$\pm$
M.R.	"	Renal calculi	62	F	Dialysis	++
R.S.	"	G/N	36	F	Dialysis	++
J.W.	"	G/N	46	M	Diet	-
T.J.	"	G/N	39	M	Dialysis	-
E.G.	"	G/N	39	F	Dialysis & 1 - OH D_3	++
P.B.	"	G/N	46	F	Dialysis & 1 - OH D_3	++
R.W.	"	Poly-cystic	45	M	Dialysis & 1 - OH D_3	++
L.B.	Hypercalcaemia		51	F	-	+
C.G.	"		49	M	-	-
K.G.	"		45	F	-	-
M.P.	"		35	M	-	-
J.K.	"		36	M	-	-
L.J.	Hyperpara-thyroidism		36	F	Parathyroid-ectomy	$\pm$
C.B.	"		57	F	"	+
M.G.	"		53	F	"	-
D.T.	"		45	F	"	$\pm$
O.P.	Osteomalacia		70	F	Vit D_2/Ca	++
B.Z.	"		23	F	"	++
D.A.	"		48	M	"	++

C.R.F. = Chronic Renal Failure

G.N. = Glomerulo Nephritis
P.N. = Pyelonephritis
H   = Hypercalcaemia of mild degree

P.H. = Primary Hyperpara-thyroidism
O.M. = Osteomalacia
1 - OH D_3 = 1 - alpha - hy-droxy Vitamin D_3

RESULTS

The changes in spinal phosphorus in the groups of patients studied are shown in Fig. 5. The changes seen in chronic renal failure under treatment with 1 alpha OH Vitamin D_3 in the three patients are seen to be significant, whilst dialysis alone was associated with a significant change in one patient only. Dietary treatment alone was not associated with significant changes.

Parathyroidectomy produced significant rises, up to 38% in one patient, indicating the phosphate depletion, characteristic of this disease, which is reversed when the parathyroid adenoma is removed. Likewise in osteomalacia all three patients showed significant increases in trunkal phosphorus.

Four of five patients with mild hypercalcaemia showed no change or a significant fall in trunkal phosphorus. Paradoxically the 5th patient showed a significant rise of 28%. This is unexplained, but was associated with a similar rise in spinal calcium measured simultaneously by in-vivo neutron activation analysis using the $^{48}Ca(n,\gamma)^{49}Ca$ reaction (3,4).

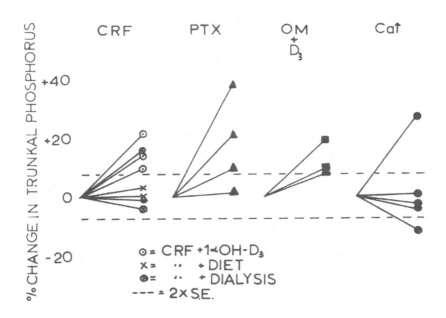

Fig. 5 Trunkal Phosphorus Changes in some Clinical Situations

The relation between spinal calcium and trunkal phosphorus is
shown in Fig. 6. Overall the phosphorus tended to rise as the calcium rose. The change in spinal calcium in one patient undergoing
regular dialysis therapy and then treated with 1 ∝ -OH D₃ was +128%
whilst the change in phosphorus was +22%. This is consistent with
high soft-tissue phosphorus content before therapy, and a marked
loss of spinal bone mineral, so that bone phosphorus changes would
be masked but bone calcium changes patent. In fact the general finding was that calcium changes tended to be greater than phosphorus
changes in the patients studied.

In 15 of the patients the relation between trunkal phosphorus
changes and serum inorganic phosphorus changes was examined, but no
correlation was found. This result was not due to inclusion of a
group of patients with chronic renal failure.

DISCUSSION

The data presented indicate that useful measurements of tissue
phosphorus content are possible using an in-vivo neutron activation

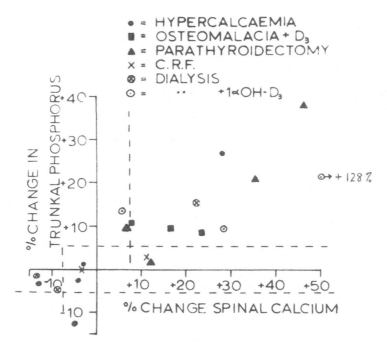

Fig. 6 Relation of Trunkal Phosphorus to Spinal Calcium

technique to measure partial body phosphorus in the thoraco-lumbar trunk. The lack of correlation between serum phosphorus concentration and tissue phosphorus content underlines the need for measurement of the latter. The use of localized irradiation limits the neutron dose which on a whole-body basis represents about 60 m Rem. The possibility of simultaneous measurement of spinal calcium and trunkal phosphorus further adds to the usefulness of the technique. The simultaneous measurement of calcium will help in differentiating soft-tissue phosphorus changes from bone phosphorus changes. The technique should prove particularly useful in investigating the importance of phosphorus in the evolution of the bone disease of renal failure.

REFERENCES

1. Report of the Task Group on Reference Man. I.C.R.P. No. 23, 1974, Pergaman Press, Oxford. p. 310.

2. KRANE, S.M. Calcium, phosphate and magnesium. In the International Encyclopaedia of Pharmacology and Therapeutics. Eds. H. Rasmussen, London, Pergamen Press Ltd.

3. DABEK, J.T., HEATH, D.A., FREMLIN, J.H., THOMAS, B.J., PRESTWICH, W.,AL-HITI, K., and HARDWICKE, J. In-vivo measurement of spinal calcium by neutron activation analysis. Clinical Science and Molecular Medicine, 47, 5, p. 22, 1974.

4. AL-HITI,K., THOMAS, B.J., AL-TIKATY,S.A., ETTINGER, K.V., FREMLIN, J.H., DABEK, J.T. Spinal calcium : Its in-vivo measurement in Man. Int. J. of Appl. Rad. and Isotopes, 27, p. 97-102, 1976.

THE INTESTINAL ABSORPTION OF PHOSPHATE IN NORMAL HUMAN SUBJECTS

M.L. Cabrejas, M.A. Méndez Falcón, Z. Man Morgenstern,
O.J. Degrossi, and C.A. Mautalen
Centro de Medicina Nuclear (CNEA) y Unidad de Osteopa-
tías Metabólicas, Sección Endocrinología
Hospital de Clínicas, Buenos Aires, Argentina

In contrast to the considerable information obtained on the intestinal handling of calcium in healthy human subjects as well as in disease states (1), there are few data concerning the gastrointestinal absorption of phosphate.

One of the reasons to explain the paucity of the studies on this area is that the most readily available radioactive isotope of phosphate - 32P - is a pure β emitter. External measurement of β rays is very difficult owing to the short range of its particles. However, from the results of different studies (2,3,4,5) it is evident that the Bremsstrahlung production by pure β emitters can be used successfully for tracing such isotopes.

The present report describes a simple technique, using a whole body counter, that permits to determine with accuracy the intestinal absorption of 32P.

MATERIAL AND METHODS

Clinical Material: Thirty subjects, 12 men and 18 women (average age 40, range 17 to 68 years old) were studied. Eighteen were hospitalized patients in the wards of the general hospital, who, despite their original reason for hospitalization, were well and in normal health at the time phosphorous absorption was measured.

Twelve non hospitalized subjects were studied daily during the performance of the procedure. Five of them were staff volunteers of the hospital, and seven were patients who showed no evidence of skeletal, endocrine, renal or gastrointestinal disease. All subjects are referred to hereafter as normal.

The hospitalized patients were on the regular hospital diet . The ambulatory subjects ate their usual home diets.

Procedure: Each subject fasted from the preceding night until 2 hours after the administration of the oral dose.

A tracer oral dose of approximately 80 uCi of 32P was added to a 25 ml solution containing different quantities of phosphrous (as PO4H2Na). Two rinses of approximately 50 ml of water were then given immediately.

Intestinal absorption of 32P was calculated adding the body retention and the urinary excretion of (absorbed) 32P, both measured seven days after the oral administration of 32P.

Urine was collected for seven days in 5 l tanks, and measured under a 8" x 4" NaI (Ta) crystal. Percent of administered dose was determined calculating the urinary activity with a suitable standard.

In order to study the fecal endogenous excretion of phosphate, six subjects received a sudden dose of 32P intravenously. The endo genous excretion of 32P at 7 days was calculated subtracting the body retention plus the urine excretion from 100 %.

Analytical methods: The patients 32P activity was measured in a whole body counter with a single 8" x 4" NaI (Ta) crystal, shadow shield, scanning bed type. The patients were measured both in the prone and supine positions on a stretcher. The detector scans above the bed at a distance of 35 cm from the centre of the plane surface of the detector to the bed.

The pulses are fed into a 400 channel analyzer. The spectrum of the Bremsstrahlung emitted from large homogenously active objects consist of energy photons up to 400 KeV. Since background contribution is very high for low energies, and 32P emission is negligible for high energies, the 60 to 210 KeV energy band was considered for 32P determination.

Several measurements of some patients, while no excretion had taken place, were made on the initial studies. Three patients were measured hourly up to a maximun of 6 hours after the administration of the dose. Since the isotope distribution changed during the first hours, the measurements in the prone and supine positions varied (prone measurements diminished and supine measurements increased) but the sum of both remained constant. This means that the determinations of 32P body activity taken in each individual during the first 2 to 6 hours after the oral dose, and before any urinary excretion, could be taken as a reliable 100 % assessment of the administered dose.

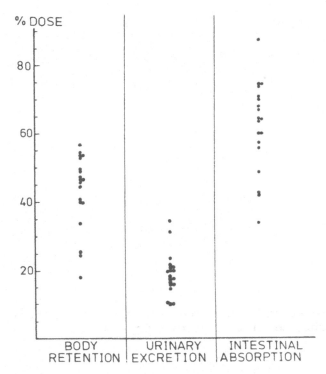

Figure 1. Body retention and urinary excretion at 7 days, and intestinal absorption of 32P in 19 control subjects which received an oral dose of tracer mixed with 1000 mg of phosphate carrier (as PO4H2Na)

Especially towards lower energies the background varies considerably with the weight of the measured object. For this reason the activity of each patient was measured before the administration of 32P and this result was used as the background counting throughout the study. For the urine, a 5 l tank containing water was placed under the counter for accurate assessment of the background activity.

The statistical error was less than 2 % for the whole body counter and less than 5 % for the urinary excretion determinations.

For accurate measurements of the used radionuclide, a dose of approximately 80 uCi had to be administered. The effective half life of 32P is 11 days (6). After 7 half lives (77 days = 11 weeks) the subjects received a whole body dose of 0.85 rads. This dose is slightly less than the weekly permissible dose for employees using radioactive materials.

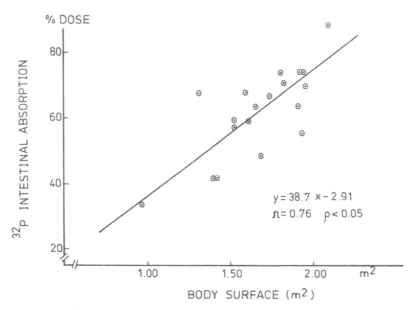

Figure 2. Correlation between the intestinal absorption of 32P and and the body surface in 19 control subjects.

RESULTS

Figure 1 shows the results obtained in 19 subjects who received the oral dose of 32P mixed with a carrier of 1000 mg of phosphate (as PO4H2Na). The body retention at 7 days was (average $\pm$ 1 SEM) 43.4 $\pm$ 2.5 % of the dose. The urinary excretion during the same period was 18.9 $\pm$ 1.5 and the intestinal absorption of 32P 62.3 $\pm$ 3.1 % of the dose.

The intestinal absorption of 32P was found to be positively correlated with the body surface of the subjects studied (r = +0.76; p < 0.05) (Figure 2). The results obtained in each subject were therefore corrected to a uniform body surface of 1.73 m2. The corrected intestinal absorption of 32P was therefore (average $\pm$ 1 SEM) 63.9 $\pm$ 2.2 % of the dose (range 49 to 87 percent).

There was no correlation between the age of the subjects and the intestinal absorption of 32P.

Five subjects received the oral tracer dose of 32P mixed with 200 - 500 mg of phosphate carrier (as PO4H2Na). The intestinal absorption of 32P in this group was higher than that observed in the controls receiving the dose with a 1000 mg phosphate carrier (72.2 $\pm$ 2.3 vs. 63.9 $\pm$ 2.2 % of the dose). The difference, however, only

Table I- Body retention (R), urinary excretion (U) and R + U, 7 days after the administration of the intravenous dose.

Patient Sex/Age	Body Retention = R (% dose)	Urinary Excretion = U (% dose)	R + U (% dose)
EL F/36	70.37	23.04	93.41
AV F/47	73.00	25.48	98.48
ME F/65	86.44	16.08	102.52
MG F/41	79.65	25.14	104.79
IL F/40	69.98	23.08	93.06
NH F/40	84.53	14.99	99.52
$\overline{X}$	77.33	21.30	98.63
σ	7.23	4.59	4.74
$\sigma_{\overline{X}}$	2.95	1.87	1.93

$\overline{X}$ = Average; σ = Standard deviation; $\sigma_{\overline{X}}$ = Standard error of the mean

approached significance ($0.05 < p < 0.1$).

In order to assess the endogenous fecal excretion of the 32P, six subjects received an intravenous dose of the isotope. Table I shows the results obtained. Average fecal excretion in 7 days was 1.37 ± 0.07 percent of the administered dose.

DISCUSSION

The present paper describes a simple method to assess the gastro-intestinal absorption of phosphate using a whole body counter. Although considerable information has been gathered by Caniggia and Gennari (7) by serial serum sampling after the oral administration of 32P, the use of a whole body counter has the advantage of of the simplicity of measurements as well as greater sensitivity and accuracy.

As suggested by the presently reported results and previous data (8) the absorption of 32P depends on the dose of phosphate carrier employed. One thousand milligrams of phosphate in the carrier has been selected hoping to allow the differentiation of high and low phosphate absorbers from normal subjects.

The fecal excretion of the intravenously injected 32P was relatively small (Table I) supporting previous studies of Erf and Lawrence (9). These authors measuring directly the 32P content of the stools found that the 6 days cumulative fecal excretion of the intravenously injected tracer was less than 2 % of the dose in a group of normal subjects and patients with leukemia. The error induced by the fecal excretion of the already absorbed 32P would be therefore relatively low and would not interfere with the clinical application of the described technique.

The use of a precise and relatively simple technique for the measurement of phosphate gastro-intestinal absorption would improve our understanding of the factors that govern it and the alterations produced in different diseases. The results obtained can be used as a provisional normal reference standard of radioactive phosphate absorption for control subjects on a regular diet.

REFERENCES

1- Mautalen, C.A., Cabrejas, M.L., and Soto, R.J.: Isotopic determination of intestinal calcium absorption in normal subjects. Metabolism 18:395,1969.

2- Liden, K.: The determination of 90Sr and other beta emitters in human beings from external measurement of the Bremsstrahlung. Proc. 2nd. U N Int. Conf.P U A E 23:133,1958.

3- Tubiana, M., Albarede, P., and Nahum, H.: Study of radioactive phosphorous (32P) distribution in man by external Bremsstrahlung measurement. Proc. 2nd. U N Int. Conf. P U A E 26:217,1958.

4- Mehl , H.G.: Kinetics and distribution of 32P as measured by Bremsstrahlung intensity and diagnosis and therapy. Proc. 2nd. U N Int. Conf. P U A E 26:224,1958.

5- Bengtsson, L.G.: Human beta Bremsstrahlung detection by means of thin and thick sodium iodide crystals. Assessment of Radioactivity in Man. I A E A. Vol 1:91,1964.

6- Quimby, E., and Feitelberg, S.: Radioactive isotopes in Medicine and Biology. Ed. Lea & Febiger. Phyladelphia, USA:122,1963.

7- Caniggia, A., and Gennari, C.: Absorption du phosphate radioactif chez l'homme et sa régulation. Symposium International sur Phosphate et Métabolisme Phosphocalcique. Paris, 1970.

8- Gennari, C., Bencini, M. Palazzuoli, V., and Cesari, L.: Influen
za di una elevata dose di "carrier" sull'assorbimento intestinale
del radiocalcio e del radiofosfato. Boll. Soc. Ital. Biol. Sper.
42:589,1965.

9- Erf, L.A., and Lawrence, J.H.: Clinical studies with the aid
of radioactive phosphrous. I) The absorption and distribution
of radio-phosphrous in the blood and its excretion by normal
individuals and patients with leukemia. J. Clin. Invest. 20:
567,1941.

EFFECT OF THE DIPHOSPHONATE EHDP ON PLASMA INORGANIC PHOSPHATE AND HEMOGLOBIN OXYGEN AFFINITY OF DIABETIC AND HEALTHY SUBJECTS

Jørn Ditzel, Chr. Hau and Niels Daugaard

Department of Medicine

Aalborg Regional Hospital, Denmark

INTRODUCTION

Red cells of patients with diabetes mellitus have been found to contain increased proportions of glyco-hemoglobins (Hb A_{Ic}) with increased oxygen affinity (1,2). Hemoglobin A_{Ic}, which comprises about 3-6 per cent of normal human hemoglobin, is elevated to 10-20 per cent in diabetes. Hemoglobin A_{Ic} concentration correlates with both glucose intolerance and fasting blood glucose (3). 2,3-diphosphoglycerate in the red cells, through its effect on the position of the oxy-hemoglobin dissociation curve, is an important regulator of oxygen transport. In patients with insulin requiring diabetes the content of red cell 2,3-diphosphoglycerate (2,3-DPG) has been found to vary much more than normally depending upon the state of metabolic control (4,5, 6,7). The variations in red cell 2,3-DPG in non-acidotic diabetics were not correlated to the blood glucose level but rather to fluctuations in plasma inorganic phosphate (7,8). In newly discovered diabetics a correlation was present between the concentration of plasma inorganic phosphate (Pi), red cell 2,3-DPG and the oxygen affinity of hemoglobin (8,9).

As red cells of diabetics contain much more hemoglobin A_{Ic} with increased oxygen affinity than red cells of healthy subjects, the red cell 2,3-DPG content has to be significantly elevated in diabetics in order to guarantee an optimal erythrocytic oxygen release

(6,7). In diabetics the oxygen release may be intermittently insufficient leading to hypoxic responses in the microcirculation and these responses may be of pathogenetic importance in the development of diabetic angiopathy (10).

It is well known that the plasma inorganic phosphate through its effect on the phosphofructokinase and glyceraldehyde-3-phosphate dehydrogenase may influence the red cell 2,3-DPG concentration and thereby the position of the oxyhemoglobin dissociation curve (ODC). In order to study pharmacologic agents, which can sustain hyperphosphatemia, we have examined the effect of the disodium ethane-1-hydroxy-1,1-diphosphonate, EHDP, on Pi, red cell 2,3-DPG and hemoglobin oxygen affinity of diabetic and healthy subjects.

PATIENTS AND METHODS

Oral disodium ethane-1-hydroxy-1,1-diphosphonate, EHDP, and placebo was given between meals in the forenoon as a single daily dose (20 mg kg^{-1} day^{-1}) for 28 days to 14 insulin-treated, non-acidotic male diabetics and 5 healthy male volunteers in a double blind trial. All subjects were non-smokers or smoked less than two cigarettes daily. The diabetics were all ambulatory and fully active with duration of their disease varying from 1 to 13 years (mean: 4,6 yrs.). The ages of the diabetic subjects varied from 18 to 43 years (mean: 30,3 yrs.) and the controls from 28 to 50 years (mean: 34,6 yrs.). None of the diabetics had severe anemia or infections, or suffered from cardiac, respiratory or renal insufficiency. Three showed minimal diabetic retinopathy.

All persons were examined after 28 days' treatment with EHDP or placebo in the morning after 12 hours of complete fasting. Arterial blood samples were drawn anerobically, immediately placed in iced-water, and assayed within 15 minutes for pH, pO_2, pCO_2, and standard bicarbonate in a BMS-3 blood gas system (Radiometer A/S, Copenhagen, Denmark). Venous blood was collected into heparinized syringes. Red cell indices were measured by means of a Coulter Counter S (Coulter Electronics Ltd., Dunstable, England). Red cell 2,3-diphosphoglycerate (2,3-DPG) concentration was determined according to Ericsson and de Verdier (11) and plasma inorganic phosphate (Pi) as described by Parekh and Jung (12).

Blood glucose measurements were performed with Technicon Auto Analyzer.

Oxyhemoglobin dissociation curves on heparinized whole blood were run in a Radiometer DCA-1 apparatus, the principles of which have been described in detail by Duvelleroy et al. (13). This method has been shown to give results which are identical with those obtained by the mixing technique (14). In addition, the pH of the blood was recorded continuously during the oxygenation procedure. Oxygen affinity was expressed as P_{50} i.e. pO_2 at 50% oxygen saturation, P_{25} and P_{75} at actual pH.

Student's t-test was used for statistical analysis. Means, standard deviation (SD) linear regressions, correlation coefficients, and significance test were performed with the Compucorp calculator Series 300 (Computer Design Corporation, Los Angeles, California, U.S.A.

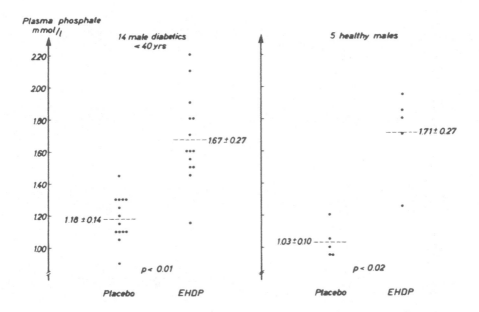

Fig. 1: The effect of EHDP and Placebo on plasma inorganic phosphate in diabetic and healthy subjects

RESULTS

Figure 1 shows the effect of EHDP on plasma inorganic phosphate (Pi) in diabetic and healthy subjects. The mean concentration of Pi increased in the diabetics from 1.18 to 1.67 mmol/l (p < 0.01) and in the healthy from 1.03 to 1.71 mmol/l (p < 0.02).

EHDP gave rise to a significant increase in the red cell 2,3-DPG content only in the diabetic subjects (15.2 vs. 16.3 µmol/g Hb, p < 0.005).

Figure 2 presents the P_{50} values of the ODC on placebo and on EHDP in diabetic and healthy subjects. In both groups the mean values significantly increased during EHDP treatment (diabetics: 25.4 vs. 26.6 mmHg, p < 0.02, healthy controls: 26.3 vs. 28.9 mmHg, p < 0.02). There was a significant relationship between the plasma inorganic phosphate concentration and the P_{50} at actual pH of the ODC in both diabetic (r = 0.58, p < 0.01) and in healthy subjects (r = 0.69, p < 0.05).

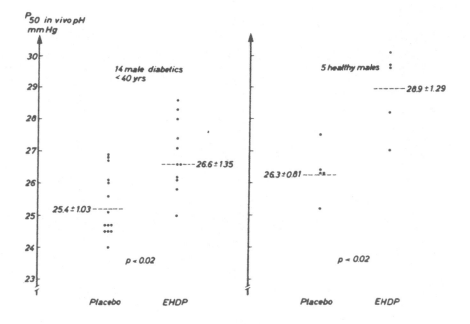

Fig. 2: The effect of EHDP and Placebo on the P_{50} at in vivo pH of the oxyhemoglobin dissociation curves in diabetic and healthy subjects

DISCUSSION

This study supports and amplifies previous reports emphasizing the importance of the level of plasma inorganic phosphate (Pi) on the oxygen transport function of red cells (4,6,7,15,16,17).

The diphosphonate EHDP when given for 28 days produced a prolonged elevation of Pi in both diabetic and healthy subjects and simultaneously a decrease in the oxygen affinity of hemoglobin. The level of Pi was significantly correlated to the position of the ODC. The hyperphosphatemia was not associated with significant changes in the level of serum calcium and the drug was well tolerated and without any toxic or side effects.

The mechanism leading to the change in oxygen affinity of the blood in the two groups of subjects appears to be different. In the diabetics the shift to the right of the ODC may be related, at least partly, to a significant increase in red cell 2,3-DPG concentration. On EHDP the mean 2,3-DPG content in the diabetics was significantly higher than normally. This tends to indicate that the 2,3-DPG compensated oxygen release prior to EHDP was not optimal in the diabetics. In the healthy subjects the increase in oxygen release capacity cannot be explained by this mechanism, since no increase in red cell 2,3-DPG occurred. However, in this group a slight but significant decrease in blood pH occurred and this might cause a decrease in the oxygen affinity of hemoglobin through the Bohr effect.

For the diabetics it may be advantageous to be able to counteract the effect of the increased amount of hemoglobin A_{IC} on the ODC. In doing so the reversible microvascular responses to decreased tissue oxygen availability may be prevented, which might postpone or prevent the development of diabetic angiopathy.

SUMMARY

The effect of oral disodium ethane-1-hydroxy-1,1-diphosphonate, EHDP (20 mg kg^{-1} day^{-1}) and placebo given for 28 days on plasma inorganic phosphate (Pi) red cell 2,3-diphosphoglycerate and oxygen affinity of hemoglobin was evaluated in 14 insulin-treated diabetics and 5 healthy volunteers. EHDP significantly increased mean

Pi (diabetics: 1.18 to 1.67 mmol/l, $p < 0.01$, controls: 1.03 to 1.71 mmol/l, $p < 0.02$) and P_{50} at in vivo pH of the oxyhemoglobin dissociation curve (diabetics: 25.4 to 26.6 mmHg, $p < 0.02$; controls: 26.3 to 28.9 mmHg, $p < 0.02$). Pi and P_{50} were correlated in both diabetics and in controls ($p < 0.05$). 2,3-DPG increased when the diabetics were on EHDP ($p < 0.005$). The study emphasizes the importance of Pi on red cell function and indicates that an elevation of Pi tends to counteract the defect in oxygen release capacity of the red cells in diabetic subjects.

ACKNOWLEDGEMENT

This study was supported by the Miami Valley Research Laboratories, Cincinnati, Ohio.

REFERENCES

1. Trivelli, L.S., Ranney, H.M. and Lai, H.T.: Hemoglobin components in patients with diabetes mellitus. New Engl. J. Med. 284: 353-357, 1971

2. Paulsen, E.P.: Hemoglobin A_{IC} in childhood diabetes. Metabolism 22: 269-271, 1973

3. Koenig, R.J., Peterson, C.M., Kilo, C., Cerami, A. and Williamson, J.R.: Hemoglobin A_{IC} as an indicator of the degree of glucose intolerance in diabetes. Diabetes 25: 230-232, 1976

4. Ditzel, J.: Effect of plasma inorganic phosphate on tissue oxygenation during recovery from diabetic ketoacidosis. Adv. Expl. Med. and Biol. 37A: 163-172, 1973

5. Standl. E. and Kolb, H.J.: 2,3-diphosphoglycerate fluctuation in erythrocytes reflecting pronounced blood glucose variations. Diabetologia 9: 461-466, 1973

6. Ditzel, J., Andersen, H. and Daugaard Peters, N.: Oxygen affinity of hemoglobin and red cell 2,3-diphosphoglycerate in childhood diabetes. Acta Paediatrica Scand. 64: 355-365, 1975

7. Ditzel, J. and Standl, E.: The problem of tissue oxygenation in diabetes mellitus II Evidence of disordered oxygen release from the erythrocytes of diabetics in various conditions of metabolic control. In: Diabetic Microangiopathy (Ditzel, J. and Poulsen, J.E. eds.). Acta med. Scand. Suppl. 578: 59-69, 1975

8. Ditzel, J. and Standl, E.: Plasma inorganic phosphate and erythrocyte 2,3-diphosphoglycerate concentrations in non-acidotic diabetics in various degrees of metabolic control. Clin. Chem. 22: 550-551, 1976

9. Ditzel, J., Jaeger, P.and Standl, E.: The oxygen transport System of red blood cells in non-acidotic diabetics in relation to metabolic control and variations in plasma inorganic phosphate. Submitted 1976

10. Ditzel, J.: The problem of tissue oxygenation in diabetes mellitus III The "three-in-one concept" for the development of diabetic microangiopathy and a rational approach to its prophylaxis. In: Diabetic Microangiopathy (Ditzel, J. and Poulsen, J.E. eds.) Acta med. Scand. Suppl. 578: 69-83, 1975

11. Ericsson, A. and de Verdier, C.H.: A modified method for the determination of 2,3-diphosphoglycerate in erythrocytes. Scand. J. clin. Lab. Invest. 29: 85-90, 1972

12. Parekh, A.C. and Jung, D.H.: Serum inorganic phosphorus determination using p-phenylene-diamine as a reducing agent. Clin. chim. Acta 27: 373-377, 1970

13. Duvelleroy, M.D., Buckes, R.C., Rosenkaimer, S., Tung, C. and Laver, M.A.: An oxyhemoglobin dissociation analyzer. J. Appl. Physiol. 28: 227-233, 1970

14. Bellingham, A.J. and Lenfant, C.: Hb affinity for O_2 determined by O_2-Hb dissociation analyzer and mixing technique. J. Appl. Physiol. 30: 903-904, 1971

15. Lichtman, M.A. and Miller, D.R.: Erythrocyte glycolysis, 2,3-diphosphoglycerate and adenosine triphosphate concentration in uremic subjects. Relationship to extracellular phosphate concentration. J. Lab. Clin. Med. 76: 267-279, 1970

16. Lichtman, M.A., Miller, D.R., Cohen, J. and Waterhouse, C.: Reduced red cell glycolysis, 2,3-diphosphoglycerate and adenosine triphosphate concentration, and increased hemoglobin-oxygen affinity caused by hypophosphatemia. Ann. Int. Med. 74: 562-568, 1971

17. Travis, S.F., Sugarman, H.J., Ruberg, R.L., Dudrick, S.J., Delivoria-Papadopoulos, M, Miller, L.D. and Oski, F.A.: Alteration of red cell glycolytic intermediates and oxygen transport as a consequence of hypophosphatemia in patients receiving intravenous hyperalimentation. New Engl. J. Med. 285: 763-768, 1971

THE ACTION OF 1αHYDROXY VITAMIN D$_3$ AND PHOSPHATE SUPPLEMENTS IN HYPOPHOSPHATAEMIC OSTEOMALACIA

M. PEACOCK, J.E. AARON, P.J. HEYBURN and B.E.C. NORDIN

M.R.C. MINERAL METABOLISM UNIT, THE GENERAL INFIRMARY,

LEEDS, LS1 3EX, YORKSHIRE, ENGLAND.

INTRODUCTION

Vitamin D resistant hypophosphataemic osteomalacia (VDRHPO) occurs as an inherited disorder or more unusually in association with certain connective tissue tumours[1]. The primary defect is considered to be a failure of phosphate transport with decreased tubular phosphate reabsorption and hypophosphataemia resulting in osteomalacia and myopathy[2].

The osteomalacia and myopathy are usually treated with a combination of phosphorus supplements and _pharmacological_ doses of vitamin D, although phosphorus supplements alone can be effective in some patients[2]. The results of such treatment however are not uniformly good and these patients remain a therapeutic challenge. Furthermore is is not clear how either of these therapies act. Phosphorus supplements may act by simply raising the plasma phosphate thus driving more phosphorus into bone. The plasma phosphate concentration however required to achieve this net transfer and the stimulus for simultaneous transport of calcium necessary for normal mineralisation are unknown. _Pharmacological_ doses of vitamin D may act directly on bone but their therapeutic effect may solely be due to their action on phosphate and calcium transport. The nature of the resistance of the bone to the action of

vitamin D remains uncertain.   It is unlikely to be due to a block
in vitamin D metabolism since the plasma concentrations of $1\alpha,25$
dihydroxy vitamin D_3 ($1\alpha,25(OH)_2D_3$) are normal in patients with
this disorder.   The resistance therefore seems to be at the receptors, and it has been postulated that since hypophosphataemia
should stimulate renal 1αhydroxylase, in VDRHPO normal concentrations of $1\alpha,25(OH)_2D_3$ represents a failure of response to hypophosphataemia.[3].

The present study details the abnormalities in a group of
patients with VDRHPO.   The effects of phosphorus supplements and
high doses of 1αhydroxy vitamin D_3 ($1\alpha OHD_3$) on the biochemical
abnormalities are described in an attempt to define firstly the
action of these therapies and secondly the biochemical defects
present in VDRHPO.

PATIENTS   The studies were performed in ten patients (6 male and
4 female) whose ages ranged from 10 to 70.   In only one patient
was there definite evidence of an inherited disorder and he and his
mother are included in the study.   In five other patients there
was a history of rickets in childhood and in three patients the
condition presented in adulthood.

METHODS   The methods used in these studies were carried out as
previously described[4]. Since the biochemistry was collected over
long time periods in all patients it has been expressed as mean
values for the various study periods.   The change in biochemistry
during treatment has been expressed as cumulative differences from
the mean untreated values (QUSUM).

RESULTS   Untreated   Table 1 shows the mean fasting plasma and
urine biochemistry in the ten patients before treatment.   The
plasma calcium, parathyroid hormone and 25 hydroxy vitamin D
concentrations were normal.   All patients had a low plasma phosphate with a decreased maximum tubular reabsorption of phosphate/L
glomerular filtrate (TmP/GFR).   The plasma alkaline phosphatase
was raised but in 4 of the 10 patients it was in the normal range.

Table 1

Plasma Ca mmol/L (2.25 - 2.60)			Plasma PO_4 mmol/L (0.8 - 1.3)			Plasma PTH ng/ml (0.5 - 1.5)		
Mean	S.D.	n	Mean	S.D.	n	Mean	S.D.	n
2.41	0.12	10	0.53	0.07	10	0.94	0.37	9

Plasma Alk. Ph. K.A/100ml (4 - 13)			TmP/GFR (0.7 - 1.4)			Urine OHP/Cr (0.022 - 0.006)		
Mean	S.D.	n	Mean	S.D.	n	Mean	S.D.	n
16.9	9.0	10	0.43	0.11	10	0.039	0.027	7

Table 2

^{45}Ca Absorption Fraction Dose Absorbed/Hour (0.3 - 1.2)			^{32}P Absorption Fraction Dose Absorbed/Hour (0.4 - 1.3)		
Mean	S.D.	n	Mean	S.D.	n
0.39	0.14	10	0.57	0.33	9

Table 3

% volume of Bone (15 - 30)			% volume of Osteoid (< 1)			% of Osteoid Surfaces (2 - 25)			% of Osteoid Surfaces with Calcification Fronts (60 - 100)		
Mean	S.D.	n	Mean	S.D.	n	Mean	S.D.	n	Mean	S.D.	n
37.9	11.5	9	13.8	11.2	8	76.8	23.4	8	28.6	11.7	8

The urine hydroxyproline/creatinine was raised but in 2 of the 7 patients it was in the normal range.

Table 2 shows the mean absorption of radiocalcium and radio-phosphorus. There was malabsorption of radiocalcium in 3 of the 10 patients and the others showed poor absorption. Of the 7 patients tested for absorption of radiophosphorus, 2 showed malabsorption.

Table 3 shows the results of histomorphometry on iliac crest biopsies. All patients showed an increase in the volume of bone and in the volume of osteoid. Almost all the surfaces were covered in thick osteoid and there was a defect in mineralisation as measured by the number of calcification fronts. Two of the

10 patients had no evidence of myopathy either clinically or on
electromyography.   These two patients had the least bone involvement as judged by the number of bone surfaces covered in osteoid.
<u>Effect of phosphorus supplements</u>   Figure 1 shows the effect of
phosphorus supplements on calcium and phosphorus balance in one
patient.   There was a rapid increase in bone turnover as measured
by radiocalcium kinetics, by plasma alkaline phosphatase and the
urine hydroxyproline/creatine ratio.   There was retention of
calcium and phosphorus and a fall in urine calcium.

A further illustration of the effect of phosphorus on one
patient established on a 6μg 1αOHD$_3$ is shown in Figure 2.   Oral
phosphorus supplements further increased the bone turnover rate,
and the retention of both calcium and phosphorus.

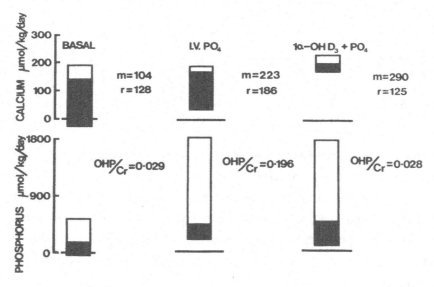

Fig. 1. The mean calcium and phosphorus balance in a patient untreated (basal), on phosphorus supplements (some given I.V.) and
on 6μg 1αOHD$_3$/day and oral phosphorus supplements. Intake is plotted positively from zero and urine (□) and faeces (■) negatively
from intake.   The corresponding data for mineralisation (m), resorption (r) and urine hydroxyproline/creatinine are shown.

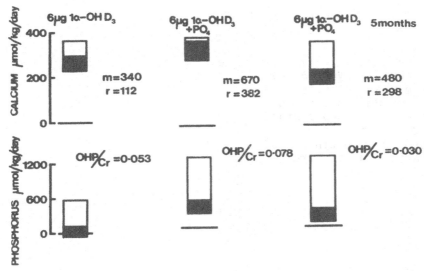

Fig. 2. The mean calcium and phosphorus balance in a patient on 6μg 1αOHD$_3$/day, immediately after the addition of oral phosphorus supplements and after 5 months of treatment. Intake is plotted positively from zero, urine (□) and faeces (■) negatively from intake. The corresponding data for mineralisation (m), resorption (r) and urine hydroxyproline/creatinine are shown.

Effect of 1 OHD$_3$ 6μg 1αOHD$_3$ increased the absorption of radio-calcium in all patients some into the hyperabsorption range, and as shown in Fig. 1 and 2 this was reflected in a large increase in calcium and phosphorus absorption, in bone turnover and net calcium and phosphorus retention.

The biochemical changes observed on treatment with 6μg 1αOHD$_3$ in one patient are shown in Fig. 3, 4 and 5. After two months there was an increase in urine hydroxyproline, which re-turned to its pre-treatment value by seven months and returned into the normal range by twelve months (Fig. 3).

The plasma alkaline phosphatase (Fig. 3) showed no change until the third month of treatment. Thereafter there was an increase which continued until the sixth month when there was a substantial decrease and by the eighth month it had fallen into the normal range and continued to fall to a low normal value.

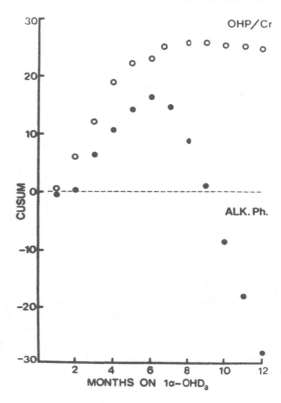

Fig. 3. Cumulative changes
from the mean untreated
values (QUSUM) in fasting
plasma alkaline phosphatase
(●) and fasting urine hy-
droxyproline/creatinine (o)
in a patient during treatment with $1\alpha OHD_3$.

The plasma phosphate (Fig. 4) showed an increase at the first
month and this continued until the sixth month when a further increase was seen which continued throughout treatment. The TmP/
GFR was unchanged until the fifth month (Fig. 5) after which it
showed a steady increase. Although this was associated with a
decrease in plasma parathyroid hormone (PTH), the fall in plasma
PTH was present even at one months treatment (Fig. 5). There was
a slight fall in plasma calcium during the first two months of
treatment. After the third month there was a small but steady
increase. Hypercalcaemia developed only after eleven months of
treatment, and was easily abolished by reducing the dose of $1\alpha OHD_3$
to 3µg/day. The urine calcium/creatinine ratio remained unchanged
until the eighth month when it increased during the course of treatment. (Fig. 5).

Fig. 4. Cumulative changes
from the mean untreated
values (QUSUM) in fasting
plasma phosphate (▲),
calcium (●) and urine
calcium/creatinine (o)
during treatment with
1αOHD₃.

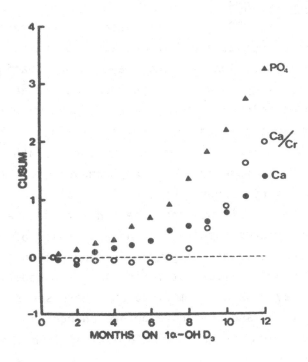

Fig. 5. Cumulative changes
from the mean untreated
values (QUSUM) in fast-
ing maximum tubular
reabsorption of phosphate
(TmP●) and fasting plasma
parathyroid hormone
(PTHo) in a patient
during treatment with
1αOHD₃.

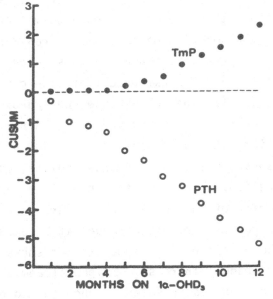

CONCLUSIONS

1.   VDRHPO is characterised by a decreased tubular reabsorption of phosphate and a low plasma phosphate.   In addition there is malabsorption of calcium and in some patients of phosphorus.   Bone histology shows severe osteomalacic changes with an increase in bone volume which may be associated with normal plasma alkaline phosphatase and urine hydroxyproline.   The more severe the osteomalacia the more severe the myopathy.

2.   Measurements of bone turnover, i.e. radiocalcium kinetics, urine hydroxyproline and plasma alkaline phosphatase indicate that in many patients the bone tends to become "aplastic".   Both phosphorus supplements and high doses of $1\alpha OHD_3$ stimulate bone turnover suggesting that in many patients phosphate depletion may be an important factor in the osteomalacia.   The stimulation however is not immediate and there seems to be a retention of calcium and phosphate before changes in bone-turnover are obvious.

3.   Treatment of VDRHPO with oral phosphorus supplements alone is difficult; very large doses are not easily tolerated by the patient, they may cause hypocalcaemia and they do not correct the malabsorption of calcium.   Treatment with high doses of $1\alpha OHD_3$ gives hyperabsorption and allows large amounts of phosphorus and calcium to be transferred from the gut.   There is an initial rise in alkaline phosphatase and hydroxyproline especially where these are suppressed.   After 6-8 months treatment there are indications of bone healing with a fall in plasma alkaline phosphatase and urine hydroxyproline, and a rise in urine calcium excretion.   The time sequence of healing varies with the severity of the condition.   There is a rise in plasma phosphate throughout treatment although it becomes more marked at the time of bone healing.   Plasma calcium shows an initial fall followed by a gradual increase.   Hypercalcaemia is never a problem as long as the bone is unhealed.   Once the bone has healed hypercalcaemia develops but can be rapidly controlled by reducing the dose of $1\alpha OHD_3$.

A rise in urine calcium always preceeds the hypercalcaemia.

4.   Tubular phosphate reabsorption shows no change with treatment in some patients.   In others there is an increase but only when the bone has almost healed.   Although this is related to a fall in PTH, the fall in PTH like the response in muscle occurs as soon as treatment with $1\alpha OHD_3$ is started.   The immediate fall in PTH secretion may represent a direct action of $1\alpha OHD_3$ on the parathyroid gland[5].

5.   The resistance to vitamin D appears more severe when assessed in the presence of untreated bone disease since patients can be managed on a much lower dose of $1\alpha OHD_3$ once the bone disease has healed.   Furthermore the malabsorption of calcium responds to $2\mu g$ $1\alpha OHD_3$ and $6\mu g$ causes hyperabsorption.   The response in absorption, PTH secretion and myopathy occur very early on treatment with $1\alpha OHD_3$ whereas the response on bone and tubular reabsorption. of phosphate occur later.   It seems that part of the resistance to vitamin D is induced by phosphate depletion.

ACKNOWLEDGEMENTS

The help of the technical and secretarial staff of the M.R.C. Mineral Metabolism Unit is gratefully acknowledged. We thank Leo Pharmaceutical Products, Copenhagen, Denmark, for providing the $1\alpha OHD_3$ used in these studies.

1.   WILLIAMS, T.F. and WINTERS, R.W.   Familial (Hereditary)
      Vitamin D - Resistant Rickets with hypophosphatemia. In
      The Metabolic Basis of Inherited Disease. Ed. Stanbury, J.B.
      Wyngaarden, J.B. and Fredrickson, D.S., McCraw-Hill, New York,
      1972.

2.   SCRIVER, C.R. Rickets and the pathogenesis of impaired
      tubular transport of phosphate and other solutes.   Amer.
      J. Med. 57, 43-49, 1974.

3.   HAUSSLER, M.R., BAYLINK, D.J., HUGHES, M.R., BRUMBAUGH, P.F.,
      WERGEDAL, J.F., SHEN, F.H., NIELSON, R.L., COUNTS, S.J.,
      BURSAC, K.M. and McCAIN, T.A. The assay of 1α,25 Dihydroxy
      Vitamin D_3. Physiologic and pathologic modulation of
      circulating hormone levels. Clinical Endocrinology 5,
      151s-165s, 1976.

4.   Calcium, Phosphate and Magnesium Metabolism: Clinical
      Physiology and Diagnostic Procedures. Ed. B.E.C. Nordin.
      Churchill Livingstone, Edinburgh, 1976.

5.   PEACOCK, M., NORDIN, B.E.C., GALLAGHER, J.C. and VARNAVIDES,
      C.   Action of 1α-Hydroxy Vitamin D_3 in Man.   pp 604-611.
      In: Vitamin D and Problems Related to Uremic Bone Disease.
      Ed. Norman, A.W., Schaefer, K. Grigoleit, H.G., Herrath,
      D.V., Ritz, E. de Gruyter, Berlin, 1975.

25-HYDROXYCHOLECALCIFEROL: HIGH AFFINITY SUBSTRATE FOR HEPATIC CYTOCHROME P-450

Dominick L. Cinti
Department of Pharmacology
The University of Connecticut Health Center
Farmington, Connecticut 06032
Francis H. Glorieux and Edgard E. Delvin
Department of Experimental Surgery
McGill University and The Shriner's Hospital
Montreal, Canada
Ellis E. Golub and Felix Bronner
Department of Oral Biology
The University of Connecticut Health Center
Farmington, Connecticut 06032

In vitro studies with hepatic microsomes showed that 25-hydroxyvitamin D_3 (25-OH-D_3) is bound tightly by the microsomal cytochrome P-450 system, with the spectral dissociation constant of 84 nM the lowest reported to-date for a natural or xenobiotic compound. Vitamin D_2 and dihydrotachysterol also were bound, but their dissociation constants were 200 - 300 times higher. Aminopyrine demethylation was competitively inhibited in the presence of 25-OH-D_3 and NADPH cytochrome. P-450 reductase activity was doubled by 25-OH-D_3 addition. Taken together these findings suggest that liver microsomes are involved in the transformation and degradation of 25-OH-D_3 and other vitamin D congeners. However, the enzyme systems are not vitamin D-dependent. Moreover, even though phenobarbital treatment led to a doubling of enzyme activity and, in animals undergoing vitamin D depletion, to a 40% faster time-dependent drop of 25-OH-D_3 plasma levels, as compared to untreated controls, the two groups had the same levels of intestinal calcium-binding protein (CaBP). If CaBP is one expression of the active metabolite, 1,25-dihydroxyvitamin D_3 (1,25-(OH)$_2$-D_3), then alterations of a substrate (25-OH-D_3)-product (1,25-(OH)$_2$-D_3) relationship at a single control point (liver), brought about by phenobarbital treatment, did not lead to detectable changes in hormone expression. The experiments underscore the stability of the calcium regulating system and point to the existence of multiple control loops.

There is now ample evidence (see 1 for review) that vitamin D
is transformed in the liver to a more polar hydroxylated metabolite,
25-hydroxyvitamin D,[1]   which in turn is transformed further in
liver and kidney. It is less certain whether or not the enzyme that
transforms vitamin D to 25-hydroxyvitamin D is a mixed function oxidase of the type that is induced by phenobarbital treatment. In subjects on chronic phenobarbital therapy the transformation of vitamin
D to 25-hydroxyvitamin D and other polar metabolites appeared to be
accelerated (2) and their 25-OH-D_3 serum levels were depressed (3).
These data are consistent with the possibility that phenobarbital and
other antiepileptic drugs like dilantin induce an enzyme that acts
directly on the transformation of vitamin D to 25-hydroxyvitamin D.
On the other hand, reports from DeLuca's laboratory (4, 5), although
indicating that 25-hydroxylation occurs in liver microsomes, state
that the reaction is not blocked by carbon monoxide, is unaffected
by inhibitors of cytochrome P-450 and is not induced by phenobarbital. It seemed of interest therefore to reinvestigate this question.
We undertook two types of studies: an analysis of the binding in
vitro of vitamin D and its congeners to liver microsome cytochrome
P-450, and a study of the effect of in vivo phenobarbital treatment
on the expression of vitamin D regulation of calcium metabolism.

MATERIALS AND METHODS

     Male Sprague-Dawley rats, purchased either from Charles River,
Wilmington, MA., or ARS, Madison, WI., were used throughout. Animals
that were used for the vitamin D-deficiency study were weanlings,
those for the other studies were young adults (150-225g). Treatment
of animals with phenobarbital consisted of an initial injection of
70 mg/kg BW, administered intraperitoneally, followed by 0.1% phenobarbital, administered in the drinking water. Stock diets consisted
of Purina Chow. Vitamin D-deficient diets were semi-synthetic, containing 28% vitamin-free test casein, 5% corn oil, 1% vitamin supplement without vitamin D, 3% salt mixture, 56% sucrose, plus cellophane
spangles (a nutrient-free filler). Diets were purchased from Teklad
Mills, Madison, WI., and contained either 0.5% Ca and 0.2% P without
(Code No. TD 67205A) or with 2200 units/kg vitamin D (Code No. TD
75095) or 0.5% Ca and 0.2% P without (Code No. TD 75096) or with
(Code No. TD 70387) vitamin D_2. Ca and P content were verified ana-
lytically (6).

     The microsomal fraction was obtained by differential ultracen-
trifugation (7) after livers had been perfused with isotonic saline
and the tissue homogenized in 0.25 M sucrose containing 1.0 mM Tris-
HCl buffer, pH 7.4. Cytochrome P-450 substrate binding was measured
by difference spectroscopy with an Aminco DW-2 UV/VIS spectropho-
tometer. Cytochrome P-450 reductase was measured at 23°C with the
Aminco-Morrow stopped-flow accessory. One syringe of the stopped
flow apparatus contained 6mM glucose, 40µl glucose oxidase (Sigma,
Type V, 1400 units/ml), 10µl catalase (22,000 Sigma units/ml), micro-

somes (3mg/ml) and 50mM Tris-HCl, pH 7.4, in a final volume of 6 ml
gassed with carbon monoxide; a 1.0mM NADPH solution containing the
glucose oxidase-catalase system and gassed with carbon monoxide was
placed in the other syringe. Aminopyrine N-demethylase activity was
determined by measuring formaldehyde (8).

Plasma calcium was measured by atomic absorption spectrophotometry with 0.1% $LaCl_3$ as diluent and an air-acetylene flame. Plasma
25-hydroxyvitamin D levels were determined by a modification of the
method of Haddad and Chyu (9). After addition to the plasma samples
of labeled $25-OH-D_3$, precipitation of the lipoproteins, and extraction with ether, the samples were dried, dissolved in N-hexane and
applied to hydroxyalkoxypropyl Sephadex prepared according to Ellingboe (10). Following equilibration with N-hexane, the columns were
eluted with N-hexane, and 25-OH-D, eluted with 20% ether-hexane, was
assayed with the aid of a rat kidney cortex cytosol binding protein
(9).

Duodenal calcium-binding protein (CaBP) content was determined
by a quantitative, competitive binding assay, utilizing Chelex resin.
Duodenal mucosa were scraped, homogenized in a modified Tris-buffer,
the homogenate centrifuged, and the supernate chromatographed on
Sephadex G-50 resin. Quantitative analysis was done on peak B and
the binding activity was expressed as nanomoles Ca bound/g mucosa.
For further details, see (11, 12).

RESULTS

Figure 1 shows the type I spectral change obtained by the addition of increasing amounts of $25-OH-D_3$ to liver microsomes from untreated rats. An absorption peak was observed at 388nm, a trough at
420nm and an isosbestic point at 407nm. Analysis of these data by
an Eadie-Hofstee plot revealed a spectral dissociation constant (K_s)
of 84nM (Figure 1, insert).

Table 1 shows that dihydrotachysterol (DHT_2) and vitamin D_2 also
bound to liver microsomes in a fashion similar to 25-hydroxyvitamin
D_2, but that their spectral dissociation constant was much higher.

Table 1 also shows that microsomes isolated from animals treated
with phenobarbital for three days prior to sacrifice gave the same
half-maximal spectral changes when reacted with $25-OH-D_3$ as microsomes from untreated animals, but that the maximal binding capacity
(B_{max}, ΔE/mg protein as derived from an Eadie-Hofstee plot, insert
Fig. 1) had tripled as a result of prior phenobarbital treatment.
This suggests that the induced enzyme is similar to the native
microsomal enzyme that binds to and presumably transforms $25-OH-D_3$.

Aminopyrine-N-demethylation, a cytochrome P-450-catalyzed oxi-
dative reaction, was competitively inhibited in the presence of 25-

TABLE 1

HALF-MAXIMAL SPECTRAL CHANGES (K_S)
AND MAXIMAL BINDING CAPACITY (B_{max})
OF VITAMIN D CONGENERS

Type I Substrate	K_S, nM	B_{max} (ΔE/mg protein)
Dihydrotachysterol (DHT$_2$)	13,500	-----
Ergocalciferol	7,100	-----
25-hydroxycholecalciferol	84	0.052
25-hydroxycholecalciferol (phenobarbital treatment)	84	0.163

Values were derived from Eadie-Hofstee plots (see text)
Phenobarbital treatment consisted of 70 mg/kg BW, administered
* intraperitoneally for three successive days.*
Protein concentration in liver microsome preparations: 2 mg/ml

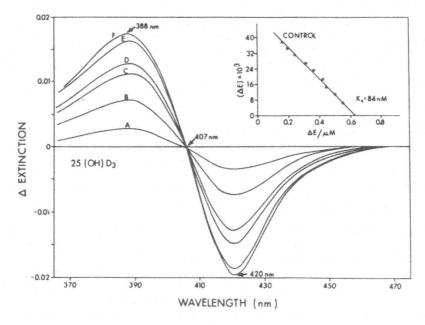

Figure 1 - 25-OH-D-induced type I spectral change. Liver micro-
somes from adults rats (2mg protein/ml in 0.1 M Tris-HCl, pH 7.4)
were distributed between two cuvettes: 25-OH-D was added to the
sample and an equivalent volume of buffer to the reference cuvette.
Final concentrations of the 25-OH-D$_3$ in a 3ml suspension: A. 11nM,
B: 33nM, C. 66nM, D. 88nM, E. 176nM and F. 242nM. Insert: Plot of
ΔE 388nM-420NM vs. ΔE/ concentration of 25-OH-D$_3$.

OH-D$_3$ (Figure 2); the Km for aminopyrine was about 0.4mM in the absence of the 25-OH-D$_3$, but was increased to 0.7 and 1.4mM in the presence of 44nM and 132nM 25-OH-D$_3$, respectively. This indicates that the 25-hydroxy metabolite may be an alternative substrate for cytochrome P-450. The calculated inhibition constant, K_i, of 25-OH-D$_3$ for aminopyrine-N-demethylation was 59nM, in good agreement with the K_s value of 84 (Table 1). Vitamin D$_2$ and DHT$_2$ also inhibited aminopyrine-N-demethylation (Figure 3), although higher concentrations were required relative to 25-OH-D$_3$.

The reduction of cytochrome P-450 by the flavoprotein reductase is the rate limiting step in microsomal mixed function oxidase reactions (13). Substrates of the P-450 system exert a positive modifier effect on this step; for example, NADPH cytochrome P-450 reductase activity is increased in the presence of substrate. Table 2 shows that a similar result was obtained by the addition of 25-OH-D$_3$ which caused the reductase activity to double.

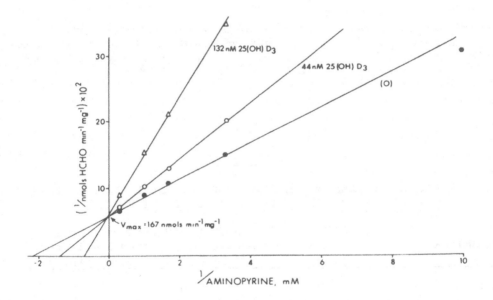

Figure 2 - Effect of 25-OH-D$_3$ addition on rat liver microsomal aminopyrine-N-demethylation. The Lineweaver-Burk plot of enzyme activity was obtained with 44nM, 132nM or no 25-OH-D$_3$. Both inhibitor and substrate were present in the assay medium which was pre-incubated for 10 min. at 37° to generate NADPH (from 0.5mM NADP$^+$). The microsomes (1mg/ml final concentration) were added to the medium and incubation continued for 5 min. at 37°C; aminopyrine concentration ranged from 0.1mM to 3mM. The Km and V$_{max}$ values were obtained by the method of least squares.

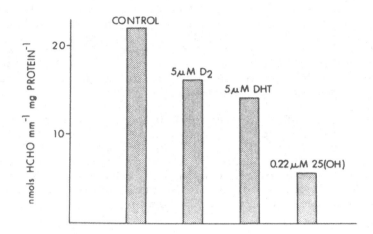

Figure 3 - Effect of various vitamin D congeners on amino-pyrine-N-demethylation by rat liver microsomes. The aminopyrine concentration was 3mM; the inhibitors were: ergocalciferol (D₂), 5μM; dihydrotachysterol (DHT₂); 5μM; 25-(OH)₂-D₃, 0.22μM.

TABLE 2

EFFECT OF 25-HYDROXYCHOLECALCIFEROL ON NADPH CYTOCHROME
P-450 REDUCTASE ACTIVITY IN RAT LIVER MICROSOMES

25-(OH)-D$_3$	NADPH P-450 reductase activity nmoles/min/mg microsomal protein	
	Exp. 1	Exp. 2
None	20	18
100nM	58	50

The fixed wavelengths were 450nm-490nm

The reductase activity was measured with the Aminco-Morrow stop-flow apparatus (see text).

TABLE 3

CYTOCHROME P-450 CONTENT
RAT LIVER MICROSOMES

	Control		Phenobarbital Treated	
	Vitamin D Replete (15)	Vitamin D Deficient (12)	Vitamin D Replete (15)	Vitamin D Deficient (12)
nanomoles mg protein	0.98	1.02	2.01	2.39
SE	0.07	0.12	0.10	0.36

Numbers in parentheses refer to the number of animals.

It seemed of interest to verify whether the liver microsomal enzyme system shows vitamin D-dependence. To this end control and phenobarbital-treated animals were raised from weaning on vitamin D-deficient or vitamin D-replete regimens (Code Nos. TD 75095 and TD 67205A, respectively) and, when the animals on the deficient regimen were hypocalcemic (< 6 mg/dl, 6, 12) microsomal cytochrome P-450 content was determined. Table 3 shows that the cytochrome P-450 levels were the same in deficient and replete animals, whether or not the animals had been phenobarbital treated.

Fig. 4 shows the time-course of the plasma 25-OH-D levels as the animals were being depleted of vitamin D. As expected, the plasma levels of this vitamin D metabolite dropped with time, but the rate of drop was 40% higher in the phenobarbital-treated animals as compared to the untreated controls, with the plasma 25-OH-D levels of the treated animals consistently lower than those of the vitamin D-deficient controls.

Notwithstanding the large difference in plasma 25-OH-D levels, there were no significant differences in the mucosal CaBP levels of the two groups of animals undergoing vitamin D-depletion. As shown by Fig. 5, CaBP dropped in both groups at the same rate. Moreover, the CaBP concentration had not yet reached undetectable levels ($\lesssim 5$ nanomoles Ca bound/gm mucosa) when the animals had been on the deficient diet 22 days. Such levels were reached two weeks later.

In contrast, plasma calcium levels [Ca_S], had reached a plateau by day 13, not decreasing thereafter (Fig. 6). In both groups the rate of drop was the same, although [Ca_S] was consistently and significantly higher in the phenobarbital-treated animals 0.4 mg/ml

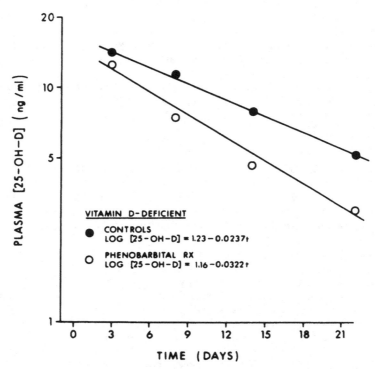

Figure 4 - Plasma 25-OH-D levels in two groups of rats undergoing vitamin D depletion, one of which had received 0.1% phenobarbital in its drinking water starting 6 days before the first measurements. Upon receipt the animals were placed on a vitamin D-replete diet (Code No. TD 67205A) and, on day 0, were shifted to an identical diet, except that it was vitamin D-deficient (Code No. TD 75095).

(SE: 0.11), significance having been determined by the Wilcoxon matched-pairs signed-ranks test (14).

DISCUSSION

When a substrate binds to the oxidized form of cytochrome P-450, a type I spectral change is elicited. This change is attributed to an absorbance shift from 420 nm to 385-390 nm. In the difference spectrum this shift is manifested as a peak at 385-390 nm and as a trough at about 420 nm, as observed in the difference spectrum displayed in Fig. 1. It has been shown (see 15 for examples) that this spectral change reflects the formation of a metabolically active cytochrome P-450 substrate complex. Such spectral changes have been observed with a solubilized, partially purified (16), as well as a homogeneous enzyme preparation (17). It therefore seems that 25-OH-D and other vitamin D congeners constitute substrates for the liver microsomal enzyme system. Furthermore, since phenobarbital treatment

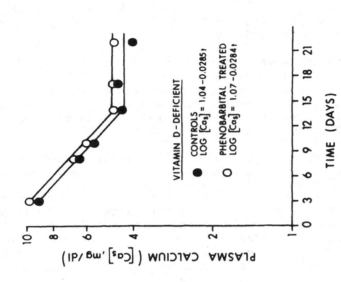

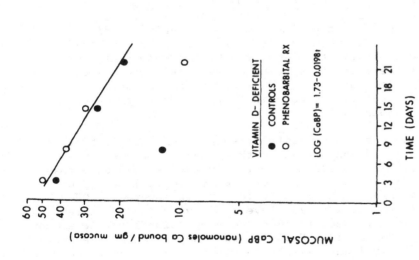

Figure 5 - Mucosal CaBP levels in two groups of rats, control and phenobarbital-treated, undergoing vitamin D-depletion. The experimental conditions are described in the legend of Fig. 4. CaBP measurements were made on pooled duodenal scrapings from 3 animals each, as described in the text.

Figure 6 - Plasma calcium levels, [Ca_s], in two groups of rats, control and phenobarbital-treated, undergoing vitamine D-depletion. The experimental conditions are described in the legend of Fig. 4. [Ca_s] was measured on the same pooled plasma taken for 25-OH-D analysis (Fig. 4)

increased both the total cytochrome P-450 activity (Fig. 4) and the maximal binding capacity, B_{max}, for 25-OH-D, while the K_s value for 25-OH-D remained the same (Table 1), it may be concluded that the native enzyme system binding and transforming 25-OH-D_3 is the same as the phenobarbital-induced one.

This conclusion is strengthened by the fact that 25-OH-D_3 competitively inhibited aminopyrine-N-demethylation (Fig. 2) and that this was also true of other vitamin D congeners, though at higher concentrations (Fig. 3). Moreover, the 25-OH-D_3 concentrations used in the competitive inhibition studies bracketed normal plasma concentrations of 20 ng/ml (Fig. 4; 20 ng/ml $\equiv$ 50 nM).

The doubling of the cytochrome P-450 reductase activity (Table 2) also provides evidence that the P-450 system binds and transforms 25-OH-D_3. Finally, the K_s value observed for 25-OH-D_3 (Table 1) is 2-3 orders of magnitude lower than that reported for any other compound, natural or xenobiotic, that interacts with the cytochrome P-450 system. The other vitamin D congeners tested, on the other hand, had K_s values 2-3 orders of magnitude higher than 25-OH-D_3 (Table 1). Thus it seems logical to conclude that the liver cytochrome P-450 is involved in the degradation of 25-OH-D, as well as of other vitamin D metabolites. Therefore, this enzyme system is probably not responsible for the specific hydroxylation of vitamin D at carbon 25.

If 25-OH-D_3 and other vitamin D congeners and metabolites are degraded by the hepatic cytochrome P-450 system, one might expect the system to exhibit vitamin D dependence. As shown in Table 3, this was not the case. In other experiments, vitamin D-deficient animals were treated with phenobarbital, but again no vitamin D-dependent differential effect on the cytochrome P-450 system was observed. It must therefore be concluded that the P-450 system, despite its high affinity for vitamin D metabolites, is not highly specific for these sterols and does in fact act on a large variety of hydroxylated compounds.

Table 3 shows that phenobarbital treatment of animals brought about an increase in an enzyme system that degrades 25-OH-D, a key compound in the pathway to the metabolically active 1,25-dihydroxy-vitamin D (1,25-$(OH)_2$-D_3). It therefore seemed logical to expect that phenobarbital-treated animals would exhibit lowered 25-OH-D plasma and diminished mucosal CaBP levels. In vitamin D-deficient animals CaBP levels have been found to be proportional to the amount of administered 25-OH-D_3 (12). Fig. 4 shows that vitamin D-depletion of phenobarbital treated animals led to a faster drop in plasma 25-OH-D levels than vitamin D-depletion in untreated controls. However, as shown in Fig. 5, this was not associated with a greater diminution in mucosal CaBP levels. Our analytical method can readily detect differences in CaBP levels of 20% or more (11). The near-identity in mucosal CaBP levels of the two groups of animals therefore is

likely to have functional significance. The most conservative interpretation is that regulation in the whole animal significantly
blunts the effect of even those maneuvers that markedly alter substrate-product relationship at a single control point.

This conclusion is also borne out quantitatively. Phenobarbital
led to a doubling of P-450 activity (Table 3), which in turn raised
the rate of disappearance of 25-OH-D from the plasma by only about
40% (Fig. 4); yet the quantitative expression of $1,25-(OH)_2-D_3$ was
completely unaffected, the CaBP concentrations having been unchanged
(Fig. 5). In this connection it is of interest that the rate at
which the plasma calcium dropped as a result of vitamin D depletion
(Fig. 6) was the same in both control and phenobarbital-treated
groups, even though the 25-OH-D plasma level dropped much faster in
the treated animals. Clearly the plasma calcium level in those
animals was not directly related to their plasma 25-OH-D levels.
This conclusion is reinforced by the fact that plasma calcium
levels plateaued on Day 13 (Fig. 6), whereas plasma 25-OH-D continued to drop throughout the experiment. Finally, the plasma calcium levels of the phenobarbital-treated animals were significantly
higher than those of the controls. This was the opposite of the
relationship of the 25-OH-D levels (Fig. 4). The significance of
the rise in $[Ca_s]$ remains obscure.

While these experiments failed to contribute to a clarification
of the interrelationships between plasma calcium, 25-hydroxyvitamin
D and 1,25-dihydroxyvitamin levels (at least as far as the mucosal
expression of the latter is concerned), they do point out that alterations of a substrate-product relationship at a single control
point do not necessarily lead to detectable changes at the level of
hormone expression. They thus underscore the stability of the calcium
regulating system and the existence of multiple control loops.

ACKNOWLEDGMENTS

Supported in part by USPHS grants AM 16678 (D.L.C.), CA 15897
(D.L.C.), AM 16408 (F.B.), AM 19439 (F.B.), General Research
Support Grant 5-S01-RR05677-07 to the School of Dental Medicine
from the National Institutes of Health (E.E.G.), and a grant from
The Shriners of North America (F.G.).

We thank Marilyn Reid, Cynthia Bossak, Lorraine Wolpert and
Mireille Dussault for their excellent assistance and Nancy Sprouse
for devoted secretarial help.

FOOTNOTES

[1] Vitamin D_3 (cholecalciferol) is thought to be the native compound,
with vitamin D_2 (ergocalciferol) the compound that is commonly ingested in the diet. Both compounds are equally effective in the

mammal. Abbreviations used: 25-hydroxyvitamin D: 25-OH-D; 1,25-dihydroxyvitamin D: 1,25-(OH)$_2$-D. D$_3$ refers to cholecalciferol or its hydroxylated derivatives. D$_2$ refers to ergocalciferol or its hydroxylated derivatives.

REFERENCES

1. Norman, A.W. and Henry, H. 1,25-dihydroxycholecalciferol - a hormonally active form of vitamin D$_3$. Recent Progr. Hormone Res. 30:431-480, 1974.

2. Hahn, T.J., Birge, S.J., Scharp, C.R. and Avioli, L.R. Phenobarbital-induced alterations in vitamin D metabolism. J. Clin. Invest. 51:741-748, 1972.

3. Hahn, T.J., Hendin, B.A., Scharp, C.R., and Haddad, J.G. Effect of chronic anticonvulsant therapy on serum 25-hydroxy-calciferol levels in adults. New Engl. J. Med. 287:900-904, 1972.

4. Bhattacharyya, M. and DeLuca, H.F. The regulation of rat liver calciferol hydroxylase. J. Biol. Chem. 248:2969-2973, 1973.

5. DeLuca, H.F. Metabolism of vitamin D: current status. Am. J. Clin. Nutr. 1976 (in press).

6. Hurwitz, S., Stacey, R.E. and Bronner, F. Role of vitamin D in plasma calcium regulation. Am. J. Physiol. 216:254-262, 1969.

7. Schenkman, J.F. and Cinti, D.L. Hepatic mixed function oxidase activity in rapidly prepared microsomes. Life Sci. 11:247-257, 1972.

8. Cinti, D.L. and Ozols, J. Binding of homogeneous cytochrome b$_5$ to rat liver microsomes: Effect on N-demethylation reactions. Biochim. Biophys. Acta 410:32-44, 1975.

9. Haddad, J.G. and Chyu, K.J. Competitive protein-binding radioassay for 25-hydroxycholecalciferol. J. Clin. Endocr. 33:992, 1971.

10. Ellingboe, J., Nyström, E. and Sjövall, J. Liquid-gel chromatography on lipophilic hydrophobic Sephadex derivatives. J. Lipid Res. 11:266, 1970.

11. Freund, Thomas and Bronner, Felix. Regulation of intestinal calcium-binding protein by calcium intake in the rat. Am. J. Physiol. 228:861-869, 1975.

12. Bronner, Felix and Thomas Freund. Intestinal CaBP: a new quantitative index of vitamin D deficiency in the rat. Am. J. Physiol. 229:689-694, 1975.

13. Gigon, P.L., Gram, T.E. and Gillette, J.R. Studies on the rate of reduction of hepatic microsomal cytochrome P-450 by reduced nicotinamide adenine dinucleotide phosphate. Effect of drug substrates. Molec. Pharmacol. 5:109-122, 1969.

14. Wilcoxon, Frank. Individual comparisons by ranking methods Biometrics 1:80-82, 1945.

15. Orrenius, S. and Ernster, L. Microsomal cytochrome P-450-linked monooxygenase systems in mammalian tissue. In: Molecular Arrangements of Oxygen Activation, ed. O. Hayaishi. Academic Press, New York, 1974, pp. 215-244.

16. Lu, A., Strobel, H. and Coon, M. Properties of a solubilized form of the cytochrome P-450-containing mixed function oxidase of liver microsomes. Molec. Pharmacol. 6:213-220, 1970.

17. Gunsalus, I.C. Soluble methylene hydroxylase system: Structure and role of cytochrome P-450 and iron-sulfur protein components. Hoppe-Seyler's Z. Physiol. Chem. 349:1610-1613, 1968.

RENAL FUNCTION IN TREATED HYPOPARATHYROIDISM

A POSSIBLE DIRECT NEPHROTOXIC EFFECT OF VITAMIN D

A.M.Parfitt, M.B., B. Chir, FRCP, FRACP, FACP
Director, Bone and Mineral Research Laboratory, Henry
Ford Hospital, Clinical Associate Professor of Medicine,
University of Michigan, Ann Arbor, Michigan.
2799 W. Grand Blvd.   Detroit, Michigan 48202, USA

Vitamin D* intoxication is a well known hazard in the treatment of hypoparathyroidism. Impaired renal function in a patient receiving vitamin D is usually attributed to hypercalcemia (1), but even in the absence of this complication, the metabolic abnormalities of parathyroid hormone (PTH) deficiency are incompletely corrected by vitamin D. The plasma phosphate usually falls to within the normal range, but the mean value remains elevated. PTH increases the tubular reabsorption of calcium; vitamin D may have a similar effect (2), but normocalcemia can often only be maintained in the absence of PTH at the expense of hypercalciuria (3). Either persistent hyperphosphatemia or hypercalciuria might conceivably result in renal injury. Finally, as in the rat, vitamin D itself may have a direct nephrotoxic effect (4). In view of these uncertainties, a detailed study was undertaken of renal function in vitamin D treated hypoparathyroidism.

CLINICAL MATERIAL

Twenty-seven patients were studied, 24 with chronic surgical hypoparathyroidism (SHP), 2 with idiopathic hypoparathyroidism (IHP), and 1 with pseudohypoparathyroidism (PHP). Twenty-three were female and 4 male. From a total population of 50 such patients, all who had received continuous treatment for five years or longer or who had experienced one or more episodes of vitamin D intoxication were selected. Both criteria were fulfilled by 11 patients, only the first by 12 and only the second by 4. Most of the patients had

----

*In this paper the term "vitamin D" is used in a generic sense to refer to all substances which are antirachitic in man.

Table 1. Characteristics of patients studied (mean $\pm$ SD)

Sex	24F, 4M
Age (years)	53.8 $\pm$ 11.8
Body Surface Area (m^2)	1.67 $\pm$ 0.20
Plasma calcium (mg/100ml)-Pretreatment	6.37 $\pm$ 0.43
-On treatment	9.34 $\pm$ 0.36
Plasma Phosphate (mg/100ml)-Pretreatment	5.10 $\pm$ 0.83
-On treatment	4.13 $\pm$ 0.43
Duration of treatment (years) with range	8.0 (3.1 - 33)
Dose of DHT (or D$_2$ equivalent)(mg/day)	0.70 $\pm$ 0.24

been treated for most of the time with encapsulated preparations of either ergocalciferol (D$_2$) or dihydrotachysterol (DHT) which were free of the defects present in commercially available preparations (5), according to the principles found to minimize fluctuations in plasma calcium and the occurrence of vitamin D intoxication (6). Many of these patients had been on exactly the same dose of vitamin D for more than 5 years prior to the study. However, about half of the patients had at some time received treatment with other preparations and according to other principles. The dosage, duration and type of vitamin D therapy, and the plasma calcium and inorganic phosphate levels at three monthly or shorter intervals during treatment were available in all cases. Pretreatment plasma calcium and inorganic phosphate levels were known in all except two cases. These data are given in Table 1.

METHODS

A Sydney Hospital one-day renal function profile (7) with slight modification was performed in each patient. The procedure comprises: basal creatinine clearance (C_{cr}), minimum urinary pH, titratable acidity (TA), bicarbonate (HCO_3) and ammonium (NH_4) excretion after acid load, maximum urinary osmolarity after pitressin, and phenolsulphonphthalein (PSP) excretion. Urine was collected from 8:30 A.M. to 11:30 A.M., 11:30 A.M. to 2:30 P.M., and 2:30 P.M. to 4:30 P.M. Ammonium Chloride 0.1g/kg BW was given as 0.5g unsealed gelatin capsules between 9:00 A.M. and 10:00 A.M. with no more than 100ml of water. Torecan 6.5mg. was given I.M. 30 minutes earlier to prevent nausea and vomiting. Five units of Pitressin Tannate in oil was given subcutaneously at 8:30 A.M. after precautions to ensure dispersion of the solid material. PSP 18mg/m^2 body surface area was given IV at 2:15 P.M. Surface area was calculated from height and weight using a standard nomogram (8). Analytical methods for pH, TA, HCO_3, NH_4 and osmolarity and PSP were as cited or described (7,9). Creatinine and phosphate were measured by standard autoanalyser methods.

Table 2. Results of Renal Function Tests (Mean ± SD)

	Observed	Age > 40 normal[1]	Age Predicted[2]
Creat. clearance[3]	78.2 ± 28.4	105.8 ± 23.6	98.6 ± 7.6
PSP_{15} excretion[4]	22.3 ± 11.5	22.7 ± 9.9	27.6 ± 2.8
PSP_{135} excretion[4]	63.4 ± 19.2	58.7 ± 11.0	----
Max. osmolarity[5]	674 ± 113.8	861.0 ± 67.3	GFR corrected
Minimum urine pH	5.28 ± 0.49	4.81 ± 0.19	(100ml C_{cr})
HCO_3 excretion[6]	2.0 ± 3.4	0.9 ± 0.5	2.8 ± 4.2
Titratable acidity[6]	23.1 ± 8.9	29.3 ± 5.1	34.4 ± 22.0
NH_4 excretion[6]	34.0 ± 8.0	38.9 ± 10.1	45.4 ± 17.4
Net acid excretion[6]	55.1 ± 19.2	67.3 ± 13.8	77.0 ± 32.9

1. Source given in text. 2. Based on formulae given in text.
3. ml/min/1.73m^2. 4. %. 5. mOsm/kg. 6. μeq/min/1.73m^2.

An intravenous pyelogram was performed in each patient and the histories and medical records were reviewed to determine the incidence of nephrolithiasis, nephrocalcinosis and other types of soft tissue calcification. The mean and SD of all plasma calcium and phosphate values during treatment were determined in each patient. Values for plasma calcium which were more than 0.5mg/100ml outside the normal hospital range of 8.7 to 10.7mg/100ml, that is, between 8.2 and 11.2mg/100ml, were included, but values outside these ranges were treated separately as episodes of hyper or hypocalcemia. These were classified on the basis of symptoms, the extent and duration of the elevation or depression of plasma calcium, changes in renal function, and the vigor with which treatment was modified as mild, moderate or severe.

The dose of the different preparations of vitamin D was expressed in mg. of DHT per day on the assumption that 3.0mg. of D_2 was equivalent to 1.0mg. of DHT (6). TmP/GFR was estimated in each patient from fasting values for plasma and urinary phosphate and creatinine by a modification of the method of Bijvoet (10).

RESULTS

The mean values for each of the indices of renal function are shown in Table 2. They are compared with mean values obtained in 20 normal persons aged 40-67 (mean 54.8 years) studied by Dr. A.Z. Gyory (personal communication). The individual results for each patient are shown in Figure 1 with normal ranges for subjects under 40 years (7) and over 40 years (A.Z. Gyory). The mean values for C_{cr} in the vitamin D treated patients was significantly lower (p< 0.001 by paired t test) than the mean of values predicted from the patients age (Table 2) by the equation: C_{cr}(ml/min/1.73m^2) = 133 - 0.64 x age(years). This equation is adjusted for use with the autoanalyser (total chromagen) method for plasma creatinine

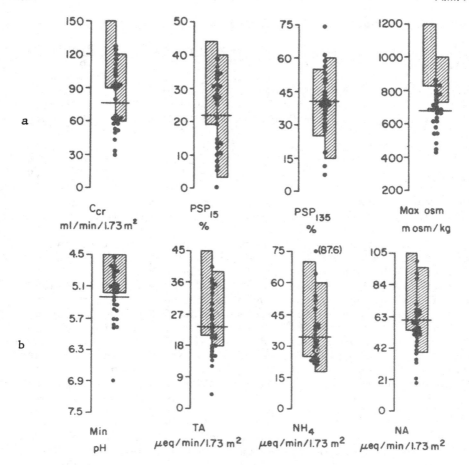

Figure 1 a and b: Renal function in vitamin D treated hypoparathyroidism. In each panel shaded areas indicate normal ranges in subjects under 40 years on the left, and over 40 years on the right.
Horizontal lines indicate mean values.

Table 3. Correlation of Renal Function with Mean Plasma Ca and P

	Ca r	Ca r_p	P r	P r_p	Explained Variation	F ratio
C_{cr}	−0.1493	−0.1021	0.3161	0.2983	0.1092	1.4710
Max. osm	−0.1275	−0.1034	0.1574	0.1388	0.0351	0.4365
Min. pH	0.0721	−0.0221	0.3012	0.2940	0.0911	1.2027

r−coefficient of correlation; r_p−coefficient of partial correlation
allowing for r of 0.1704 between Ca and P, F−variance ratio.

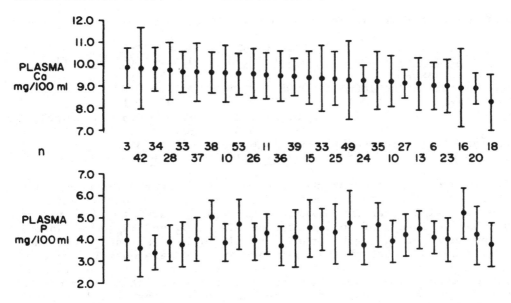

Figure 2: Plasma calcium and phosphate levels during vitamin D treatment in hypoparathyroidism. Closed circles represent individual mean values, ranked in descending order of plasma Ca. Vertical lines represent individual ± 2SD, n indicates number of observations in each case. There was no significant correlation between mean Ca and mean P (r = -0.1704).

(11), rather than the true creatinine method (7). The mean 15 minute PSP excretion in the vitamin D treated patients was significantly lower (P < 0.01 by paired t test) than the mean of values calculated from the age predicted C_{cr} using the equation (9): PSP = (1.08C_{cr}-19.42/3.14, but did not differ significantly from the over 40 normal values (Table 2). This discrepancy suggests that PSP excretion was relatively less impaired than C_{cr}. However, the observed PSP excretion did not differ significantly from the mean

Table 4. Effect of Severity of Vitamin D Intoxication (means ± SE)

Characteristic	Mild	Severe	Significance
No. of cases	12	15	
Mean Plasma Ca(mg/100ml)	9.25 ± 0.12	9.40 ± 0.08	ns
Mean Plasma P (mg/100ml)	4.08 ± 0.14	4.17 ± 0.10	ns
C_{cr} (ml/min)	87.8 ± 7.4	70.5 ± 7.5	P < 0.10
PSP_{15}	22.9 ± 3.4	22.3 ± 2.2	ns
Max. osmolarity (m. osm/kg)	677 ± 28	672 ± 33	ns
Minimum pH	5.23 ± 0.18	5.31 ± 0.10	ns

Table 5. Effect of Mean Plasma Calcium Level (means ± SE)

Characteristic	Mean Ca < 9.4mg/100ml	Mean Ca > 9.4mg/100ml	Significance
No. of cases	13	14	
Mean Plasma Ca (mg/100ml)	9.08 ± 0.08	9.62 ± 0.04	–
Mean Plasma P (mg/100ml)	4.27 ± 0.11	3.99 ± 0.11	ns
C_{cr} (ml/min)	86.2 ± 7.5	69.8 ± 7.5	P < 0.10
PSP_{15}	22.3 ± 3.3	22.2 ± 4.5	ns
Max. osmolarity (m.osm/kg)	690 ± 30	657 ± 33	ns
Minimum pH	5.28 ± 0.11	5.28 ± 0.11	ns

of values calculated from the observed C_{cr} using the above equation
(20.7%), and the observed and C_{cr} predicted values for PSP excretion were significantly correlated (r=0.61, p < 0.001). When values
for the components of acid excretion (TA, HCO_3 and NH_4)were expressed per unit of C_{cr} rather than per unit of body surface area, the
mean values and most of the individual values were normal (Table 2).
This suggests that the observed reductions were entirely explained
by the reduction in C_{cr}. However, the impairment of maximum urinary concentration was more severe than could be explained in this
way, suggesting an additional defect in distal tubular and collecting duct function. The impairment in acidification probably has a
similar explanation, but significant bicarbonate wasting was present
in five patients, suggesting a proximal lesion also.

The relationship of the renal functional abnormalities to the
biochemical state during vitamin D treatment (Figure 2) was examined in two ways. First the correlation of C_{cr}, minimum pH and maximum osmolarity with the two independent variables of mean plasma
calcium and mean plasma phosphate was calculated. Second, the
patients were partitioned into two groups in three different ways.
These were on the basis of the level of the mean plasma calcium
(above or below 9.4mg/100ml), the level of the upper 2SD boundary
of plasma phosphate (above or below 5.0mg/100ml)and the severity
of vitamin D intoxication. In twelve cases either no episode of
vitamin D intoxication (7 cases) or a single mild episode lasting
less than one week (5 cases) occurred. In the remaining 15 cases

Table 6. Effect of Mean Plasma Phosphate (means ± SE)

Characteristic	P + 2SD < 5.0mg/100ml	P + 2SD > 5.0mg/100ml	Significance
No of cases	14	13	
Mean Plasma Ca (mg/100ml)	9.39 ± 0.12	9.29 ± 0.07	ns
Mean Plasma P (mg/100ml)	3.81 ± 0.05	4.48 ± 0.09	–
C_{cr} (ml/min)	71.4 ± 8.1	85.6 ± 7.8	ns
PSP_{15}	19.6 ± 3.1	25.2 ± 3.0	ns
Max. osmolarity (m.osm/kg)	637 ± 32	714 ± 26	ns
Minimum pH	5.30 ± 0.10	5.26 ± 0.17	ns

Table 7.   Differences Between Low and High P Groups (means $\pm$ SE).

Characteristic	Low P	High P	Significance
Age (years)	53.4 $\pm$ 3.7	54.2 $\pm$ 2.7	ns
Body surface area (m^2)	1.62 $\pm$ 0.06	1.74 $\pm$ 0.05	ns
Pre-treatment Ca (mg/100ml)	6.12 $\pm$ 0.28	6.63 $\pm$ 0.23	ns
Pre-treatment P (mg/100ml)	5.08 $\pm$ 0.28	5.11 $\pm$ 0.22	ns
Rise in mean Ca (mg/100ml)	+3.21 $\pm$ 0.27	+2.64 $\pm$ 0.23	ns
Fall in mean P (mg/100ml)	−1.27 $\pm$ 0.24	−0.63 $\pm$ 0.22	$p < 0.05$
Duration of treatment (yrs)	9.2 $\pm$ 1.9	6.7 $\pm$ 0.9	ns
Dose of DHT (mg/day)	0.67 $\pm$ 0.07	0.74 $\pm$ 0.05	ns
Urine P (24 hr P/Cr)	0.606 $\pm$ 0.044	0.683 $\pm$ 0.065	ns
(fasting mg/100mlC_{cr})	0.569 $\pm$ 0.108	0.483 $\pm$ 0.117	ns
TmP/GFR (mg/100ml)	3.27 $\pm$ 0.22	4.20 $\pm$ 0.31	$p < 0.02$

one or more episodes of more severe or prolonged vitamin D intoxication occurred, the overall experience being judged moderate in 7 and severe in 8. None of the correlations were significant (Table 3). The severe hypercalcemic and high Ca groups had lower values for mean creatinine clearance (Table 4 and 5), but these differences were only significant at the 10% level with a one-tailed test. In both the low calcium and mild intoxication groups the mean C_{cr} was significantly below the mean of the age predicted values ($p < 0.05$ by one-tailed t test). None of the other renal function tests were even remotely different between the two groups for any of the three partitions, and in the high P group, the mean C_{cr} was actually higher than in the low P group (Table 6). There was no significant difference in mean plasma Ca and P levels between any two groups except when used as the basis of the partition. It is unfortunate that data for urinary calcium excretion was too incomplete for a similar analysis.

The difference between the high P and low P groups was examined in more detail. There was no significant difference in pretreatment plasma calcium or phosphate level, age, body surface area, dura-

Table 8.   Incidence of Renal and Other Calcifications.

		Nephro-lithiasis	Nephro-calcinosis	Calcific Periarthritis
Total No. of cases	(27)	5	3	3
Severe intoxication	(15)	5	2	3
Mild intoxication	(12)	0 $p < 0.10$	1	1
High Calcium	(13)	2	1	1
Low Calcium	(14)	3	2	2
High Phosphate	(13)	2	2	3
Low Phosphate	(14)	3	1	0 $p < 0.10$

tion of vitamin D therapy, dose of vitamin D therapy, 24 hour P/Cr ratio or fasting P excretion in mg/100ml C_{cr}, but TmP/GFR was higher in the P group (Table 7). There was also a significant difference in response to treatment for P but not for Ca. The occurrence of nephrolithiasis, radiographic nephrocalcinosis and extra renal soft tissue calcification is shown in Table 8. Nephrolithiasis could have been due to analgesic nephropathy in one case, who passed calcified papillae (12), but no cause other than prolonged vitamin D therapy was evident in the other four, or in the three cases of nephrocalcinosis. The only other type of soft tissue calcification was periarthritis of the shoulder noted in three patients. There was a probable association ($p < 0.10$ by Chi-squared with Yates correction) between severe vitamin D intoxication and nephrolithiasis, and between high plasma P and calcific periarthritis, but nephrocalcinosis was not significantly associated with any of the three partitions.

DISCUSSION

The results indicate a significant reduction in renal function, both glomerular and tubular, after prolonged treatment with vitamin D. Contrary to expectation, this impairment was only marginally related to severity of vitamin D intoxication. All indices studied were sometimes significantly reduced even in the complete absence of vitamin D intoxication and when plasma Ca levels were persistently normal. Mild hyperphosphatemia prolonged for up to 8 years had no detectable effect on the kidney. The results suggest that either prolonged hypercalciuria or vitamin D itself may have caused nephrocalcinosis by a direct effect. If the site at which PTH stimulates calcium reabsorption is proximal to the major site of concentration and acidification (13), it is conceivable that a lack of PTH stimulated calcium reabsorption (2) and consequent increase in urinary calcium concentration could have led to impairment of collecting duct function. However, it is difficult to conceive how such an abnormality could reduce the glomerular filtration rate, and it seems more likely that this is a direct consequence of vitamin D when given in a high pharmacologic dose for a prolonged period of time. This suggestion was first made many years ago (14) on very flimsy evidence. Subsequent commentators have discounted the idea, but not presented any additional data. In the hypoparathyroid rat, vitamin D administration leads to histologic nephrocalcinosis even though the plasma calcium remains subnormal (4), and the present study suggests that the same may occur in man.

The difference in plasma P between the high and low P groups was not due to a difference in the severity of hypoparathyroidism as judged by pretreatment plasma calcium (15), in the adequacy of treatment or in renal function. Although the difference in 24 hour

P/Cr did not quite achieve statistical significance, it seems likely that the diet made some contribution, although the difference in TmP/GFR was mainly responsible. The latter difference presumably reflected a difference in renal tubular responsiveness to the phosphaturic effect of vitamin D therapy, whether this is achieved directly or as a result of restoring normocalcemia.

Hyperphosphatemia possibly predisposed to calcific periarthritis of the shoulder in three patients but may have merely determined the radiographic visibility of the lesion rather than its initiation, since two of the three lesions were asymptomatic and were discovered accidentally. Lowering the plasma phosphate by dietary phosphate restriction has only a trivial effect on both total and ionised calcium (10) and the therapeutic value of such restriction remains unestablished.

SUMMARY AND CONCLUSIONS

1. Creatinine clearance, maximum urine osmolarity and minimum urine pH were all significantly reduced in 27 hypoparathyroid patients after long term vitamin D therapy.

2. When the patients were partitioned into two groups on the basis of severity of vitamin D intoxication, mean plasma Ca or +2SD upper boundary of plasma P, there was no significant difference between the two groups in any of the indices of renal function tested, although the mean creatinine clearance was more severely reduced in the high plasma Ca and the severe vitamin D intoxication groups. Differences in urinary calcium may have accounted for differences in urinary concentration and acidification, but not for differences in C_{cr}.

3. Nephrolithiasis occurred in five patients and was correlated with the frequency and severity of vitamin D intoxication. Nephrocalcinosis occurred in three patients but could not be correlated with any of the three partitions. Calcific periarthritis occurred in three patients in the high P group.

4. In patients with vitamin D treated hypoparathyroidism, as in normal subjects, TmP/GFR is the major determinant of plasma P.

5. The difference in plasma P between the high and low P groups was probably due to difference in renal tubular responsiveness to treatment and in diet, rather than in severity of hypoparathyroidism, adequacy of treatment or GFR.

6. Moderate hyperphosphatemia continued for up to 8 years had no detectable effect on renal function, but may have predisposed to soft tissue calcification.

7. The value of dietary P restriction as an adjunct to vitamin D therapy in hypoparathyroid remains unestablished.

8. In man, as previously found in the rat, vitamin D may have a direct effect to cause nephrocalcinosis and impaired renal function in the absence of hypercalcemia.

REFERENCES

1. Parfitt, A.M.: Hypercalcaemic nephropathy., Med. J. Aust., 2: 127-134, 1964.
2. Peacock, M., Nordin, B.E.C.: Plasma calcium homeostasis. Hard tissue growth, repair and mineralization. Ciba Foundation Symposium 11 (New series). Associated Scientific Publishers Amsterdam, 1973.
3. Hunt, G., Morgan, D.B.: The early effects of dihydrotachysterol on calcium and phosphorus metabolism in patients with hypoparathyroidism. Clin. Sci. 38: 713-725, 1970.
4. Mathieu, M., et al: Action toxique de la vitamine D sans hypercalcémie chez le rat parathyroidectomise. I Etude des lesions anatomiques. Path. Biol. 12: 674-687, 1964.
5. Parfitt, A.M., Frame, B.: Treatment of rickets and osteomalacia. Seminars on Drug Treatment. 2: 83-115, 1972.
6. Parfitt, A.M.: Idiopathic, surgical and other varieties of parathyroid hormone deficient hypoparathyroidism. in: The Metabolic Basis of Endocrinology, ed. L. DeGroot, (in press).
7. Gyory, A.Z., Edwards, K.D.G., Stewart, J.H., Whyte, H.M., Comprehensive one-day renal function testing in man. J. Clin. Path. 27: 382-391, 1973.
8. Documenta Geigy Scientific Tables. Sixth ed. J.R. Geigy, Basle, 1962.
9. Healy, J.K.: Clinical assessment of glomerular filtration rate by different forms of creatinine clearance and a modified urinary phenosulphonthalein excretion test. Amer. J. Med. 44: 348-358, 1968.
10. Parfitt, A.M., Frame, B.: Phosphate loading and depletion in vitamin D treated hypoparathyroidism. Implications for different physiological models of phosphate reabsorption. in: Proceedings of Second International Workshop on Phosphate (in press).
11. Rowe, Z.W., Andres, R., Tobin, J.D., Norris, A.H., Schock, N.W., Age adjusted standards for creatinine clearance. Ann. Int. Med., 84: 567-569, 1976.
12. Blackman, J.E., Gibson, G.R., Lavan, J.W., Learoyd, H.M., Posen, S. Urinary calculi and the consumption of analgesics. Brit. Med. J. 800-802, 1967.
13. Sutton, R.A.L., Dirks, J.H.: The renal excretion of calcium: a review of micropuncture data. Canad. J. Physiol. Pharmacol. 53: 979-988, 1975.
14. Steck, I.E., Deutsch, M., Reed, C.I., Struck, H.C.: Further studies on intoxication with vitamin D. Ann. Int. Med. 10: 951-964, 1937.
15. Parfitt, A.M.: The spectrum of hypoparathyroidism. J. Clin. Endocr. 34: 152-158, 1972.

Phosphate and Renal Osteodystrophy

THE ROLE OF PHOSPHATE AND OTHER FACTORS ON THE PATHOGENESIS OF RENAL OSTEODYSTROPHY

E. Slatopolsky, W.E. Rutherford, K. Martin, and K. Hruska

Washington University School of Medicine, Department of

Medicine, 4550 Scott Avenue, St. Louis, Missouri 63110

Renal osteodystrophy is a serious complication of chronic renal disease, characterized by several alterations in bone structure. This includes osteitis fibrosa cystica, representing the effects of secondary hyperparathyroidism; and osteomalacia, representing defective bone mineralization secondary to abnormalities in the metabolism of vitamin D and other substances induced by renal failure. Less commonly, osteosclerosis and osteoporosis are also seen.

The pathogenetic mechanisms responsible for the development of renal osteodystrophy are not fully understood; thus, a unified therapeutic approach is not available. However, in the past ten years, investigators have clarified some of the factors involved in the development of renal osteodystrophy. The manifestations of disordered mineral metabolism in chronic renal disease include hyperphosphatemia, hypocalcemia, hypermagnesemia, hyperplasia of the parathyroid glands, elevated serum levels of immunoreactive PTH, skeletal resistance to the action of parathyroid hormone (PTH), decreased renal degradation of PTH, abnormal vitamin D metabolism, defective intestinal absorption of calcium and abnormal collagen metabolism. The main known pathogenetic factors responsible for the development of renal osteodystrophy are summarized in Figure 1.

SECONDARY HYPERPARATHYROIDISM

Secondary hyperparathyroidism is a frequent complication of chronic renal disease. It appears early in the course of renal failure (1), at which time phosphate retention is the major patho-

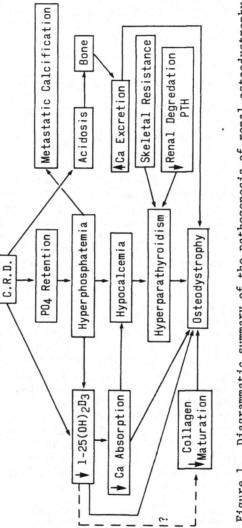

Figure 1. Diagrammatic summary of the pathogenesis of renal osteodystrophy.

genetic mechanism involved in its production (2-3). The kidney plays an important role in the regulation of phosphate. Approximately 70% of the phosphate that is ingested in the diet is excreted by the kidneys. To effect this rate of excretion within normal renal function approximately 10 to 20% of the filtered phosphate must be excreted. However, in chronic renal disease the number of excretory units decreases and as the number of nephrons diminish, if phosphate balance is to be maintained, each nephron must increase the rate of phosphate excretion. The lower the number of excretory units, the greater the amount of phosphate excreted per unit (4). This adaptation is sufficiently precise to permit phosphate balance so plasma phosphorus remains close to normal unless the glomerular filtration rate decreases below 25 ml/min. We have demonstrated (4) that this phosphaturia per nephron is mediated in part by an increase in the levels of parathyroid hormone. During the evolution of chronic renal disease recurrent periods of phosphate retention occur each time the glomerular filtration rate falls. This phosphate retention, even though it may be small in magnitude, will lead to an increased plasma phosphate concentration and produce a reciprocal decrease in serum calcium concentration. The fall in ionized calcium will be sensed by the parathyroid glands which will respond by increasing the rate of parathyroid hormone secretion. The increase in parathyroid hormone levels will promote an increase in the rate of phosphate excretion in the remaining nephrons. Thus, total phosphate excretion will rise and serum phosphorus concentration will return to normal. As we mentioned before, when the glomerular filtration rate falls below 25 ml/min the number of excretory units are too small and constant hyperphosphatemia develops. Thus, severe phosphorus retention should be avoided to prevent changes in ionized calcium with a consequent development of secondary hyperparathyroidism.

With the progression of renal disease, calcium malabsorption in the gastrointestinal tract becomes unavoidable and a second important factor is added to the pathogenesis of secondary hyperparathyroidism.

VITAMIN D RESISTANCE

Alterations in the metabolism of vitamin D in chronic renal disease plays an important factor in the development of renal osteodystrophy. Vitamin D is normally produced in the skin when ultraviolet radiation is absorbed by a pro-vitamin, 7-dehydrocholesterol. However, for cultural reasons, the exposure of man's skin to sunlight is insufficient to allow the synthesis of this compound in sufficient quantities to regulate mineral metabolism; thus, dietary supplementation in the form of either vitamin D_3, cholecalciferol or vitamin D_2 ergocalciferol are necessary to meet the demands of the body.

Dietary vitamin D is absorbed in the small intestine and is transported in lymph by chylomicrons and stored in the body in the muscles and adipose tissue serving as a reservoir during periods of deprivation or decreased exposure to sunlight. Vitamin D is transported into the liver for further changes in its molecular composition. The first step in the metabolism of vitamin D is the addition of an hydroxyl group in the 25 position, thus the first metabolite of vitamin D is known as 25-hydroxycholecalciferol (25-OH D_3).

Recently, 25-hydroxycholecalciferol has been shown to undergo further hydroxylation in the kidney to 1,25-dihydroxycholecalciferol (1,25-OH$_2$D$_3$). Evidence from different laboratories (5-6) clearly indicates that the kidney is the only organ responsible for the formation of 1,25-dihydroxycholecalciferol. This metabolite is responsible for all the known actions of vitamin D.

Patients with chronic renal disease have low levels of 1,25-dihydroxycholecalciferol in blood. Thus, they develop severe calcium malabsorption. The decrease of 1,25-OH$_2$D$_3$ in blood also may be responsible for some of the osteomalacic changes that are present in bones. If a normal individual is fed a low calcium diet, the percentage of calcium absorbed increases and calcium balance is maintained. This adaptative mechanism is mediated by the formation of 1,25-dihydroxycholecalciferol; however, this control mechanism is lost in patients with chronic renal disease. Thus, if a uremic patient is placed on a diet that contains less than 1.5 grams of elemental calcium per day, the patient develops negative calcium balance, which will aggravate the hypocalcemia.

ABNORMAL RENAL DEGRADATION OF PARATHYROID HORMONE

The kidney plays an important role in the degradation of parathyroid hormone. Recently Hruska and collaborators (7) have studied the contribution of the kidney to the metabolism of parathyroid hormone. In normal dogs, the kidney extracted approximately 20% of the C-terminal immunoreactive parathyroid hormone (PTH) delivered to it and the renal clearance of immunoreactive PTH was 60 ml/min. The participation of the kidney accounted for 2/3 of the total metabolic clearance for PTH. When the dogs were rendered uremic by ligation of most of the branches of left renal artery and right nephrectomy, there was a remarkable decrease in the metabolic clearance rate of PTH mainly accounted for by the decrease in the renal clearance of PTH. Analysis of the disappearance curves of immunoreactivity following injection of

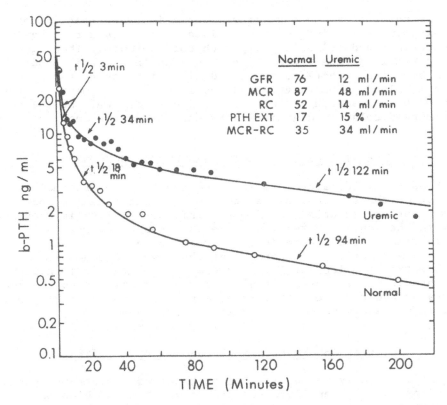

Figure 2. Disappearance curves of immunoreactive PTH after
injection of b-PTH in a dog studied when normal
(o——o) and after the induction of uremia (●——●).
(Reproduced with permission from Reference 7)

b-PTH 1-84 (Figure 2), demonstrated that the major effect of
chronic renal disease became apparent after 10-15 minutes post-
injection. At these times, the predominant forms of circulating
PTH were C-terminal PTH fragments. This suggested that impaired
renal degradation was especially important to the genesis of the
high levels of PTH fragments seen in chronic renal failure. In
subsequent studies, we have demonstrated lack of detectable uptake
of PTH fragments by organs other than the kidney, again calling
attention to the role of impaired renal degradation in producing
high circulating levels of PTH fragments in renal failure.

The results of these studies clearly indicate that in dogs
with experimentally induced renal disease there is a remarkable
decrease in the degradation of parathyroid hormone. Thus, in
chronic renal disease, there is not only an increase in production
of PTH but also a decrease in degradation with consequent accumulation in blood. The exaggerated levels of PTH fragments in the
blood of patients with chronic renal disease may well be due to
their marked delay in degradation by the diseased kidney.

SKELETAL RESISTANCE TO PARATHYROID HORMONE

Massry and collaborators (8) have reported an abnormal
response of the skeletal system to the calcemic action of parathyroid hormone in uremic patients. This abnormality is seen
early in the course of renal disease and is not reversed by
hemodialysis. Since there is a synergistic action between
vitamin D and parathyroid hormone at the level of bone, it is
possible that the lack of 1,25-dihydroxycholecalciferol in patients
with chronic renal disease renders the bone resistant to the action
of parathyroid hormone. Therefore, a greater amount of PTH in
blood is necessary to mobilize calcium from bone.

SKELETAL ABNORMALITIES IN CHRONIC RENAL DISEASE

Until recently the evaluation of renal osteodystrophy through
bone biopsies has been neglected and in general the biopsies,
when obtained, were decalcified prior to microscopic examination.
Thus, differentiation between unmineralized osteoid and mineralized
bone was impossible. New techniques have been developed (9) for
histological evaluation of bone pathology. The calcified bone
can be cut in thin sections, allowing the study of the mineralized
bone and the osteoid tissue. When osteomalacia is the primary
pathological process, the histological findings are an increase in
the total volume of osteoid matrix and an overall decrease in
bone apposition rate. In patients with severe osteomalacia the
osteoid seams are wider than 20 microns and there is a failure in
the uptake of tetracycline label; thus, this results in an
inability to demonstrate a calcification front (9). When the main
component is osteitis fibrosa cystica, the number of osteoclast is
increased and usually there is marrow-fibrosis.

SOFT TISSUE CALCIFICATION

The most important predisposing factor to soft tissue calcification in chronic renal disease is an increased phosphate-calcium
product in blood. Hyperphosphatemia is responsible for the precip-

itation of calcium usually seen around the joints; mainly shoulder,
hip, wrist and fingers. Vascular calcification sometimes may
produce ischemic changes with necrosis and gangrene of the
extremities. Slit lamp examination may disclose ocular calcification and some patients may develop a syndrome characterized by
an acute conjunctivitis, a syndrome called "the red eye of uremia."
Precipitation of calcium in the skin may be responsible for pruritus.

<u>TREATMENT</u>

In view of the pathophysiological events which take place in
the course of renal insufficiency, general guidelines for the
treatment of renal osteodystrophy can now be proposed (Table I).
Phosphate retention should be avoided early in the course of
chronic renal disease. Phosphate restriction should begin when
the levels of serum creatinine are between 3 and 4 mg/100 ml in
order to prevent the development of severe secondary hyperparathyroidism. Dietary phosphate restriction, especially dairy
foods, and the addition of phosphate binders are means of achiev-
ing a proper phosphate intake. Phosphate depletion should also
be avoided and serum phosphorus levels should be maintained in
the range of 3 to 4 mg/100 ml.

Most of the diets prescribed for uremic patients are low in
calcium in the order of 300-400 mg/24 hrs. Thus, calcium supplementation is strongly recommended. Approximately 1 to 1.5 gms of
elemental calcium per day should be administered orally as
calcium carbonate (40% is calcium) or calcium lactate (13% is
calcium) or calcium gluconate (9% is calcium). The concentration
of calcium in the dialysate is extremely important. Patients
dialyzed with a bath containing less than 6 mg/100 ml will develop
negative calcium balance. The amount of calcium in the dialysate
should be increased to 6.5-7 mg/100 ml. The use of a high calcium
concentration in the dialysate without appropriate control of
serum phosphorus would cause severe soft tissue calcification.
Thus, before calcium is supplemented into diet or increased in
the dialysate, phosphorus must be under control.

Since uremic patients retain magnesium, and plasma concentrations of 2-3 mg/100 ml are not unusual, the amount of magnesium in
the dialysate should not be greater than 1.5 mg/100 ml. Phosphate
binders containing magnesium should not be prescribed to patients
with chronic renal disease.

There are now several new metabolites of vitamin D. These
are 25-hydroxycholecalciferol, 1-alpha-hydroxycholecalciferol and
1,25-dihydroxycholecalciferol. All of these three metabolites are

TABLE I

Guidelines for the treatment of renal osteodystrophy

1. Early treatment
   GFR 30 to 40 ml/min

2. Phosphate restriction
   a. Diet
   b. Binders

3. Calcium supplementation
   1 g daily as:

   a. Carbonate (40%)
   b. Lactate (13%)
   c. Gluconate (9%)

4. Calcium in dialysate
   6.5 to 7.0 mg/100 ml

5. Magnesium in dialysate
   1.0 to 1.5 mg/100 ml

6. Administration of vitamin D metabolites
   a. 25-hydroxycholecalciferol
   b. 1-alpha-hydroxycholecalciferol
   c. 1,25-dihydroxycholecalciferol

7. Parathyroidectomy
   a. Persistent hypercalcemia
   b. Intractable pruritus associated with high PTH
   c. Severe soft tissue calcification or necrosis unrespon-
      sive to effective control of PO_4

potent drugs which can correct calcium malabsorption in a relatively short period of time and produce an improvement in the
histology of the bones. If these metabolites are used the serum
calcium should be monitored frequently since patients may develop
severe hypercalcemia. The daily recommended doses for these
metabolites are: 25-hydroxycholecalciferol, 50 to 150 µg; 1-alpha-
hydroxycholecalciferol, 1 to 2 µg; and 1,25-dihydroxycholecalciferol,
0.25 to 0.75 µg. Regardless of the metabolite used, all of these
three drugs are extremely potent and the patient should be followed
very closely. These drugs should not be given in the presence of
hyperphosphatemia. Finally, the role of surgical parathyroidectomy
in the treatment of renal osteodystrophy is somewhat controversial;
however, certain conditions such as 1) persistant hypercalcemia
(before vitamin D is given to the patient), 2) severe pruritus

unresponsive to conservative treatment especially in association with high levels of parathyroid hormone, 3) severe progressive soft tissue calcification or tissue necrosis unresponsive to effective control of serum phosphorus in association with high levels of parathyroid hormone, are indications for surgical parathyroidectomy.

REFERENCES

1. Reiss, E., Canterbury, J.M., and Egdahl, R.H. Experience with a radioimmunoassay of parathyroid hormone in human sera. Trans. Assoc. Am. Phys. 81: 104, 1968.

2. Bricker, N.S., Slatopolsky, E., Reiss, E., and Avioli, L.V. Calcium, phosphorus and bone in renal disease and transplantation. Arch. Int. Med. 123: 543, 1969.

3. Slatopolsky, E., Caglar, S., Pennell, J.P., Taggart, D.D., Canterbury, J.M., Reiss, E., and Bricker, N.S. On the pathogenesis of hyperparathyroidism in chronic experimental renal insufficiency in the dog. J. Clin. Invest. 50: 492, 1971.

4. Slatopolsky, E., Robson, A.M., Elkan, I., and Bricker, N.S. Control of phosphate excretion in uremic man. J. Clin. Invest. 47: 1865, 1968.

5. Fraser, D.R., and Kodicek, E. Unique biosynthesis by kidney of a biologically active vitamin D metabolite. Nature 228: 764, 1970.

6. Gray, R., Boyle, I., and DeLuca, H.F. Vitamin D metabolism: The role of kidney tissue. Science 172: 1232, 1971.

7. Hruska, K.A., Kopelman, R., Rutherford, W.E., Klahr, S. and Slatopolsky, E. Metabolism of immunoreactive parathyroid hormone in the dog: The role of the kidney and the effects of chronic renal insufficiency. J. Clin. Invest. 56: 39, 1975.

8. Massry, S.G., Coburn, J.W., Lee, D.B.N., Jowsey, J., and Kleeman, C.R. Skeletal resistance to parathyroid hormone in renal failure. Study in 105 human subjects. Ann. Int. Med. 78: 357, 1973.

9. Bordier, P., Marie, P.G., and Arnaud, C.A. Evolution of renal osteodystrophy: Correlation of bone histo-morphometry and serum mineral and immunoreactive parathyroid hormone values before and after treatment with calcium carbonate or 25-hydroxycholecalciferol. Kidney International 7: s102, 1975.

ULTRASTRUCTURAL ASPECTS OF BONE MINERA-
LIZATION IN RENAL OSTEODYSTROPHY

BONUCCI E.

Institute of Pathological Anatomy

University of Rome, Rome, Italy

It has repeatedly been shown that chronic renal failure almost constantly induces the development of "renal osteody-strophy" (1), that is of skeletal changes characterized by the contemporaneous occurrence of osteomalacia and secondary hyperparathyroidism. While these changes have repeatedly been studied with the light microscope, they have not been extensively studied with electron microscopy.

Recently, we have had the opportunity of examining bone biopsies taken from the iliac crest of 80 unselected patients suffering from chronic renal failure; 40 of them were treated conservatively and received low protein diet (24-35 g protein/ day), 40 were treated with hemodialysis and received a free diet. The needle biopsies of all of these patients were fixed in paraformaldehyde and post-fixed with osmium tetroxide, both buffered to pH 7.2 with phosphate buffer, and were then embedded in an epoxy resin (Araldite). Serial semithin (about 1 u thick) and ultrathin (about 800 Å thick) sections were studied comparatively with light and electron microscopy. The former were stained with Azure II - Methylene blue and with von Kossa method; the latter were examined unstai-ned and after staining with uranyl acetate and lead citrate. Detailed descriptions of the results of these investigations, showing that all of the patients had a variable degree of hyper-parathyroidism and osteomalacia, have been reported else-where (2-5).

In all of the patients, and especially in the youngest
and in those submitted to maintenance   dialysis, the most
evident abnormality was represented by the presence of exces-
sively thick and wide borders of osteoid tissue on the trabecular surface (Fig. 1). No quantitative measurement   was
attempted, but a semiquantitative evaluation of the amount of
osteoid tissue showed that it was from 3 to 6 times more
abundant than in normal subjects.   Moreover, the osteoid
borders were sometimes so thick that one or many osteocy-
te-like cells were present in them.

Under the electron microscope, the osteoid tissue was
characterized by the presence of loosely arranged collagen
fibrils which were sometimes collected in lamellae and very
often were irregularly oriented. The single collagen fibrils
did not appear abnormal: they had a periodic banding of
about 640 Å and a thickness of about 700 Å. However, some
of them were more than 2000 Å thick, apparently because of
the lateral aggregation of two or three thin fibrils.

The osteoid tissue was in contact with both roundish,

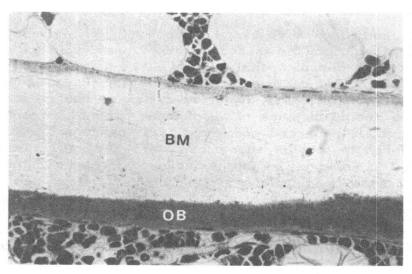

Fig. 1. Detail of an undecalcified bone trabecula stained
with Azure II - Methylene blue; BM: calcified bone matrix.
A thick osteoid border (OB) is present along the lower
margin of the trabecula. x 350.

plump osteoblasts and with spindle-shaped cells. The former were frequently found in the youngest subjects. Under the electron microscope, they showed a developed rough ergastoplasmic reticulum and wide Golgi areas and on the whole they had the same structure as that of normal osteoblasts (6). The spindle-shaped cells had very few cytoplasmic organelles and frequently contained aggregates of glycogen. They were like the cells described as "resting osteoblasts" (7).

A few osteoblast-like cells placed near and in contact with the osteoid tissue contained intracytoplasmic clusters of inorganic crystals which seemed to be contained within mitochondria.

The collagen fibrils of the osteoid tissue were usually completely uncalcified. However, in some cases small, roundish clusters of needle-shaped crystals were randomly scattered through the osteoid matrix (Fig. 2). These clusters were especially found near the fully calcified matrix, where

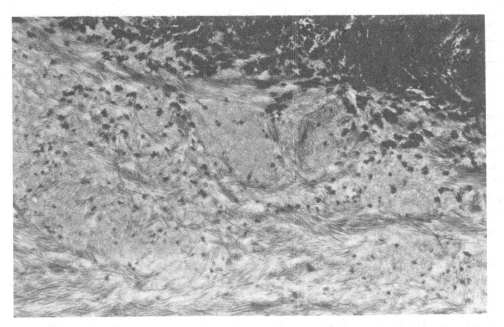

Fig. 2. Electron micrograph showing a detail of the osteoid tissue in a zone adjacent to the fully calcified matrix (above). Very small clusters of crystals are scattered through the osteoid matrix. Uranyl acetate and lead citrate, x 7000.

they gave rise to the formation of a thin calcification front, and around the osteocytes. Moreover, a few crystals were found near and within roundish, electron-dense bodies which were sometimes surrounded by a membrane and consisted of homogeneous matrix. These bodies, comparable with those described as matrix vesicles (8) and calcifying globules (9) and found in both calcifying cartilage (8-10) and bone (9, 11-14), were numerous near a few of the plump osteoblasts and were usually lacking in the inner zone of the uncalcified osteoid tissue.

The degree of calcification of the bone matrix was variable. Chiefly in proximity to the osteoid tissue, the mineral substance was not uniformly distributed through the bone matrix. In these zones, roundish and elongated areas of calcification separated by uncalcified zones were present. Moreover, in the calcified areas the mineral substance consisted of very small granules rather than of needle-shaped crystals and the granules were collected in bands of intrinsic electron density closely related to the periodic banding of the collagen fibrils. As previously reported (9,15,16), these pictures are typically found in early calcifying and low calcified bone matrix and show that in renal osteodystrophy wide areas of bone matrix remain hypocalcified.

All of the patients, and especially those submitted to hemodialysis, showed evident enhancement of the osteoclastic bone resorption. The osteoclasts were often smaller than those found in normal subjects. Frequently, they were collected in clusters (Fig. 3). Moreover, osteoclastic bone resorption was occurring not only on the surface of the trabeculae; in some cases, osteoclasts were present also within the trabeculae which consequently were more or less completely dissected. Where osteoclasts were not present, empty Howship's lacunae, and lacunae filled by osteoid tissue showed that the bone matrix had previously been reabsorbed by them.

Under the electron microscope, the osteoclasts were similar to those found in normal subjects (6, 17-21). They looked like very active cells as shown by their developed ruffled border, by the disaggregated appearance of the adjacent bone matrix, and by the numerous cytoplasmic vacuoles containing phagocytosed crystals. Occasionally, osteoclasts were placed between osteoblasts and were in close contact with

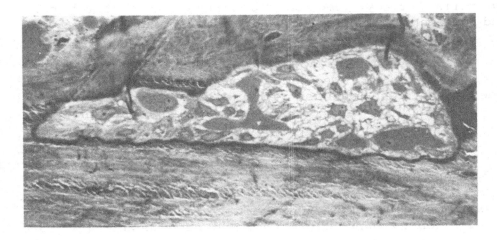

Fig. 3. Osteoclasts within a wide lacuna of a trabecula. Azure II - Methylene blue, x 550.

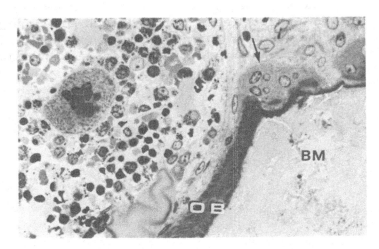

Fig. 4. Detail of an osseous trabecula in an undecalcified section stained with Azure II - Methylene blue. A wide osteoid border (OB) is present in the lower left part of the trabecula, which is undergoing osteoclastic resorption in its upper part. Note that an osteoclast (arrow) is at the same time in contact with the osteoid border and the bone matrix (BM). x 500.

the osteoid tissue (Fig. 4) which seemed to be reabsorbed by them. Actually, electron microscopy showed that uncalcified collagen fibrils were present between the infoldings of the brush borders of these osteoclasts.

Osteoclasts were not the only cells engaged in bone resorption; in fact, also the osteocytes were very active. They were often contained within enlarged and irregular lacunae which in many cases seemed to be coalescing (Fig. 5). These pictures are considered typical modifications occurring on the wall of the lacunae of the osteocytes engaged in osteocytic osteolysis (22). There is no doubt that osteolysis was responsible of the enlargement and irregularity of the lacunae of most of the osteocytes found in the present series of biopsies. However, as previously underlined by Sissons (23), when hyperparathyroidism and osteomalacia are found together in the same subjects, osteolytic-like changes of the lacunae can be produced by defective calcification of the perilacunar matrix rather than by periosteocytic osteolysis.

This was in fact confirmed by electron microscopy. Under the light microscope, almost all of the osteocytes placed in hypomineralized areas had enlarged and irregular lacunae. Under the electron microscope, these osteocytes often showed an osteoblastic structure because of the presence in their cytoplasm of a developed rough ergastoplasmic

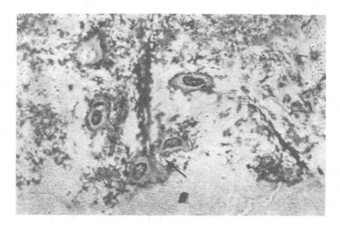

Fig. 5. Osteocytes with irregular and enlarged lacunae; two of them (arrow) seem to be coalescing. Also osteocytic canaliculi are enlarged and coalescing. Azure II - Methylene blue, x 850.

reticulum and of wide Golgi areas. Moreover, their peripheral membrane was in direct contact with the collagen fibrils of the surrounding matrix. This was uncalcified, or contained only small, roundish clusters of needle-shaped crystals like those which can be found in calcifying matrices. All of these findings show that these osteocytes were still in a formative phase and that the wall of their lacunae appeared irregular under the light microscope because it was not yet completely calcified. These findings underline the necessity of always evaluating the degree of calcification of the bone matrix when bone sections are to be examined for osteocytic osteolysis.

Most of the osteocytes found in fully calcified bone matrix had enlarged and irregular lacunae (Fig. 5). Electron microscopy showed that these osteocytes had an irregular shape because of the arched outline of their peripheral membrane and of the presence of many cytoplasmic processes protruding from them into the pericellular space and eventually penetrating the bone matrix in every direction. Moreover, these osteocytes were not in direct contact with the wall of their lacunae because of the interposition of a space which contained granular and flocculent material, very thin filaments, and small fragments of collagen fibrils (Fig. 6). Clusters of inorganic crystals were sometimes present in the mitochondria of these osteocytes. All these findings are considered to be indicative of the occurrence of osteocytic osteolysis (24-31), so that the conclusion must be drawn that in renal osteodystrophy most of the osteocytes placed in fully calcified matrix are engaged in this process. This conclusion is in agreement with the results of previous investigations (32) carried out by differential count of osteocytes in femoral bone of normal and uremic subjects.

The mechanism of the osteocytic osteolysis is still unknown. Because phagocytosed crystals, like those present in osteoclasts, have never been found in the cytoplasm of the activated osteocytes, it is possible to speculate that the mineral substance is solubilized extracellularly and that the breakdown   products are collected in the pericellular space which is formed in consequence of the matrix demolition. Successively, the solubilized mineral substance could be reabsorbed by the osteocyte. When, as in the present series of cases, a condition of severe hyperparathyroidism leads to excessive osteolytic activity and, consequently, to excessive

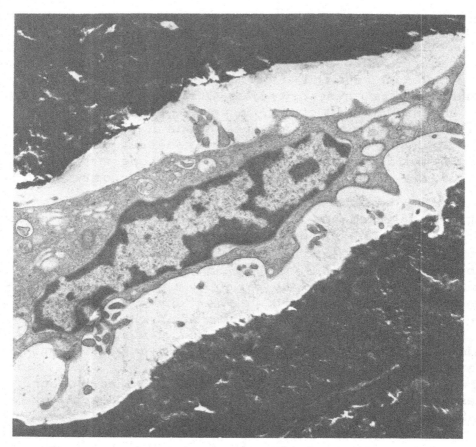

Fig. 6. Electron micrograph showing an osteocyte placed in an enlarged and irregular lacuna; note the pericellular space, the arched outline of the cell membrane, the numerous cell processes and the material around the cells. Uranyl acetate and lead citrate, x 15,000.

intracytoplasmic calcium and phosphate concentration, the mineral substance can be accumulated in mitochondria, as frequently observed in renal osteodystrophy.

Not all of the osteocytes placed in fully calcified matrix were contained within enlarged and irregular lacunae. Some of them were placed in small, roundish and elongated lacunae having a regular, apparently smooth wall. Under the electron microscope, these osteocytes had a "mature" appearance, that is they had a reduced cytoplasm with few organelles and

very few rough cysternae of the ergastoplasmic reticulum.
Usually, these small osteocytes were directly in contact with
the wall of their lacunae.

Electron microscopy showed that the walls of these
lacunae were not as smooth as they appeared under the
light microscope. In fact, many needle- and filament-like
crystals protruded from the calcified matrix in the direction
of the osteocytes, forming a more or less continuous crystal
layer all around the lacunae. These crystals were almost
perpendicular to the osteocyte peripheral membrane and were
often placed side-to-side like the bristles of a brush (Fig. 7).
Similar structures have previously been described in the
lacunae of the osteocytes of medullary bone of pigeons (33).

No direct evidence has been obtained that the crystals
which protrude from the lacunar wall can be reabsorbed by
the osteocytes. However, indications that this resorption
could occur were furnished by the following observations.

A few of the small osteocytes showed evidence of early

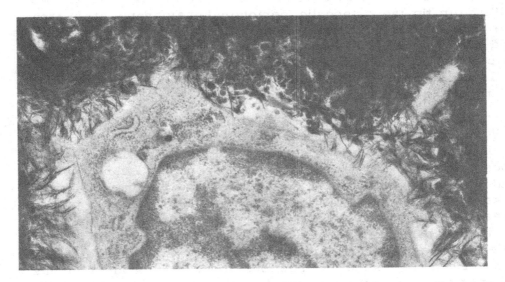

Fig. 7. Electron micrograph showing part of a small osteocyte found in fully calcified bone. Note the crystals protruding
from the bone matrix in the direction of the osteocyte and
touching its peripheral membrane in many places; also note
the reduced amount of cytoplasm and the very few cytoplasmic
organelles. Uranyl acetate and lead citrate, x 29,000.

osteolytic activity, that is the initial formation of a space was recognizable around them, and this space contained granular and flocculent material and very thin filaments, as happens in periosteocytic osteolysis. In these osteocytes, the crystals protruding from the lacunar wall were still present where, the pericellular space had not yet been formed, were disarranged and often lacking where the pericellular space had already been formed, and were present but contained into cytoplasmic invaginations where the space was in the initial phase of formation (Fig. 8).

Little is known about the role of the crystals which protrude from the lacunar wall into the lacunar space. In the present material, they did not appear to be firmly bound to collagen fibrils, although calcified collagen fibrils could be found between them. Moreover, they were loosely arranged. These characteristics are like those of the so-called "coastal crystal", that is crystals placed on the border of the osteocytic lacunae and considered to represent a labile, readily available fraction of mineral substance (34). The present findings, and the observation that many of the protruding crystals touch with their tip the osteocytic peripheral membrane, strengthen the concept that they can be easily removed by the osteocytes and can represent a disposable, easily utilizable reservoir of calcium and phosphate ions. The resorption of these crystals could occur without evident changes of the shape and width of the lacunae.

A particular structure, the so-called "osmiophilic lamina", has frequently been described around osteocyte lacunae in decalcified and stained sections (25,26,28, 31,34). It is possible that the crystals protruding from the lacunar wall and the osmiophilic lamina are coincident, as previously suggested by Wassermann and Yaeger (34) for their coastal crystals. On this regards, it is interesting that the osmiophilic lamina has been described also on the border of the calcified cartilage (35) where protruding crystals are also present (10). No decalcified sections have been studied in this investigation and consequently it has not been possible to ascertain if there is a relationship between the protruding crystals and the osmiophilic lamina.

The present results confirm that the development of renal osteodystrophy is the rule in uremic subjects. It

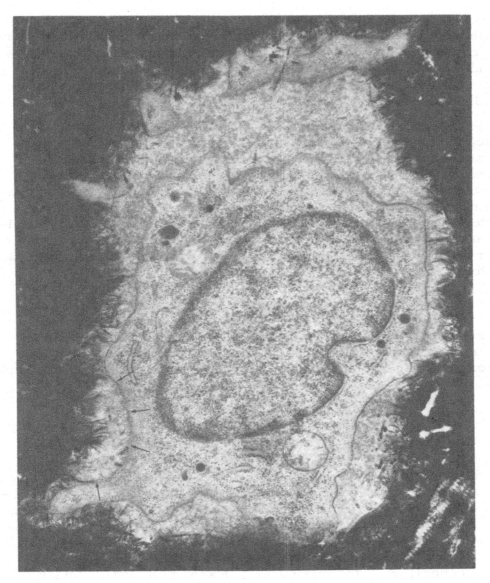

Fig. 8. A small osteocyte probably in early stage of osteolytic activity. A pericellular space of variable width is visible;
it contains flocculent and granular material. Crystals protruding from the bone matrix are still present on the lacunar
wall while are lacking on its upper side. Arrows point to a
cytoplasmic invagination which surrounds a cluster of protruding crystals. Uranyl acetate and lead citrate, x 23,000.

consists of osteomalacia and hyperparathyroidism, and these pathological conditions are not different from those which occur in nutritional osteomalacia (7) and in primary hyperparathyroidism (36), respectively. However, the skeletal changes are usually more severe in hemodialyzed patients than in patients treated conservatively.

Electron microscopy has been useful under many respects, but chiefly to determine the role of the osteocytes in bone resorption. On this regard, it has been possible to confirm that many of the osteocytes placed in fully calcified matrix are engaged in osteolytic activity and that, on the contrary, many of those found in hypomineralized matrix have osteoblastic properties. This shows that the degree of calcification of the bone matrix should always be taken into consideration when bone sections are to be examined for osteolytic osteolysis.

Acknowledgements

The investigations mentioned in this paper have been carried out with the financial support of the Italian National Research Council. The assistance of Giuliana Silvestrini, Giorgio Gherardi and Lucio Virgilii are gratefully acknowledged.

References

1. Stanbury, S.W.: Azotaemic renal osteodystrophy. Brit. Med Bull. 13, 57-60, 1957.
2. Bonucci, E., Maschio, G., D'Angelo, A., Ossi, E., Lupo, A., Valvo, E.: Morphological aspects of bone tissue in chronic renal disease. In: Vitamin D and problems related to uremic bone disease (A.W. Norman, K. Schaefer, H.G. Grigoleit, D.v. Herrath, E. Ritz, eds.). Berlin, New York: W. de Gruyter 1975, p. 523.
3. Bonucci, E., Gherardi, G., Faraggiana, T., Mioni, G., Cannella, G., Castellani, A., Maiorca, R.: Bone changes in hemodialyzed uremic subjects: comparative light and electron microscope investigation. Virchows Arch. Abt. A Path. Anat. Histol., in press.
4. Maschio, G., Bonucci, E., Mioni, G., D'Angelo, A., Ossi, E., Valvo, E., Lupo, A.: Biochemical and morphological aspects of bone tissue in chronic renal failure.

Nephron 12, 437-448, 1974.

5. Mioni, G., Cecchettin, M., Castellani, A., Cannella, G., Cristinelli, L., D'Angelo, A., Maiorca, R., Bonucci, E., Gherardi, G., Heynen, G., Franchimont, P.: Hormonal and metabolic investigations on renal osteodystrophy of uremic dialyzed subjects. Europ. J. Clin. Invest., in press.

6. Cameron, D.A.: The ultrastructure of bone. In: The biochemistry and physiology of bone, 2nd ed., v. I, p. 191. G.H. Bourne, ed. New York, London, Academic Press 1972.

7. Bonucci, E., Denis-Matrajt, H., Tun-Chot, S., Hioco, D.J.: Bone structure in osteomalacia, with special reference to ultrastructure. J. Bone Joint Surg. 51 B, 511-528, 1969.

8. Anderson, H.C.: Vesicles associated with calcification in the matrix of epiphyseal cartilage. J. Cell Biol. 41, 59-72, 1969.

9. Bonucci, E.: Fine structure and histochemistry of "calcifying globules" in epiphyseal cartilage. Z. Zellforsch. 103, 192-217, 1970.

10. Bonucci, E.: Fine structure of early cartilage calcification. J. Ultrastruct. Res. 20, 33-50, 1967.

11. Bonucci, E.: The locus of initial calcification in cartilage and bone. Clin. Orthop. Relat. Res. 78, 108-139, 1971.

12. Bonucci, E.: The organic-inorganic relationships in calcified organic matrices. In: Physico-chimie et cristallographie des apatites d'intérêt biologique, Coll. Intern. du Centre Nat. de la Recherche Scientifique n. 230, Paris 1975, p. 231.

13. Anderson, H.C.: Calcium-accumulating vesicles in the intercellular matrix of bone. In: Hard tissue growth, repair and remineralization. Ciba Found. Symp. 11, Elsevier, Excerpta Medica, North-Holland 1973, p. 213.

14. Bernard, G.W., Pease, D.C.: An electron microscopic study of initial intramembranous osteogenesis. Am. J. Anat. 125, 271-290, 1969.

15. Ascenzi, A., Bonucci, E., Steve-Bocciarelli, D.: An electron microscope study of the osteon calcification. J. Ultrastruct. Res. 12, 287-303, 1965.

16. Glimcher, 1959. Molecular biology of mineralized tissues with particular reference to bone. Rev. Mod. Phys. 31, 359-393, 1959.

17. Bonucci, E.: The organic-inorganic relationships in bone matrix undergoing osteoclastic resorption. Calcif. Tiss. Res. 16, 13-36, 1974.

18. Dudley, H.R., Spiro, D.: The fine structure of bone cells. J. biophys. biochem. Cytol. 11, 627-649, 1961.

19. Gonzales, F., Karnovsky, M.J.: Electron microscopy of osteoclasts in healing fractures of rat bone. J. Biophys. Biochem. Cytol. 9, 299-316, 1961.

20. Hancox, N.M., Boothroyd, B.: Motion picture and electron microscope studies on the embryonic avian osteoclast. J. biophys. biochem. Cytol. 11, 651-661, 1961.

21. Scott, B.L., Pease, D.C.: Electron microscopy of the epiphyseal apparatus. Anat. Record 126, 465-495, 1956.

22. Bélanger, L.F.: Osteocytic osteolysis. Calcif. Tiss. Res. 4, 1-12, 1969.

23. Sissons, H.A.: Les changements péri-ostéocytaires dans l'ostéomalacie. Rev. Chir. Orthop. App. Moteur (Paris) 55, 284, 1969 (abstr.).

24. Baud, A.: Morphologie et structure inframicroscopique des ostéocytes. Acta Anat. 51, 209-225, 1962.

25. Jande, S.S.: Fine structural study of osteocytes and their surrounding bone matrix with respect to their age in young chicks. J. Ultrastruct. Res. 37, 279-300, 1971.

26. Jande, S.S., Bélanger, L.F.: Electron microscopy of osteocytes and the pericellular matrix in rat trabecular bone. Calcif. Tiss. Res. 6, 280-289, 1971.

27. Jande, S.S., Bélanger, L.F.: The life cycle of the osteocyte. Clin. Orthop. Rel. Res. 94, 281-305, 1973.

28. Luk, S.C., Nopajaroonsri, C., Simon, G.T.: The ultrastructure of cortical bone in young adult rabbits. J. Ultrastruct. Res. 46, 184-205, 1974.

29. Remagen, W., Caesar, R., Heuck, F.: Elektronenmikroskopische und mikroradiographische Befunde am Knochen der mit Dihydrotachysterin behandelten Ratte. Virchows Arch. Abt. A Path. Anat. Histol. 345, 245-254, 1968.

30. Remagen, W., Höhling, H.J., Hall, T.T., Caesar, R.: Electron microscopical and microprobe observations on the cell sheath of stimulated osteocytes. Calcif. Tiss. Res. 4, 60-68, 1969.

31. Tonna, E.A.: Electron microscopic evidence of alterna-

ting osteocytic-osteoclastic and osteoplastic activity in the perilacunar walls of aging mice. Connect. Tiss. Res. 1, 221-230, 1972.

32. Krempien, B., Geiger, G., Ritz, E., Büttner, S.: Osteocytes in chronic uremia. Virchows Arch. Abt. A Path. Anat. 360, 1-9, 1973.

33. Bonucci, E., Gherardi, G.: Histochemical and electron microscope investigations on medullary bone. Cell Tiss. Res. 163, 81-97, 1975.

34. Wassermann, F., Yaeger, J.A.: Fine structure of the osteocyte capsule and of the wall of the lacunae in bone. Z.Zellforsch. 67, 636-652, 1965.

35. Scherft, J.P.: The ultrastructure of the organic matrix of calcified cartilage and bone in embryonic mouse radii. J. Ultrastruct. Res. 23, 333-343, 1968.

36. Bonucci, E., Lo Cascio, V.: Electron microscope study of bone biopsies of patients with primary hyperparathyroidism. In preparation.

RENAL OSTEODYSTROPHY STUDIES WITH SCANNING AND TRANSMISSION ELECTRON MICROSCOPY

B. Krempien, G. Friedrich, G. Geiger, E. Ritz

Depts. of Pathol. and Int. Med., University
of Heidelberg, 6900 Heidelberg, Germany (FRG)

Ultrastructural analysis of bone cell function and bone
cell - bone matrix interaction gives valuable insights
into the formal pathogenesis of uremic osteodystrophy.
The histological changes susceptible to investigation
by light microscopy have been studied in great detail.
In contrast, there is a dearth of information on the
ultrastructural aspects of metabolic bone disease in
renal insufficiency.
The following paper reviews our investigations by transmission and surface scanning electron microscopy in clinical and experimental renal insufficiency. In the first
part, we describe our studies on the architecture of cortical bone and remodelling activity at the endosteal surface of the femur of uremic patients. In the second part,
we review our findings on endosteal cell morphology (rat
calvarium) in experimental renal failure and after PTH
administration. Particular emphasis will be placed upon
the relation between ultrastructural abnormalities of
endosteal cells on the one hand and disturbances of matrix deposition and mineralization on the other hand.

Methods:

Transmission (TM) electron microscopical studies were
performed with undecalcified ultrathin sections. Surface
scanning (SEM) electron microscopy was performed with two
different methods: the structure of mineral was studied
after digestion of organic material with hypochlorite.
Cellular details were evaluated after fixation with glu-

taraldehyde - cacodylate butter and preparation by the
critical point method.

Scanning electron microscopy of cortical bone

In polished and etched surfaces of <u>patients without skeletal disease</u>, a regular lamellar pattern of cortical
bone is evident (fig.1). Collagen fibers are seen to meet
in clearly delineated warps. Between the warps, collagen
fibers of neighbouring lamellae mingle in a regular pattern. This regular lamellar pattern must be the result of
the concerted action of collagen secreting osteoblasts
which results in a highly ordered texture of the collagen
fiber network.

<u>In uremic patients</u>, a clearly delineated texture of warps
is no longer recognizable in newly formed bone tissue
(fig.2). The lamellar structure is blurred. If a residual
lamellar pattern is existing, collagen fibers mingle haphazardly between adjacent lamellae without any recognizable periodicity.

Surface electron microscopy at the endosteal surface

In SEM studies of the endosteal surface of human femura,
the <u>resting surfaces</u> of uremic patients were reduced in
extent at the cost of apposition and resorption surfaces;
resting surfaces differed from those of controls by the
presence of woven bone without recognizable formation of
domains (fig. 3). Domains are areas where collagen fibers
and mineral crystals are orientated along one preferential direction. This concerted orientation is thought to
result from the concerted action of one clone of cells.

<u>Resorption areas</u> of control patients were sharply deli-
neated (fig. 4); their depth was uniform; their bottom
smooth. This implies that osteoclasts resorb sequential-
ly one lamellar stratum after the other. The resorption
areas of individual osteoclasts were in close juxtaposi-
tion and separated only by shallow ridges. The direction
of the ridges appeared to be determined by and to run
perpendicular to the preferential direction of collagen
fibers.
In contrast, resorption areas of patients with uremia
were irregularly delineated and often resembled traces
of woodworms, penetrating deeply into bone without re-
specting lamellar boundaries (fig. 5). Resorption areas
of individual osteoclasts were represented by narrow deep
excavations, presumably resulting from the resorptive action of single (or few) osteoclasts, thus indicating loss

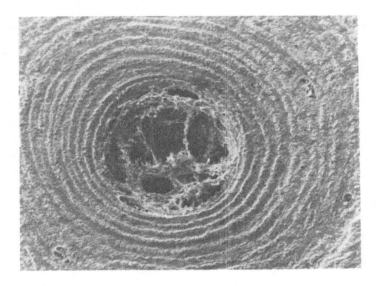

Fig. 1

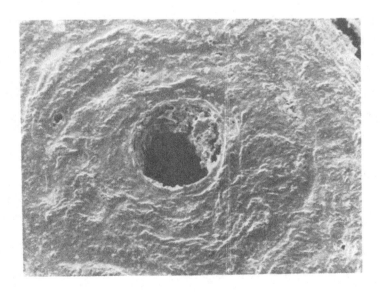

Fig. 2

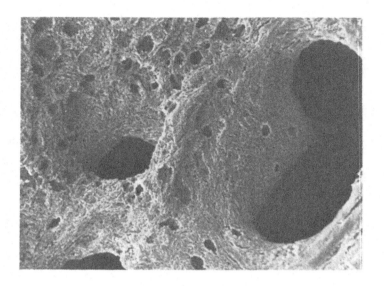

Fig. 3

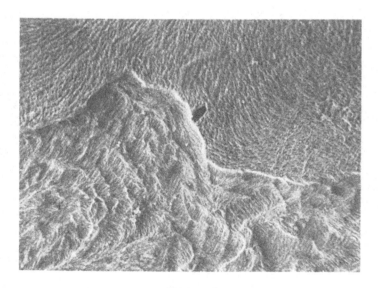

Fig. 4

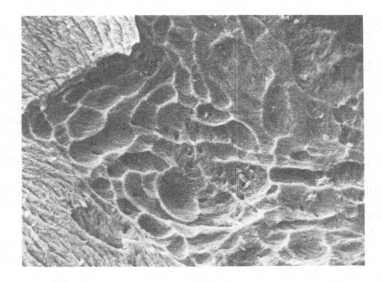

Fig. 5

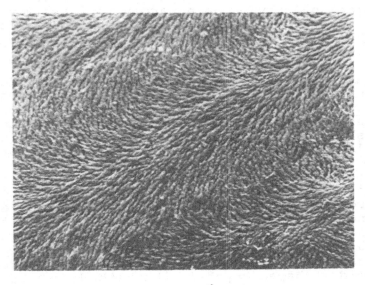

Fig. 6

of cell interaction.

The resorption of osteoclasts at the endosteal surface of uremic patients without spatial orientation and without cell interaction is thought to result from excessive stimulation by PTH.

Apposition surfaces in controls showed domain formation. This is well visible in figure 6. The calcospherites represent mineral corpuscles, approximately 4-1.5 A across of cylindrical shape, the orientation of which closely follows that of collagen fibers. In normal individuals, calcospherites were of uniform size and regular cylindrical shape. Within each domain, collagen fibers (indicated by the orientation of calcospherites) ran in parallel direction.

In contrast, in uremia, domain formation was no longer recognizable (fig. 7). The texture of collagen fibers showed various degrees of irregularity: calcospherites differed extremely in size and shape. These findings document that uremia causes loss of intercellular coordination not only in resorption surfaces, but also in apposition surfaces. We would like to suggest the loss of physical cell contact (vide infra) as a possible explanation for the lack of coordination in osteoblasts.

Some peculiarities of macroscopic bone structure in uremic osteodystrophy are the direct consequence of the microscopical derangement of collagen texture. Since the biomechanical quality of haphazardly textured woven bone is inferior to the one of lamellar bone, increased amounts of woven bone must be deposited when lamellar bone is replaced by woven bone. This causes the well known osteosclerosis in the skeleton of uremic individuals.

In lamellar bone, stress sensing osteocytes are "sandwiched" in between strain transducing lamellae. Osteocytes in woven bone, devoid of strain transducing lamellae, can no longer respond to mechanical strain like osteocytes in lamellar bone. Therefore the functional trajectorial structure of spongy bone tissue is gradually lost.

The abnormalities of collagen texture are also responsible for the diminished biomechanical quality of bone in uremia. Previous studies of our group (1) showed diminished bone hardness (Vicker's bone hardness) at the macroscopical (femoral cortex) and the microscopical (individual osteones) level. This mechanical quality is measured as the resistance bone offers to the intrusion of a pyramid – shaped crystal; the method consists in measuring the area of penetration. In addition, breaking strength of bone, measured in chips of cortical bone, was strikingly diminished in renal insufficiency (control:

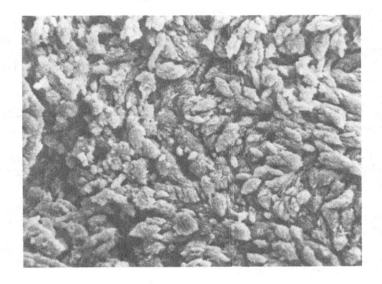

Fig. 7

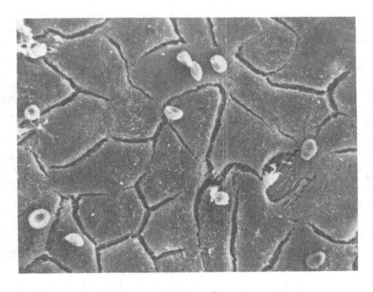

Fig. 8

19 +1,8Kp; uremia 15 +1,9Kp; p < 0,05).
Studies in fractured surfaces of cortical bone show a
different fracture profile in uremic patients (2). The
fracture surface was highly irregular, with osteones at
times completely torn out and at times protruding over
the fracture surface. This was interpreted as evidence
of osteon strength heterogeneity.

Evaluation of endosteal cells at the inner surface of rat calvaria by SEM and TEM
Effects of parathyroid hormone

The normal endosteal surface is covered by pseudoepithe-
lial, polygonal endosteal cells with narrow intercellular spaces connected by numerous tight junctions (fig. 8).

Administration of PTH in pharmacological doses leads to
characteristic changes, which depend both on the dose and
the duration of action of PTH.
Ten minutes after PTH (60 IU/100 g bw) cells retract, exhibiting a cobble stone pattern and denuding part of the
underlying secretory area (fig. 9).
After 60 minutes, characteristic "blebs" appear on cytoplasmic processes; in addition, a marked reduction of the
number of tight junctions is seen (fig. 10). Extremely
high doses cause disruption of cellular surfaces and loss
of cell integrity. When PTH was given for 3 - 6 days, (100
IU/100 g bw/day) endosteal cell surfaces became entirely
smooth; individual cells were completely isolated and exhibited no more intercellular connections; cells were separated by large areas of bone matrix, denuded from endosteal cells.
The reasons for the changes of cell surface morphology
under the influence of PTH are unknown. They might be due
to osmotic effects or due to contraction of contractile
fibers in the cell cytoplasm under the influence of raised intracellular calcium concentrations (3). Involvement
of cellular contractile mechanisms is suggested by the
observation that under long term administration of PTH,
increased numbers of microfilaments can be demonstrated
by TEM in osteocytes and osteoblasts (4).
Administration of PTH for three weeks (100 IU/day/100g bw)
resulted in noticeable irregularity of the calcospherites.
Calcospherites no longer exhibited orderly preferential
orientation along collagen fibers running in parallel.

When studied by TEM, normal endosteal cells were characterized (fig. 11) by cellular processes protruding towards the matrix, by narrow intracellular spaces, by the
close contact of osteoblasts with the collagen surface

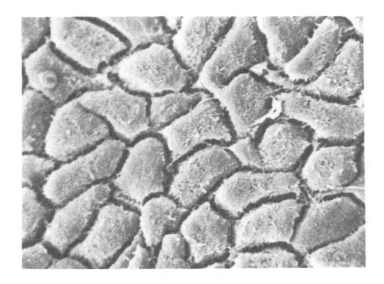

Fig. 9

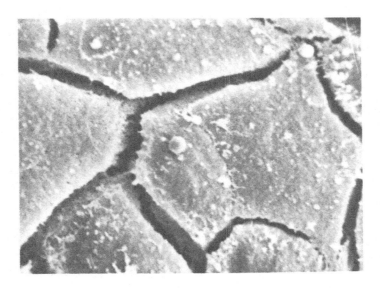

Fig. 10

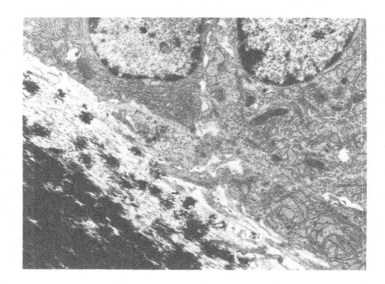

Fig. 11

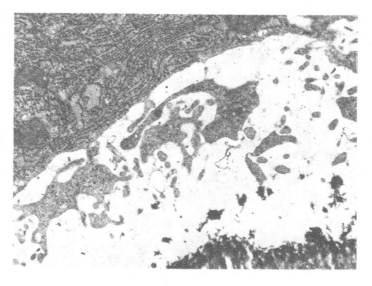

Fig. 12

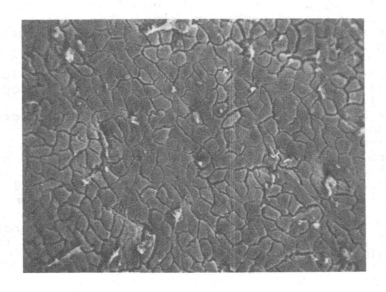

Fig. 13

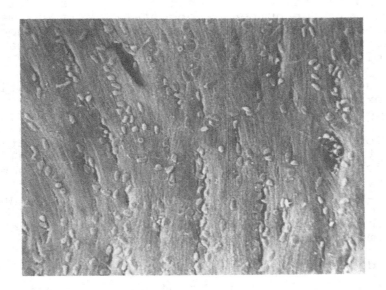

Fig. 14

and finally by the presence of endoplasmic reticulum
with closely spaced membranes within the cell cytoplasm.
Collagen exhibited a plaited texture, the direction of
collagen fibers alternating in regular intervals.

In contrast, when PTH was administered for a prolonged
period (fig. 12), cellular processes were shortened and
reduced in number. Osteoblasts seemed to have retracted
from the collagen surface thus reducing their secretion
area. The ergastoplasm was no longer composed of tightly
packed membranes, but appeared to be a loose sacculated
structure. These changes suggest reduced protein synthesis. Osteocytes, normally isotropic with respect to the
surrounding bone, became polarized under the influence
of PTH, i.e. exhibited exocytosis of lysosomes and pro-
trusion of cytoplasmic processes, filled with vacuoles
and microfilaments as well as microtubules, towards the
one cell pole and a resting cell surface towards the
other cell pole. In addition, the characteristic "plaited" texture of orderly arranged collagen fibers was no
longer visible (5).

Findings in chronic experimental renal insufficiency

After chronic uremia of 4 weeks duration (s. Ritz et al.,
this volume), the number of endosteal cells was markedly reduced (fig. 13,14). Endosteal cells with smooth
surfaces were separated by large areas of bone matrix
completely denuded of covering cells.

We conclude from our studies both from uremic patients
and in experimental animals that bone cells under the
influence of large doses of PTH escape from control mechanisms that normally regulate bone remodelling. The
separation of individual endosteal cells (retraction,
loss of tight junctions) may be the morphological equivalent for the loss of cell interaction. Consequently,
collagen, deposited by osteoblasts under the influence
of PTH, looses its regular supramolecular structure. The
resorption by osteoclasts under the influence of PTH is
an anarchical haphazard process. As a consequence, skeletal homeostasis is progressively disturbed.

Acknowledgement:

We thank Ms. I. Schütz and Ms. M. Petri for skilful
technical assistance.

With the support of "Deutsche Forschungsgemeinschaft".

REFERENCES

1. Krempien, B., Geiger, G., and Ritz, E.: Hardness of bone in in various ages and diseases. Proc. 9th Europ. Symp. Calc. Tiss. Czitober H., Eschberger S. (eds.) Facta Publication Wien. p. 95-99, 1973.

2. Krempien, B., Geiger G., and Ritz, E.: Alteration of bone tissue structure in secondary hyperparathyroidism. A scanning electron microschopical study. In: Vitamin D and problems related to uremic bone disease. A.W. Norman et al (eds.), Gruyter, p. 157-165, 1975.

3. Rasmussen, H., Bordier, P.H.: The physiological and cellular basis of metabolic bone diseases. Williams and Wilkins, Baltimore, 1974.

4. Krempien, B., Friedrich, G., Ritz, E.: Ultrastructural studies of bone cells. Proc. Europ Symp. Calc. Tissues, Leeds, 1976 (in press).

5. Boyde, A. and Jones, S.J.: Osteoblasts and bone collagen orientation. Intern. Workshop Calc. Tiss. Gesher Haziv, Israel, 1974.

CONTROVERSIES REGARDING INTESTINAL PHOSPHATE TRANSPORT AND ABSORPTION

Louis V. Avioli and Stanley J. Birge

The Jewish Hospital of St. Louis

St. Louis, Missouri

Phosphate balance is ultimately dependent upon the relationship between the intestinal absorption of ingested phosphate, the skeletal affinity for mineral and the degree of phosphaturia. Although inorganic phosphate is usually considered a hand-maiden to calcium, it should be emphasized that a variety of disease entities which are characterized by disturbances in calcium absorption also present with alterations in intestinal phosphate transport. Hyperabsorption of phosphate, although uncommon, has been noted in primary hyperparathyroidism, idiopathic hypercalciuria, normal subjects given an excess of vitamin D, and in sarcoidosis. Phosphorus malabsorption has been documented in vitamin D deficiency (both in the absence or presence of dietary calcium), chronic renal failure, hepatic cirrhosis, glucocorticoid excess syndrome, hyperthyroidism, hypoparathyroidism and in an inherited vitamin D-resistant form of hypophosphatemic rickets. Despite these observations, there are a variety of conflicting reports of experiments conducted in a variety of animal species regarding: 1) the intestinal site of phosphate absorption, 2) factors which initiate and perpetuate its transport across the mucosal barrier, and 3) the relationship between intestinal calcium and phosphate transport.

It has been well demonstrated that in normal individuals, a linear relationship exists between the intake and net absorption of phosphorus. Although absorption in man appears to be controlled primarily by a non-saturable, passive process, the active transport of phosphate may become significant in states of dietary phosphorus deficiency. The existence of an intestinal transport process for phosphate against a thermodynamic gradient was demonstrated in 1961 by Harrison and Harrison (1). Using everted rat intestinal segments, these authors reported that phosphate transport was inhibited by

metabolic poisons and anerobiosis and, dependent on potassium as
well as calcium. Subsequently, Helbock et al also demonstrated
active phosphate transport by rat duodenum in a short-circuited
system (2), and observed that phosphate had a significant effect
on calcium translocation across the rat intestine in vitro.
Wasserman and Taylor (3) also provided evidence that phosphate
transport across the chick intestine was a metabolically dependent
saturable process. In contrast to earlier studies, these authors
(3) noted that phosphate transport in the chicken was independent
of luminal calcium concentrations, but correlated directly with
the level of serum calcium in response to vitamin D loading.
Wasserman and Taylor (3) could only conclude from their observations
that intenstinal phosphate and calcium transport were independent
and, that unlike calcium transport, phosphate absorption obtained
in the absence of a specific mucosal-binding protein. Kowarski
and Schachter (4) and Hurwitz and Bar (5) also concluded that
calcium and phosphate absorption represented mutually exclusive
transport parameters since, in their studies, vitamin D enhanced
phosphate transport to a greater extent in the jejunum than in the
duodenum. In contrast to these observations, maximal stimulation
of calcium transport occurred in the duodenum of vitamin D-treated
animals. In 1974, Chen et al (6) reported that phosphate transport
in the rat was highest in the upper deodenum in the presence of
calcium. In this intestinal segment, phosphate transport was
dependent on calcium,whereas in the jejunum, phosphate transport
was independent of calcium (6). In these experiments they noted
that vitamin D and its biologically active metabolites, 25-hydroxy-
cholecalciferol (25OHD$_3$) and 1,25-dihydroxycholecalciferol (1,25
(OH)$_2$D$_3$) stimulated jejunal phosphate transport. These same
authors concluded that jejunal phosphate transport was energy-
dependent since glucose was an essential substrate in this regard
(6). These observations were contrary to those of Neville and
Holdsworth who has previously reported that in the chick ileum,
vitamin D increased phosphate transport only in the presence of
calcium (7). Cramer (8) noted that the greatest effective reabsorption of ^{32}P-labeled inorganic phosphate occurred in the rat ileum
(38%) followed by the duodenum (29%), jejunum (25%) and colon (8%).
He also reporeted that ^{32}PO$_4$ absorption was limited by the movement
of the isotope into gut segments with slower absorption rates. In
view of these observations, it should be noted that in the pig,
calcium absorption is most active in the proximal fourth of the
small intestine and phosphate from the proximal half (9). In
this animal the most intensive absorption of calcium and phosphate
from the small intestine takes place at a point where the solubility
of these elements in the contents of the small intestine is greatest
(9). This observation is consistent with the hypothesis that both
the mucous coating of the mucosal cells and the preferential release
of hydrogen ions on the mucosal side of the jejunum, as a result
of lactic-acid production, most probably play an important role in
phosphate transport and net absorption (10).

The relationship between calcium and phosphate transport by
the intestine and the presence or absence of an active phosphate
transport process are still controversial at best. Using in vivo
perfusion of Thiry-Vella jejunal fistuals of dogs, Cramer reported
that phosphate absorption was primarily passive and that phosphate
actually enhances calcium absorption (11). These observations
should be contrasted with those of Wrobel et al (12), and Walling
and Rothman (13), who reported that active calcium transport in
rat duodenal segments was totally independent of the phosphate ion.
More recently, Taylor (14) observed that the omission of calcium
from the incubation medium or the addition of a calcium chelator
partially reduced the vitamin D-stimulated serosal transport of
$^{32}PO_4$ in chicken intestine. In this species, phosphate transport
may be, in fact, independent of calcium transport but may be, in
part, dependent on the presence of the calcium ion.

In addition to the partial dependence of intestinal transport
on the calcium ion, potassium (1) and sodium (14) appear essential
for the stimulated response to vitamin D. Taylor also observed
that in the chick, ethacrynic acid but not ouabain inhibited intestinal mucosal phosphate uptake, although both substances inhibited
the transfer of phosphate from the serosal surface of the intestine.
This response to ouabain may be attributed, in part, to a reduction
in the electrical potential gradient across the cell membrane which
would facilitate phosphate entry and retard its efflux. Our own
experience indicates that the initial rate of phosphate uptake by
chick intestinal mucosal explants is inhibited by ouabain (15), an
observation consistent with the response of renal tubular cells to
cardiac glycosides (16). The cardiac glycosides may be inhibiting
an ATPase which modulates phosphate transport into the cell (17).
Although the observations of Taylor (14) in chick intestine do not
support the requirements of sodium for phosphate uptake, data
derived from renal phosphate transport studies suggest that sodium
and phosphate transport are linked, since volume expansion inhibits
the calcium-sensitive phosphate transport process (18). In prokary-
otic (19) and eukaryotic cells (20-22), phosphate transport has
also been linked to membrane alkaline phosphatase(s). Phosphate
deprivation results in concomitant decreases in alkaline phospha-
tase(s) activity and the activity of high affinity phosphate transport systems. In the rat, a decrease in dietary phosphate results
in a two-fold increase in renal cell alkaline phosphatase activity
although at least ten other renal enzyme systems are unaffected (23).
Similar observations have been reported to characterize the chick
intestinal response to phosphate deprivation (24). Both mouse and
chick intestine accumulate phosphate at a rate which parallels
concomitant changes in intestinal alkaline phosphatase activity

*See Avioli, L.V. Intestinal Absorption of Calcium, Arch. Intern.
Med. 129:345, 1972 for detailed review

under a variety of experimental conditions. It has also been
established by Holdsworth (25) and Normal et al (26)* that vitamin
D stimulates intestinal alkaline phosphatase activity. These
collective observations, although limited, suggest that alkaline
phosphatase(s) may also condition or modulate the intestinal
transport of phosphate.

The dependence of phosphate absorption on vitamin D was demonstrated by Nicolaysen in 1937 (27) and Carlsson in 1954 (28). As
noted earlier in this review, following the demonstration by Harrison
and Harrison that vitamin D activated a phosphate transport system
in the rat, Chen et al (6) proved that vitamin D stimulated phosphate transport throughout the entire length of small intestine
and that calcium enhances this transport only in the duodenum in
which there is a very active vitamin D-dependent calcium transport
mechanism. More recently, Peterlik and Wasserman (29), studying
unidirectional phosphate fluxes across the mucosal side of the
epithelial layer of chick jejunum, reported that vitamin D enhances
the maximal transport velocity with no apparent effect on Km. They
also observed that phosphate efflux from the cell was not affected
by vitamin D and that protein synthesis was essential to the active
transport process. Although it has been established that vitamin
D stimulates the intestinal absorption of phosphate in man (30),
the nature of this response is still virtually unknown. In
studying patients with an inherited form of vitamin D resistant
rickets which is characterized by defects in the intestinal (31)
and renal (32) phosphate transport systems, Short et al demonstrated
a defect in phosphate transport in the absence of calcium by intestinal mucosa from affected individuals (33). These investigators
identified two phosphate transport systems in human intestinal
mucosa with Km's of 0.006 mM and 0.6 mM. Since the high affinity
transport system was malfunctioning in hypophosphatemic patients
with intestinal phosphate malabsorption who were resistant to
vitamin D, it is tempting to postulate that in normal man, a vitamin
D-dependent, high affinity and rate limited transport systems is
essential for maximal absorption of dietary phosphate. Until more
definitive studies are available from experiments in human subjects,
we must rely on what is presently a disarray of conflicting data
collected from in vitro and/or in vivo experiments in a variety of
animal species, some of whom (chicken) lay eggs and others who are
either nocturnal eaters and normally hyperphosphatemic (rat), or
normally subjected to a diet which is characterized by a very high
phosphorus content (dog).

REFERENCES

1. Harrison, H.E. and Harrison, H.C.: Intestinal transport of phosphate: Action of vitamin D calcium and potassium. Am. J. Phys. 201:1007, 1961.

2. Helbock, H.J., Fork, J.G., and Saltman, P.: The mechanism of calcium transport by rat intestine. Biochim. Biophys. Acta. 126:81, 1966.

3. Wasserman, R.H., and Taylor, A.N.: Intestinal absorption of phosphate on the chick: Effect of vitamin D3 and other parameters. Nutr. 103:586, 1973.

4. Kowarski, S., and Schachter, D.: Effect of vitamin D on phosphate transport and incorporation into mucosal constituents of rate intestinal mucosa. J. Biol. Chem. 244:211, 1969.

5. Hurwitz, S., and Bar, A.: Site of vitamin D action in chick intestine. Am. J. Phys. 222:761, 1972.

6. Chen, T.C., Castillo, L., Koryeka-Cahl, M., and DeLuca, H.F.: Role of vitamin D metabolites in phosphate transport of rat intestine. J. Nutr. 104:1056, 1974.

7. Neville, E., and Holdsworth, E.S.: Phosphorus metabolism during transport of calcium. Biochim. Biophys. Acta 163:362, 1968.

8. Cramer, C.F.: Progress in rate of absorption of radiophosphorus through the intestinal tract of rats. Canad. J. Biochem. Physiol. 39:499, 1961.

9. Moore, J.H., and Tyler, C.: Studies on the intestinal absorption and excretion of calcium and phosphorus in the pig. Brit. J. Nutr. 9:81, 1955.

10. Clarkson, T.W., Rothstein, A., and Cross, A.: Transport of monovalent anions by isolated small intestine of the rat. Am. J. Physiol. 200:781, 1961.

11. Cramer, C.F.: Effect of Ca/P ratio and pH on calcium and phosphorus absorption from dog gut loops in vivo. J. Physiol. Pharmacol. 46:171, 1968.

12. Wrobel, J., Michalska, L., and Niemiro, R.: The requirements of anions for transport of calcium in rats duodenum. FEBS Letter 29:121, 1973.

13. Walling, M.W., and Rothman, S.S.: Phosphate-independent, carrier-mediated active transport of calcium by rat intestine. Am. J. Physiol. 217:1144, 1969.

14. Taylor, A.N.: In vitro phosphate transport in chick ilium: Effect of cholecalciferol, calcium, sodium and metabolic inhibitors. J. Nurt. 104:489, 1974.

15. Birge, S.: Personal observations.

16. Kupfer, S., and Kosorsky, J.D.: Effect of cardiac glycosides on renal tubular transport of calcium, magnesium, in organic phosphates and glucose in the dog. J. Clin. Invest. 44:1132, 1965.

17. Kupfer, S., and Kosorsky, J.D.: Renal intracellular phosphate and phosphate excretion: The effect of digoxin in parathyroid hormone. Mount Sinai J. Med. 37:357, 1970.

18. Popovtzer, M.D., Robinette, J.B., MacDonald, K.M., and Kuruvila, C.K.: Effect of Ca^{++} on renal handling of PO_4^{---}: Evidence for two reabsorptive mechanisms. Am. J. Physiol. 229:901, 1975.

19. Torriani, A.: Influence of inorganic phosphate in the formation of phosphatasis by escherichio coli. Biochim. Biophys. Acta 38:460, 1960.

20. Koyerma, H., and Ono, T.: Further studies on the induction of alkaline phosphatase by 5-bromodeoxyurioadine in a hybrid line between mouth and chinese hamster in culture. Biochim. Acta 264:497, 1972.

21. Ihlenfeldt, M.J.A. and Gibson, J.: Phosphate utilization and alkaline phosphatase activity in anacystis tridalans (synechococcus). J. Arch. Microbiol. 102:23, 1975.

22. Bayinet, G.F., Jr., and Slayman, C.W.: Phosphate transport in neurospora. Depression of a high affinity transport system during phosphorus starvation. Biochim. Biophys. Acta 389:541, 1975.

23. Gunitore, A.: Regulation by phosphate of alkaline phosphatase in rat kidney. Biochim. Biophys. Acta 138:411, 1967.

24. McCudig, L.W., and Motzok, I.: Regulation of intestinal alkaline phosphatase by dietary phosphate. Canad. J. Physiol. Pharm. 50:1152, 1972.

25. Holdsworth, E.S.: The effect of vitamin D on enzyme activities in the mucosal cells of the chick small intestine. J. Mem. Biol. 3:43, 1970.

26. Norman, A.W., Mirchoff, A.K., Adams, T.H., and Spielvogel, A.: Studies on the mechanisms of action of calciferol. III. Vitamin D-mediated increase of intestinal brush border alkaline phosphatase activity. Biochim. Biophys. Acta 215:348, 1970.

27. Nicolaysen, K.: Studies upon the mode of action of vitamin D. III. The influence of vitamin D on absorption of calcium and phosphorus. Biochem. J. 31:122, 1937.

28. Carlsson, A.: The effect of vitamin D on the absorption of inorganic phosphate. Acta Physiol. Scand. 31:301, 1954.

29. Peterlik, M., and Wasserman, R.H.: Effect of vitamin D3 and 1,25-dihydroxy vitamin D3 on intestinal transport of phosphate. Abstracted in the Workshop Proceedings of the 2nd International Workshop on Phosphate, Heidelberg, Germany, 1976 (this volume).

30. Cannagia, A., Gennari, C., Bencini, M., and Palazzouli, V.: Intestinal absorption of radiophosphate in osteomalacia before and after vitamin D treatment. Calc. Tiss. Res. 2:299, 1972.

31. Condon, J.R., Nassim, J.R., and Rutter, A.: Defective intestinal phosphate absorption in familial and non-familial hypophosphataemia. Brit. Med. J. 3:138, 1970.

32. Glorieux, F., and Scriver, C.R.: Loss of a parathyroid hormone sensitive component of phosphate transport in x-linked hypophosphatemia. Science 175:977, 1972.

33. Short, E.M., Binder, H.J., and Rosenberg, L.E.: Familial hypophosphatemic rickets: Defective transport of inorganic phosphate by intestinal mucosa. Science 179:700, 1973.

SKELETAL GROWTH IN UREMIA

E. Ritz, O. Mehls, B. Krempien, G. Gilli,
H. Udes, W. Harendza
Depts. Internal Medicine; Pediatrics, Patholo-
gy, Versuchstierzentrale des Theoretikums
Heidelberg University, 6900 Heidelberg (FRG)

Retardation of growth continues to be the single most
important unsolved problem in the treatment of renal
failure of children. Chronic renal insufficiency is usually associated with a diminished growth rate, which is not
completely reversed by hemodialysis. The following paper
reviews our clinical, histological and experimental studies on growth failure in uremia.

Clinical observations

In 64 children in end stage renal failure, studied by
one of us (OM), bone age was less than expected for
chronological age, but height age was again less than
expected for bone age (fig.1). This indicates that the
rate of bone maturation exceeds the rate of longitudinal
growth, but is less than expected for age (1-2). Therefore, final height is bound to be inadequate.
At the beginning of hemodialysis, body height is below
the third percentile in one third of the children (3-6).
After the beginning of hemodialysis, the growth rate
(corrected for bone age) tends to increase initially and
to fall again after one to two years (6). We attribute
the temporary growth spurt primarily to improved calorie
and protein intake after the beginning of hemodialysis.
It should be mentioned, however, that in addition, the
clinical severity of renal osteodystrophy is less in dialysed as opposed to non-dialysed uremic children. We
found slipped epiphysis — which is the severest expression
of renal osteodystrophy — in 12 out of 56 non-dialysed,
but only in 1 out of 82 dialysed uremic children (7).

Histological observations

There is a dearth of information on the histology of the
growth zone in renal failure. Our studies showed (7,8)
that the cartilagenous growth zone is rather narrow,
albeit irregular, and devoid of chondroosteoid. This
finding is in contrast to what is ordinarily seen in
vitamin D deficiency rickets, where disorderly accumu-
lating cartilage increases the width of the epiphyseal
growth cartilage. Perhaps the growth cartilage is nar-
rowed down by chondroclastic cartilage removal once
growth arrest has occured. Alternatively, hyperparathyroidism, which is more intensive in uremia than
in nutritional vitamin D deficiency, may stimulate chon-
droclasts to resorb chondroid more avidly particularly
so since chondroid is well mineralized.
It is also remarkable that the zone of primary mineralization in uremic children with growth arrest is densely
sclerotic and does not exhibit signs of defective mineralization as usually seen in vitamin D deficiency. The
good mineralization of chondroid in the provisional zone
of calcification is paradoxical in view of the common
mineralization block in uremia. Possibly, mineralization
is preserved as a consequence of hyperphosphatemia or mineralization - though delayed - is adequate in relation
to the slow growth rate.
A quantitative study was designed to differentiate the
cellular and architectural responses of bone to growth
arrest in uremic osteodystrophy as opposed to growth
arrest from non-renal disease and immobilization. The
distal femoral growth zone was studied in 8 children with
terminal renal failure, 11 children without skeletal disease dying suddenly from accident or intoxication, 21
children with growth arrest from heart failure and 14
children suffering from brain tumor who were both immobilized and malnourished (Krempien et al., in preparation).
Quantitative micromorphometry documented the failure of
epiphyseal width to be increased; active osteoid was diminished in immobilized and malnourished children with
brain tumor but unchanged in uremia. There was, however,
an increase of inactive osteoid in uremic children,
pointing to the presence of a mineralization block.
There was a tendency for the surface/volume ratio of
metaphyseal trabecules to fall. Since the surface/vol-
ume ratio of a cylinder decreases as the diameter increases, the finding points to the presence of plump coarse
trabecules in uremia. Bone density, i.e. the fraction of
spongy bone occupied by bone mass, decreased in immobilized children with growth arrest, but failed to fall in

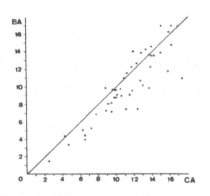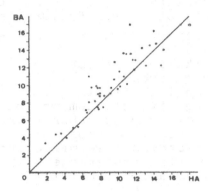

Fig. 1

Bone Age (BA) and Chronological Age (CA) in Children with End Stage Renal Failure.

Bone Age (BA) and Height Age (HA) in Children with End Stage Renal Failure.

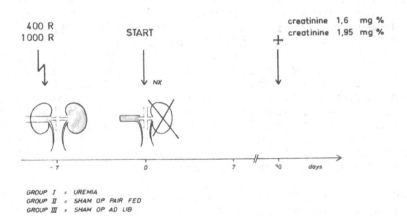

Fig. 2. Experimental Protocol

uremic children in spite of growth arrest, pointing to
some degree of osteosclerosis.

Experimental observations

A variety of factors has been implicated in the pathogenesis of growth failure in uremia (9):

- malnutrition (i.e. diminished intake of protein and
  calories)
- vitamin D resistance as a result of disturbed vitamin
  D metabolism
- genuine vitamin D deficiency in malnourished children
- negative calcium balance
- secondary hyperparathyroidism
- metabolic acidosis
- somatomedin insufficiency
- insulin resistance
- hyperadrenocorticism

The experimental study reported in the following addres-
sed itself exclusively to the roles of calorie malnutrition and bone disease in the growth failure of uremia.

Simons (10) showed that a daily supplementation with
calories improved growth velocity in uremic dialysed
children. This has subsequently been verified in the
experimental model of rats with mild chronic uremia.
Correlating food intake and growth rate, Chantler (11)
showed that moderately uremic rats grow less than non-
uremic rats. This he attributed to diminished intake of
food. However, pairfeeding was not done in these studies.
Diaz et al. (12) could show that the rate of growth in
uremic rats was less than in control rats with free access to food and water, but identical with pairfed rats.
These experiments identified diminished intake of calories and protein as the primary cause of growth retardation in uremia. However, they failed to answer the
question, whether uremic osteodystrophy in itself inter-
feres with growth, since skeletal pathology was not observed with the relatively limited reduction of GFR
achieved by these investigators.

Therefore, we chose the model of stable advanced chronic
renal failure after subtotal nephrectomy in 60 g Sprague
Dawley rats. The experimental protocol is evident from
fig. 2. After two stage nephrectomy and extracorporal
irradiation of the remaining renal parenchyma (400 R in
the first series and 1000 R in the second series of experiments), GFR, measured by the endogenous creatinine
clearance, fell to 20% of the control values of sham-
operated pairfed rats in the first series and 12% in

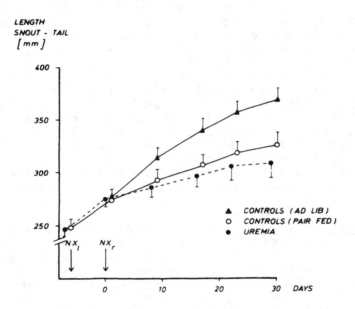

Fig. 3. Longitudinal growth in experimental uremia.

the second series of experiments. The animals were kept
on a 12 h on, 12 h off light cycle and at constant temperature and humidity. Food was offered for 4 h; spill-
age, negligible in extent, was corrected for by weighing
and refeeding. The two stage procedure which dissociates
operative stress from the acute brunt of uremia appears
essential, since other authors were unable to achieve a
comparable degree of uremia because the animals died.
The limiting factor for survival in our model is the
development of malignant hypertension (4th week: Co 122
$\pm$ 8 mmHg; U 168 $\pm$ 18 mmHG; tail plethysmography).

The findings in animals with preterminal uremia (i.e.
uremia of 4 weeks duration and a final GFR 20% of the
control value) have been described in detail elsewhere
(13). In spite of severe bone disease in these non-vi-
tamin D deficient animals (serum 25-OH-vitamin D3 in
controls 6,1 $\pm$ 3,0 nM/l; uremia 16,9 $\pm$ 6,4, p < 0,01),
no difference in longitudinal growth rate was found
between uremic animals and sham-operated pairfed control
animals. The length of ad lib fed animals, however, exceeded that of both uremic and pairfed control animals.
This suggests that uremic bone disease is not responsible
for retardation of growth in preterminal renal failure
of the rat. The rate of growth in uremic animals is only
diminished with respect to ad lib fed control animals
and must thus be attributed exclusively to diminished
intake of food.

In terminal uremia of 4 weeks duration (serum creatinine
1,99 $\pm$ 4,1 mg%; serum urea 411 $\pm$ 36,8 mg%) longitudinal
growth was clearly impaired in uremic animals as compared to sham-operated pairfed animals. As shown in fig.
3, longitudinal growth almost ceases after nephrectomy
and lags behind the pairfed controls throughout the experiments. This suggests that in terminal - as opposed
to preterminal - renal failure, renal insufficiency in
itself and/or renal osteodystrophy interfere with longitudinal growth by mechanisms other than protein/calorie
malnutrition.
As previously shown by Russell (14), marked abnormalities
in the growth zone of the tibia were present: compared
with findings in the sham-operated pairfed controls
(fig. 4), the zone of growth cartilage in uremic animals
(fig. 5) was irregularly outlined and broadened. The zone
of degenerative cartilage was enlarged and the transformation of cartilage into primary spongiosa markedly disturbed. The width of primary spongiosa was increased. Its
texture was irregular and the fraction of bone volume

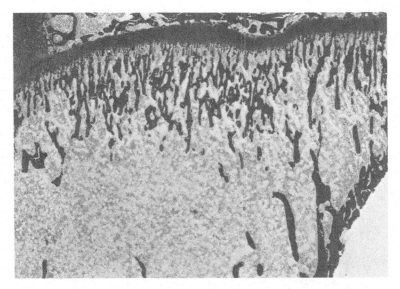

Fig 4.   Tibia, pairfed sham-operated control animal undecalcified section, v. Kossa stain, enlargement x 25 growth cartilage on top, metaphysis on bottom.

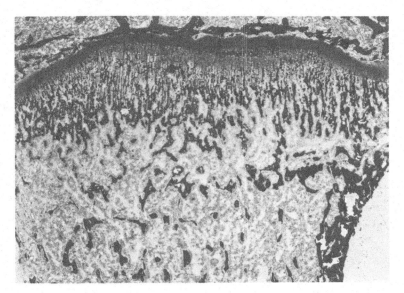

Fig 5.   Tibia, uremic animal (conditions as Fig 4) note
broadening of zone of degenerative cartilage (s. Fig 5a),
widened zone of primary spongiosa, delayed transformation of
cartilage into spongiosa, as evident from persistance of
chondroid in bone travecules.

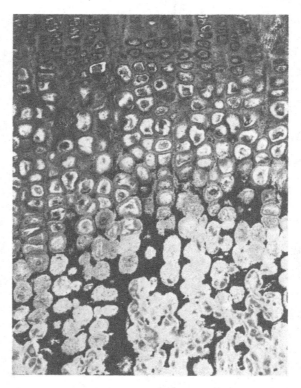

Fig 5a.   Detail of Fig 5, enlargement x 250, note long columns
of degnerative cartilage and well preserved provisional
calcification.

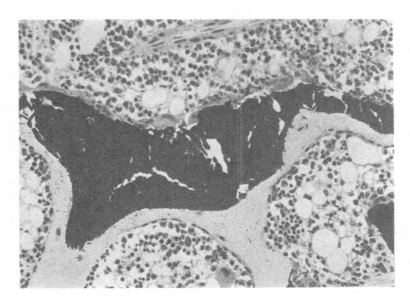

Fig 6. Osteoid seam of uremic animal (spongy bone in tibia
epiphysis; enlargement x 250). Note broad unmineralized
osteoid seam covering trabecular surface.

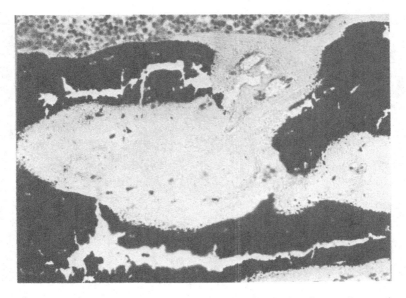

Fig 6a. Osteoid filled cavity within metaphyseal cortex
(uremic animal) enlargement x 250.

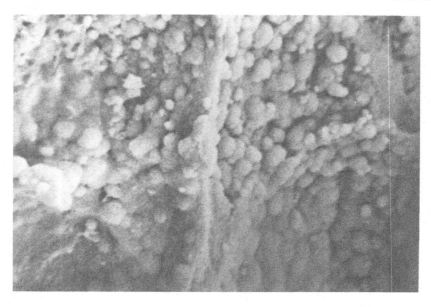

Fig 7. Zone of provisional calcification; control animal
(SEM, hypochlorite digestion, micrograph x 3000) note
globiform mineral deposits.

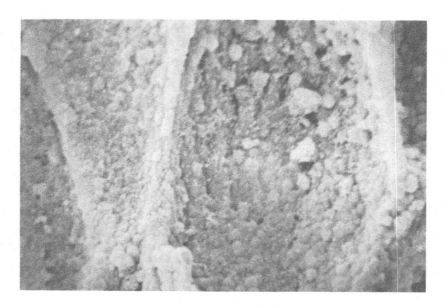

Fig. 8. Zone of provisional calcification, uremic animal
conditions as in Fig. 7. Note smaller and more varied size
and indistinct outlines of globiform mineral deposits.

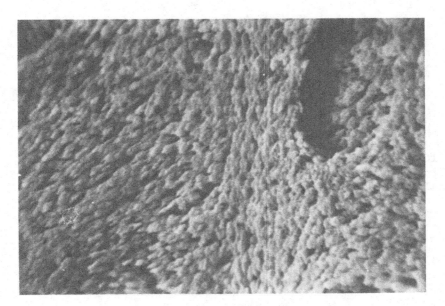

Fig 9. Metaphyseal spongiosa; sham-operated pairfed control
animal. (SEM, hypochlorite digestion, micrograph x 3000).
Clearly recognizable regular pattern of calcospherites of
uniform size and shape on surface of spongiosal trabecule
(secondary spongiosa); calcospherites follow the direction
of collagen fibers.

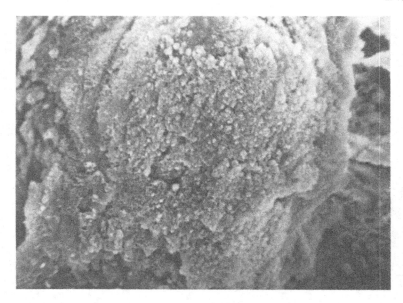

Fig 10. Metaphyseal spongiosa; uremic animal conditions as
in Fig 9. Irregular granular mineralization without formation
of calcospherites.

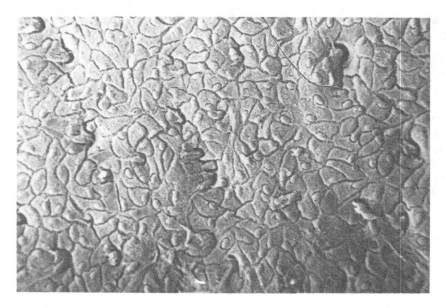

Fig 11. Inner surface of rat calvarium control animal (SEM,
critical point drying method, micrograph x 1000) pseudoepithe-
lial polygonal cells covering bone matrix; narrow intercellular
spaces.

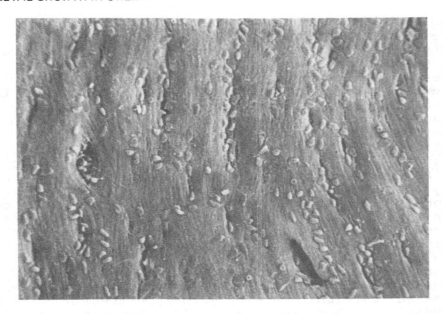

Fig 12. Inner surgace of rat calvarium, uremic animal. (SEM, critical point drying method, micrograph x 300) isolated smooth rounded-off cells leaving large areas of matrix denuded from cells.

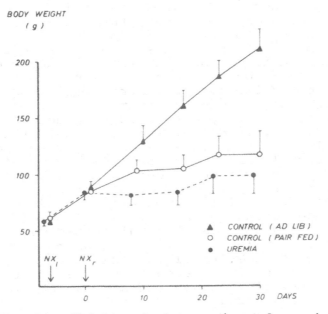

Fig. 13. Weight gain in experimental uremia.

occupied by bone matrix was increased, documenting the presence of osteosclerosis.

Persistance of osteoid was seen in various skeletal sites, e.g. epiphysis (fig. 6), metaphyseal trabecules and cavities within metaphyseal cortical bone. Defective mineralization of osteoid and chondroid was also documented by the diminished calcium content of the tibia, measured by neutron activation analysis.

Defective mineralization in the provisional zone of mineralization is suggested by diminished size and blurred outlines of the globiform mineral deposits in uremic animals as demonstrated by surface scanning electron microscopy (fig. 7,8).

A highly irregular criss-cross haphazard pattern of collagen fibers in uremic animals – as opposed to the regular collagen pattern in normal animals – agrees with the finding of disturbed collagen maturation (14) found by Russell (fig. 9,10).

Secondary hyperparathyroidism was documented by the increased number of osteoclasts per unit area and by an increased fractional rate of urinary excretion of cAMP. In addition, smooth rounded-off isolated endosteal cells in the rat calvaria could be demonstrated by SEM microscopy (fig. 11,12), a finding which is analogous to what is seen after prolonged PTH administration (s. Krempien in this volume).

Chantler (11) suggested that weight gain per calorie ingested was lower in uremic rats than in ad lib fed control rats. Using a pairfeeding procedure, Diaz (12) was unable to confirm this in rats with moderate renal failure. In contrast, in our rats with advanced renal failure, the rate of weight gain was significantly diminished as compared to pairfed control rats (fig. 13). The higher weight of the control animals was the more surprising, since pairfed control rats tended to be hungry, aggressive and hyperactive. The diminished rate of gain of weight in uremic animals is not the result of diminished intracellular or extracellular water. Intracellular water content was unchanged in muscle, heart, spleen and liver. Extracellular space, measured by Br 82, was even increased. Fecal nitrogen was not raised.

The diminished weight gain of uremic animals is therefore most likely the result of disturbed net synthesis of body mass in malnourished uremic animals. Preliminary findings suggest that total body nitrogen is decreased in uremic animals as compared to pairfed control animals. There is apparently an inefficiency of calorie utilisation for growth, suggesting that the calorie cost of growth is increased.

Summary

Stable long-term chronic renal failure in the growing
Sprague Dawley rat causes marked bone disease with impaired mineralization (i.e. rickets) and evidence of
increased parathyroid hormone activity.

Although significant bone disease is present, the rate
of longitudinal growth is not diminished in preterminal
renal failure. However, it is significantly diminished
in terminal renal failure, when uremic rats are compared
with sham-operated control rats at identical levels of
food intake.
At identical levels of food intake, weight gain is also
diminished in rats with terminal uremia as compared with
sham-operated control rats, suggesting increased calorie
cost for growth.

Acknowledgement:

With the support of "Deutsche Forschungsgemeinschaft".

We thank Mr. Kourist and Ms. Sis for skilful technical
assistance.

We thank Dr. Wesch (DKFZ Heidelberg) for performing the
neutron activation analysis and Dr. Schmidt-Gayk (Krehl-
Klinik Heidelberg) for measurements of 25-OH-vitamin D
levels.

Literature

1. Broyer, M., Kleinknecht, C., Loirat, C., Marti-Hen-
   neberg, C., Roy, M.P.: Maturation osseuse et déve-
   loppement pubertaire chez l'enfant et l'adolescent
   en dialyse chronique. Proc. Eur. Dial. Transpl. Ass.
   9:181, 1972

2. Gusmano, R., Gilli, G., Perfumo, F.: Valutazione
   critica dei risultati del trattamento emodialitico
   in eta pediatrica. Minerva Nefrologica 19:60, 1972

3. Schärer, K., Chantler, C., Bruner, F.P. et al.:
   Combined report on regular dialysis and transplan-
   tation of children in Europe 1974
   Proc. Europ. Transpl. 12:65, 1975

4. Potter, D., Larsen, D., Leuman, E., Perin, D.,
   Simmons, J., Piel, C.F., Holliday, M.A.: Treatment
   of chronic uremia in childhood: II Hemodialysis
   Pediatrics 46:678, 1970

5. Fine, R.N., Korsch, B.M., Grushkin, C.M., Liebermann, E.: Hemodialysis in children. Am. J. Child.
   118:498

6. Gilli, G.: Therapie der Wachstumsstörung bei chroni-
   scher Niereninsuffizienz. Mschr. Kinderheilkunde
   123:772, 1975

7. Mehls, O., Ritz, E., Krempien, B., Gilli, G., Schärer, K.: Slipped epiphysis in renal osteodystrophy
   in: Vitamin D and Problems related to Vitamin D
   A.W. Norman, K. Schaefer, H.G. Grigoleit, D. v. Herrath, E. Ritz, eds.
   W. de Gruyter, Berlin-New York 1975, 553

8. Krempien, B., Mehls, O., Ritz, E.: Morphological
   studies on pathogenesis of slipping in uremic children. Virchows Archive A Path. Anat. Histol. 362:129,
   1974

9. Holliday, M.A.: Calorie intake and growth in uremia
   Kidney Int. 7 (suppl):73, 1975

10. Simmons, J.M., Wilson, C.J., Potter, D.E., Holliday,
    M.A.: Caloric intake and linear growth of children
    on hemodialysis. N. Eng. J. Med. 285:653, 1971

11. Chantler, C., Liebermann, E., Holliday, M.A.: A rat
    model for the study of growth failure in uremia.
    Pediatr. Res. 8:109, 1974

12. Diaz, M., Kleinknecht, C., Broyer, M.: Growth in ex-
    perimental renal failure: role of calorie and amino
    acid intake. Kidney Int. 8:349, 1975

13. Mehls, O., Ritz, E., Krempien, B. et al.: Growth in
    experimental uremia. Nephron, in press

14. Russell, J.E. and Avioli, L.V.: Effect of chronic
    experimental renal insufficiency on bone mineral
    and collagen maturation. J. Clin. Invest. 51:3072,
    1972

THE MANAGEMENT OF RENAL OSTEODYSTROPHY

H. E. de WARDENER and J. B. EASTWOOD

PROFESSOR OF MEDICINE and LECTURER IN MEDICINE

Department of Medicine, Charing Cross Hospital Medical School, Fulham Palace Road, London, W6 8RF.

Renal osteodystrophy is so transfixed by semantic confusion and traditional myths that I would like to start with a few definitions. We would define renal osteodystrophy as the presence in the bone of a patient with chronic renal failure, of histological evidence of hyperparathyroidism with or without co-existing evidence of osteomalacia. Hyperparathyroidism consists of erosions and tunnelling of bone trabeculae, osteocytic osteolysis and marrow fibrosis. Osteomalacia consists of a diminution in mineralisation of the osteoid lamella lying closest to the calcified bone as revealed by tetracycline labelling and toluidine blue stain. Both conditions are associated with an increase in osteoid volume which is greatest with osteomalacia. The evidence suggests that all the lesions of hyperparathyroidism described above are due to an increase in the circulating concentration of parathyroid hormone which acts directly on the bone stimulating both osteoclasts and osteoblasts. The aetiology of the osteomalacia is less certain but would appear to be due to a diminished circulating concentration of one or more Vitamin D metabolites, some of which are known to act directly on the bone[1].

PREVENTION AND TREATMENT OF RENAL OSTEODYSTROPHY
BEFORE MAINTENANCE HAEMODIALYSIS

The incidence of renal osteodystrophy in 38 patients with terminal renal failure using the criteria detailed above is shown in Table 1[2].

This evidence suggests that the onset of the hyperparathyroidism precedes that of the osteomalacia. It is in keeping with the

TABLE 1

QUANTITATIVE BONE HISTOLOGY IN 38 PATIENTS WITH

TERMINAL RENAL FAILURE

Normal	6%
Hyperparathyroidism with normal calcification front	54%
Hyperparathyroidism with decreased calcification front but normal volume of osteoid	30%
Hyperparathyroidism with decreased calcification front and increased volume of osteoid	10%

findings of Ellis & Peart 1973[3] who found a similar distribution of abnormalities.   The findings also suggest that the severity of the bone lesion is related to the duration of the renal failure.

Prevention and Treatment of Hyperparathyroidism

There is substantial evidence that the raised concentration of plasma parathyroid hormone is due at least in part to the retention of phosphate, the associated tendency for hyperphosphataemia leading to hypocalcaemia [4].   There is also some suggestive evidence that the rise in serum parathyroid hormone concentration might also be due to a diminution in the circulating concentration of one of the metabolites of Vitamin D.   Prevention and treatment of hyperparathyroidism in chronic renal failure therefore should consist of trying to lower the plasma level of parathyroid hormone by raising the plasma calcium, lowering the plasma phosphate, and perhaps by the administration of a suitable preparation of Vitamin D.

Patients with renal failure on a low dietary intake of calcium are in negative calcium balance because of an impairment in calcium absorption.   If however, the calcium intake is raised to 2,000mg/day or more, calcium absorption becomes normal, the calcium balance is positive and the plasma calcium rises [5,6,7] (Fig.1).The overall effect in acute studies is to lower plasma parathyroid hormone concentration [8], which in its turn probably causes the accompanying fall in plasma phosphate[9].   Calcium carbonate also significantly raises plasma total CO_2.   The control of plasma

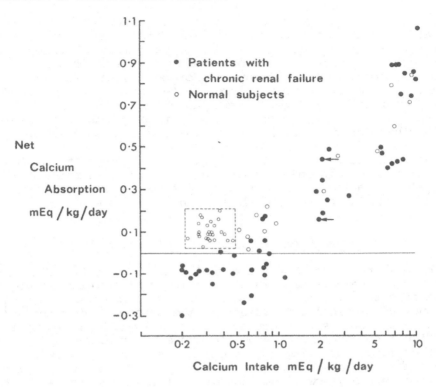

Fig. 1 Relation between calcium intake and calcium absorption in patients with chronic renal failure (•) and normal subjects (o). The circles (o) in the area bounded by the interrupted line represent Malm's (1958) 26 normal subjects on an experimental low calcium diet. The other circles (o) and solid dots (•) below 1.1 mEq/kg/day calcium intake and the two arrowed solid dots represent 29 patients with chronic renal failure (CRF) and 7 normal subjects on their usual intake of calcium. The remaining circles and dots, that is all those above 1.1 mEq/kg/day calcium intake (except the two arrowed dots), represent 21 of the 29 patients with CRF and the 7 normal subjects when taking supplementary calcium.[5]

phosphate ingestion is difficult and may give rise to a reduced intake of protein which has its own complications. Nevertheless it has been claimed that where the indigenous phosphate intake is low the incidence of renal osteodystrophy is also low[10]. Plasma phosphate is more easily controlled by the administration of aluminium hydroxide or other aluminium preparations. These preparations also lower plasma parathyroid hormone[11] acutely but there is little evidence of what occurs with prolonged use of either calcium carbonate or aluminium preparations. Johnson et al's[12] study over a period of three years is the most comprehensive but unfortunately there are no controls.   Mean glomerular filtration rates remained unchanged throughout this time.   Plasma parathyroid hormone levels were raised throughout and did not change though it is possible that without treatment plasma parathyroid hormone would have risen further.   There are certain hazards in the continuous use of aluminium preparations to lower plasma phosphate which will be discussed later.   The use of Vitamin D preparations to treat the hyperparathyroidism of chronic renal failure is also discussed later.

The ultimate weapon in the treatment of hyperparathyroidism before or during maintenance haemodialysis is parathyroidectomy. In undialysed patients it is usually confined to patients whose hypercalcaemia is not controllable in any other way.

Prevention and Treatment of Osteomalacia

There is no doubt that the administration of $1,25-(OH)_2 D_3$ to patients with the osteomalacia of chronic renal failure before they are placed onto maintenance haemodialysis will cause both histological and radiological improvement in the osteomalacic bones[13,14,15]. Nevertheless there is a reluctance to use $1,25-(OH)_2 D_3$ because it is difficult to obtain and is apt to cause hypercalcaemia.   There is another more compelling objection in that there is growing evidence that the osteomalacia of chronic renal failure is not due to the demonstrably low plasma levels of $1,25-(OH)_2 D_3$[16,17].   As the enzyme necessary for the conversion of $25-OH D_3$ to $1,25-(OH)_2 D_3$ has only been found in the kidney[18], the hypothesis that the defect in bone mineralisation is caused by a low plasma concentration of $1,25-(OH)_2 D_3$ became untenable when it was demonstrated that anephric patients do not have a higher incidence of osteomalacia than other patients on maintenance haemodialysis[19,20].   There is increasing evidence that the determining abnormality of Vitamin D metabolism which triggers off the defect in mineralisation is the low circulating concentration of plasma $25-OH D_3$[21,22,23]. We have recently compared the histological appearances on quantitative bone biopsy in 22 patients with chronic renal failure[23] with the plasma level of $25-OH D_3$.   Osteomalacia only occurred when the concentration of plasma $25-OH D_3$ was either below normal or in the low normal range.   The cause of this reduced concentration of plasma $25-OH D_3$ in only a proportion of patients includes a diminished intake of Vit. D associated with a low protein intake, and hepatic induction of microsomal enzymes.   The latter increases the rate of conversion of cholecalciferol to $25-OH D_3$ and also to other inactive conjugated metabolites which are excreted in the bile[24,25,26].   This state of affairs is exactly comparable to that of anti convulsant osteomalacia where the hepatic induction is due to barbiturates.   In chronic renal failure it is presumably due to the retention of end products of protein metabolism.

The administration of 20 to 40 μg of 25-OH D3 intravenously causes a rise in plasma 25-OH D3 to levels above normal within 28 days, together with a significant increase in the extent of mineralisation in the osteoid lamella next to the trabecular bone[27]. The prevention and treatment of osteomalacia would appear to consist of ensuring an adequate intake of Vitamin D in the diet and therefore restricting the use of low protein diets.   Ideally it would be best to monitor the plasma level of 25-OH D3 to make certain that it remains greater than 15 ng/ml with the judicious use of about 50 - 100μg of cholecalciferol, or 20 μg of 25-OH D3 per day, from time to time. It would also seem reasonable to prevent or reduce the intake of known inducers of hepatic microsomal enzymes such as barbiturates and alcohol.   The administration of calcium carbonate on its own without Vitamin D is unsatisfactory.   It causes a patchy irregular calcification of the osteoid which is quite abnormal[1,28], and which is accompanied by an incomplete radiological and clinical improvement[29].   Finally as there is some suggestion that the increased bone activity associated with hyperparathyroidism increases consumption of Vitamin D[30] it is possible that lowering the plasma parathyroid hormone level may also help to prevent the onset of hyperparathyroidism.

PREVENTION AND TREATMENT OF RENAL OSTEODYSTROPHY DURING MAINTENANCE HAEMODIALYSIS

Prevention and Treatment of Hyperparathyroidism (Table 2)

We have the impression that it is the general experience that whereas in the first few years of dialysis the radiological appearances of hyperparathyroidism may sometimes improve there is subsequently an increasing tendency for it to become more marked.   The rate of events varies widely between units and between patients in the same units.   There seems a measure of agreement that the more severe the hyperparathyroidism at the onset of haemodialysis the quicker the rate of deterioration.

The aims and methods of treatment are the same as those used before dialysis, with certain modifications.   The most notable is that the plasma calcium can be raised by raising the concentration of calcium in the dialysate to between 7 and 8 mg/100ml.   This causes a see-saw effect on plasma calcium with a varying period of hypercalcaemia after each dialysis.   The originators of this manoeuvre[31] were insistent that its capacity to lower plasma parathyroid hormone levels was effective only if it was accompanied by a strict control of plasma phosphate which in practice usually meant the simultaneous use of aluminium hydroxide or an alternative aluminium compound.   This is consistent with the findings of Bordier et al[28] who showed that though, in patients with chronic renal failure

TABLE 2

T R E A T M E N T   A N D   P R E V E N T I O N   O F   H Y P E R P A R A T H Y R O I D I S M

D U R I N G   D I A L Y S I S

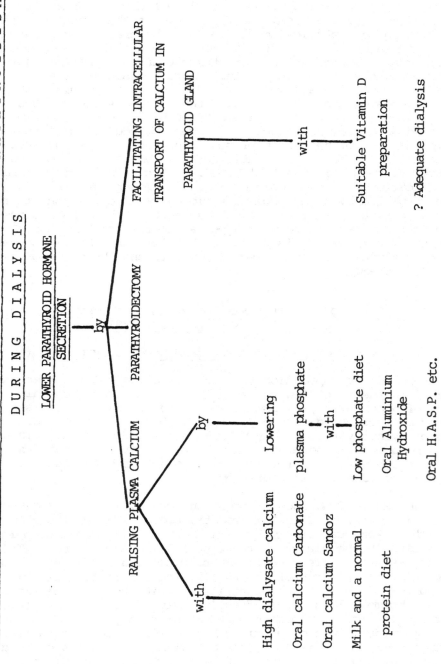

LOWER PARATHYROID HORMONE SECRETION

by

RAISING PLASMA CALCIUM

PARATHYROIDECTOMY

FACILITATING INTRACELLULAR TRANSPORT OF CALCIUM IN PARATHYROID GLAND

with

with

by

Lowering plasma phosphate

with

Suitable Vitamin D preparation

? Adequate dialysis

High dialysate calcium

Oral calcium Carbonate

Oral calcium Sandoz

Milk and a normal protein diet

Low phosphate diet

Oral Aluminium Hydroxide

Oral H.A.S.P. etc.

with plasma phosphate values below 4.5 mg/100ml the concentration
of parathyroid hormone is moderately raised, with higher levels
of plasma phosphate the rise in parathyroid hormone concentration
is very sharp.   There have now been several trials of this treatment and on the whole it has been uniformally disappointing.
Bouillon et al[30] found that though raising the dialysate calcium
produced an initial fall in plasma parathyroid hormone it did not
reach normal levels, and that within a few months the concentration
of parathyroid hormone had returned to the pre-treatment level.
Johnson et al[12] also were not able to reduce the plasma parathyroid
hormone level to normal.   We ourselves raised the dialysate calcium
to 7.5 mg/100ml for three years.   The incidence and progression of
hyperparathyroidism was unchanged and the necessity to perform parathyroidectomies for unrelenting radiological hyperparathyroidism is
the same.   There seems little doubt that the control of plasma
phosphate slows the rate of hyperparathyroidism but the value of
raising the dialysate calcium is less certain.

These relatively unsuccessful attempts to control parathyroid
hormone secretion have been accompanied by a growing realisation
that though it is essential to try and control plasma phosphate it
may be dangerous to do so.   Phosphate depletion and its ultimate
effect in causing "phosphate depletion osteomalacia" has been a
recognised complication of maintenance haemodialysis for some years
33,34,35.   This syndrome is easily avoided by continuously monitoring plasma phosphate, and when necessary giving calcium phosphate,
unless the patient is hypotensive, when sodium phosphate is more
suitable.   The potential hazard of aluminium toxicity[36] has usually
been ignored though Clarkson et al[11] did demonstrate that, in
contrast to normal subjects, patients with chronic renal failure
ingesting 100ml of aluminium hydroxide per day absorb substantial
amounts of aluminium.   Recently however, Alfrey et al[38] have
measured the aluminium content of the brain, muscle and bone of
patients on maintenance haemodialysis, all of whom have been given
aluminium hydroxide every day as a routine procedure.   There was a
significant correlation between the content of aluminium in the bone
and the number of months the patient had been dialysed.   The highest
concentration of aluminium was found in the grey matter of the
cerebral cortex from patients who had died of "dialysis dementia".
These observations suggest that to rely on the routine use of
aluminium hydroxide to control plasma phosphate, and thus hyperparathyroidism,may be unwise and that it may be better to attempt to do
so by dietary means, a greater number of hours per week on dialysis,
and by the earlier use of parathyroidectomy.

Various Vitamin D preparations have been used in the treatment
of hyperparathyroidism in patients both before and after being
placed onto maintenance haemodialysis.   The rationale behind this
approach has not usually been made clear.   If the purpose was to
depress parathyroid hormone secretion by increasing calcium

absorption and thus increasing plasma calcium there is little reason to believe that the administration of Vitamin D should be any more beneficial than raising the dialysate calcium or giving calcium carbonate by mouth.   On the other hand if the aim was to facilitate calcium transport in the cell of the parathyroid gland so as to raise the calcium concentration at some critical site which is involved in the control of parathyroid hormone secretion, then it is possible that the administration of some metabolite of Vitamin D might be much more effective than raising the plasma calcium.   The possibility that Vitamin D acts directly on the parathyroid cell is mainly based on observations recorded by Rasmussen and Bordier[39]. They demonstrated that in patients with dietary Vitamin D deficiency osteomalacia and normal renal function the administration of Vitamin D causes the concentration of plasma parathyroid hormone to fall before there is a rise in the plasma calcium.   In two of their patients the fall in parathyroid hormone was accompanied by a simultaneous fall in plasma calcium.   These observations give rise to the hypothesis that Vitamin D metabolites may act directly on the parathyroid gland and control its rate of hormone secretion. If it is true, then it is probable that part of the rise in plasma parathyroid hormone in chronic renal failure may be due to Vitamin D deficiency.   It is surprising that there do not seem to have been one animal experiment to examine this point.   It would be of immense clinical value to find that such a phenomenon exists and to know which Vitamin D metabolite was the most active in the parathyroid gland.

The preparations of Vitamin D which have been used to treat hyperparathyroidism include ergocalciferol and cholecalciferol[30,40,41], dihydrotachysterol[42,43], 25-OH D_3[28,44], 1,25-$(OH)_2$ D_3 [14,15,45,46], 1α-OH D_3 [15,47,48,49], and 5,6 Trans Vitamin D_3 [50].   With the exception of the last it has been claimed that the others have increased calcium absorption, raised plasma calcium, and improved the bone lesions.   One gets the impression that the bone lesions were initially so severe that any reduction in serum parathyroid hormone would be of obvious benefit.   Where serum levels of parathyroid hormone have been measured the concentration fell during the administration of the particular metabolite of Vitamin D and rapidly returned to the control levels thereafter.   In a few patients in whom the parathyroid hormone concentration was only moderately increased it fell to normal, sometimes without a rise in plasma calcium.   The most striking and well documented example of this phenomenon is that of Henderson et al[14] in whom the administration of 1,25-$(OH)_2$ D_3 for several months produced a radiological improvement in severe hyperparathyroidism without any accompanying rise in plasma calcium.   In most reports however, the hypercalcaemia which was probably being courted has been a nuisance, and the dose has had to be adjusted continuously.   Without it being explicitly stated one has the impression that most workers have assumed that any beneficial affect that the administration of Vitamin D might have on the hyperparathyroidism would be secondary to raising plasma

calcium.   Naturally enough therefore, most workers have used doses
of Vitamin D which manifestly did this and this is presumably why
they have been beset by hypercalcaemia.   We have not found one
report that specifically states that an attempt was made to treat
the hyperparathyroidism without raising the plasma calcium.   There
is already sufficient evidence available however, to suggest that
this might be worth doing.   The evidence also suggests that it will
take a considerable time for the serum plasma parathyroid concentration to return to normal; perhaps a year or two.

Salmon Calcitonin (100 M.R.C. units/day) for 4 to 11 weeks has
been used by Delano et al[51] to treat severe hyperparathyroidism.
The authors considered that there was no evidence of improvement,and
that there was even some suggestion that the hyperparathyroidism
became more pronounced.   The indications for parathyroidectomy vary
widely.   We would suggest that the aim is to prevent symptomatic
bone disease.   We monitor the radiological appearances of the bones
at least once a year and examine the progress of events in the distal
phalanx.   A parathyroidectomy is performed if there is a steady
deterioration with increasing evidence of erosions.   We have
performed 16 parathyroidectomies in 200 patients on maintenance haemodialysis over a period of 12 years for advancing radiological
hyperparathyroidism.   Four patients were symptomatic before operation including one who refused operation until he fractured both
scapulae when he slipped in the bath.   At one time we used to
perform parathyroidectomies for patients on maintenance haemodialysis
if the plasma calcium was persistently raised.   Now we only do so
if the hypercalcaemia is associated with symptoms such as red eyes,
for on the whole we find that the plasma calcium tends eventually
to return to normal.

Prevention and Treatment of Osteomalacia (Table 3)

In our experience the incidence of osteomalacia in patients on
maintenance haemodialysis is low and it hardly ever causes symptoms.
This is not surprising in view of Offerman et al's[22] evidence that
when patients are placed on maintenance haemodialysis and have a
normal intake of protein the plasma level of $25-OH D_3$ returns to
normal.   The administration of $25-OH D_3$ [1], $1,25-(OH)_2 D_3$ and
cholecalciferol[1] in small doses all appear to have a direct effect
on bone mineralisation.   If the patient is eating well however,
there does not appear to be any need to supplement the diet with
Vitamin D preparations to prevent the onset of osteomalacia.   It
is more important to make sure that appetite is maintained by
adequate dialysis, that barbiturates are not prescribed and that the
intake of alcohol is kept within reasonable proportions.   On the
other hand small supplements of the animal forms of Vitamin D are
probably needed when the patient suffers from some prolonged
clinical disaster such as a failed transplant.

TABLE 3

TREATMENT AND PREVENTION OF OSTEOMALACIA
DURING DIALYSIS

1.   Adequate dialysis.

2.   Cholecalciferol (50 μg/day) or 25 HCC (20 to 40 μg/day).

3.   Avoid barbiturates and high alcohol intake.

4.   Eat normal protein diet.

5.   Control hyperparathyroidism.

CONCLUSION

Hyperparathyroidism is the main cause of renal bone disease.
At the moment its progress can be retarded by controlling plasma
calcium and phosphate.   But the prevention and cure of hyperparathyroidism without surgery eludes us.   There is a suggestion
that the administration of some metabolite of Vitamin D may be more
successful.   Osteomalacia on the other hand does not appear to be
an important problem and is easily prevented and cured.

REFERENCES

1.   Eastwood, J.B., Bordier, Ph.J., Clarkson, E.M., Tun Chot, S.
     H. and de Wardener, H.E.: The contrasting effects on bone
     histology of vitamin D and of calcium carbonate in the
     osteomalacia of chronic renal failure. Clin. Sci. 47:23,1974.

2.   Eastwood, J.B.: Observations on renal osteodystrophy with
     special reference to the action of vitamin D on bone
     mineralisation. M.D. Thesis, University of London, 1974.

3.   Ellis, H.A., and Peart, K.M.: Azotaemic renal osteodystrophy:
     a quantitative study on iliac bone.   J. Clin.Path. 26:83,1973.

4.   Slatopolsky, E., Caglar, S., Pennell, J.P., Taggart, D.D.,
     Canterbury, J.M., Reiss, E., and Bricker, N.S.: On the patho-
     genesis of hyperparathyroidism in chronic experimental renal
     insufficiency in the dog. J. Clin. Invest. 50:492, 1971.

5.   Eastwood, J.B., and de Wardener, H.E.: Renal Osteodystrophy
     In: Recent Advances in Renal Disease. Ed. N.F. Jones,
     Churchill Livingstone, p.177, 1975.

6. Clarkson, E.M., Eastwood, J.B., Koutsaimanis, K.G., and de
    Wardener, H.E.: Net intestinal absorption of calcium in
    patients with chronic renal failure. Kidney Int.3:258, 1973.

7. Clarkson, E.M., McDonald, S.J., and de Wardener, H.E.: The
    effect of a high intake of calcium carbonate in normal subjects
    and patients with chronic renal failure. Clin. Sci. 30:425,
    1966.

8. O'Riordan, J.L.H. (Personal Communication).

9. Massry, S.G., Coburn, J.W., Popovtzer, M.M., Shinaberger, J.H.,
    Maxwell, M.H., and Kleeman, C.R.: Secondary hyperparathyroid-
    ism in chronic renal failure. Arch. Int. Med. 124:431, 1969.

10. Berlyne, G.M., Ben-Arie, J., Epstein, N., Booth, E.M., and
    Yagil, R.: Rarity of renal osteodystrophy in Israel due to
    low phosphorus intake. Nephron, 10:141, 1973.

11. Clarkson, E.M., Luck, V.A., Hynson, W.V., Bailey, R.R.,
    Eastwood, J.B., Woodhead, J.S., Clements, V.R., O'Riordan,J.
    L.H., and de Wardener, H.E.: The effect of aluminium hydroxide
    on calcium, phosphorus and aluminium balances, the serum
    parathyroid hormone concentration and the aluminium content
    of bone in patients with chronic renal failure. Clin. Sci.
    43:519, 1972.

12. Johnson, W.J., Goldsmith, R.S., Jowsey, J., Fronhert, P.P.,
    and Arnaud, C.D.: The influence of maintaining normal serum
    phosphate and calcium on renal osteodystrophy. In: Vitamin
    D and Problems to Uremic Bone Disease, Walter de Gryter & Co.,
    Berlin, 1975.

13. Eastwood, J.B., Phillips, M.E., de Wardener, H.E., Bordier,
    Ph.J., Marie, P., Arnaud, C.D., and Norman, A.W.: Biochemical
    and histological effects of 1,25 dihydroxycholecalciferol
    (1,25-DHCC) in the osteomalacia of chronic renal failure. In:
    Vitamin D and Problems to Uremic Bone Disease, Walter de
    Gruyter & Co. Berlin, 1975.

14. Henderson, R.G., Russell, R.G.G., Ledingham, J.G.G., Smith,R.,
    Oliver, D.O., Walton, R.J., Small, D.G., Preston, C., Warner,
    G.T., and Norman, A.W.: Effects of 1,25-DHCC on calcium
    absorption muscle weakness and bone disease in chronic renal
    failure. Lancet, 1:379, 1974.

15. Brickman, A.S., Sherrard,D.J., Coburn, L.S., Poelns, L.S., Baylink, D.J., Friedman, G.S., Massry, S.G., and Norman, A.W.: Management of renal osteodystrophy with 1,25 (OH)$_2$ and 1α(OH)-vitamin D$_3$: Experience with 36 patients. Abstract. Kidney Int. 8:407, 1975.

16. Mawer, E.B., Backhouse, J., Taylor, C.M., Lumb, G.A., and Stanbury, S.W.: Failure of formation of 1,25-dihydroxychole-calciferol in chronic renal insufficiency. Lancet, 1:626,1973.

17. Haussler, M.R.: Vitamin D: Mode of action and biomedical applications. Nutrition Reviews. 32:257, 1974.

18. Fraser, D.R., and Kodicek, E.: Unique biosynthesis by kidney of a biologically active Vitamin D metabolite. Nature, 228:764, 1970.

19. Bordier, Ph.J., Tun Chot, S., Eastwood, J.B., Fournier, A.E., and de Wardener, H.E.: Lack of histological evidence of Vitamin D abnormality in the bones of anephric patients. Clin. Sci., 44:33, 1973.

20. Ritz, E., Krempien, B., Mehl, S and Malluche, H.: Skeletal abnormalities in chronic renal insufficiency before and during haemodialysis. Kidney Int. 4:116, 1973.

21. Bayard, F., Bec, P., Ton That, H., and Louvet, J.P.: Plasma 25-hydroxycholecalciferol in chronic renal failure. Eur. J. Clin. Invest. 3:447, 1973.

22. Offermann, G., von Herrath, D., and Schaefer, K.: Serum 25-hydroxycholecalciferol in uraemia. Nephron, 13:269, 1974.

23. Eastwood, J.B., Stamp, T.C.B., and de Wardener, H.E.: Bone mineralisation and plasma 25 OH-D in chronic renal failure. In preparation.

24. Fine, A., and Sumner, D.: Alteration in hepatic acetylation in uraemia. In: Proceedings of the European Dialysis and Transplant Association, XI:433, 1974.

25. Maddocks, J.L., Wake, C.L., and Harber, M.J.: Plasma half life of antipyrine in chronic renal failure. Abstract, Kidney Int. 7:360, 1975.

26. Avioli, L.V., Birge, S., Lee, S.W., and Slatopolsky, E.: The metabolic fate of Vitamin D$_3$ - ^{3}H in chronic renal failure. J. Clin. Invest. 47:2239, 1968.

27. Eastwood, J.B., Stamp, T.C.B., de Wardener, H.E., Bordier, Ph. J., and Arnaud, C.D.: Effect of 20 - 40 ug of 25 OH Vitamin D_3 in the osteomalacia of chronic renal failure. In preparation.

28. Bordier, Ph.J., Marie, P.J., and Arnaud, C.D.: Evolution of renal osteodystrophy: correlation of bone histomorphometry and serum mineral and immunoreactive parathyroid hormone values before and after treatment with calcium carbonate or 25-hydroxycholecalciferol. Kidney Int. Suppl.2:102, 1975.

29. Snodgrass, G.J.A.I., and de Wardener, H.E.: The effects of oral calcium on renal rickets. Abstracts of Free Communications, IVth International Congress of Nephrology, Stockholm, p.78, Basle, Karger, 1969.

30. Woodhouse, N.J.Y., Doyle, F.H., and Joplin, G.F.: Vitamin D deficiency and primary hyperparathyroidism. Lancet, 2:283, 1971.

31. Goldsmith, R.S., Furszyfer, J., Johnson, W.J., Fournier, A.E., Sizemore, G.W., and Arnaud, C.D.: Etiology of hyperparathyroidism and bone disease during chronic haemodialysis. J. Clin. Invest. 52:173, 1973.

32. Bouillon, R., Verberckmoes, R., and De Moor, P.: Influence of dialysate calcium concentration and vitamin D on serum parathyroid hormone during repetitive dialysis. Kidney Int. 7:422, 1975.

33. Curtis, J.R., de Wardener, H.E., Gower, P.E., and Eastwood, J.B.: The use of calcium carbonate and calcium phosphate without Vitamin D in the management of renal osteodystrophy. In: Proceedings of the European Dialysis and Transplant Association, VII:141, 1970.

34. Baker, L.R.I., Ackrill, P., Cattell, W.R., Stamp, T.C.B., and Watson, L.: Iatrogenic osteomalacia and myopathy due to phosphate depletion. B.M.J., 3:150, 1974.

35. Bishop, M.C., Ledingham, J.G.G., and Oliver, D.O.: Phosphate deficiency in haemodialysed patients. In: Proceedings of the European Dialysis and Transplant Association, VIII:106, 1971.

36. Berlyne, G.M., Yagil, R., Ben Ari, J., Weinberger, G., Knopf, E., and Danovitch, G.M.: Aluminium Toxicity in Rats. Lancet, II:564, 1972.

37. Cam, J.M., Luck, V.A., Eastwood, J.B., and de Wardener, H.E.:
     The effect of aluminium hydroxide orally on calcium phosphorus
     and aluminium metabolism in normal subjects. Clin. Sci.
     (In press).

38. Alfrey, A.C., Gendre, G.R., and Kaehny, W.D.: The Dialysis
     Encephalopathy Syndrome: Possible aluminium intoxication.
     N. Eng. J. Med. 294:184, 1976.

39. Rasmussen, H., and Bordier, Ph.J.: The physiological and
     cellular basis of metabolic bone disease. Williams and
     Wilkins, Baltimore, 242, 1974.

40. Dent, C.E., Harper, C.M., and Philpot, G.R.: The treatment
     of renal-glomerular osteodystrophy. Quart, J. Med. New
     Series XXX, 117:1, 1961.

41. Stanbury, S.W., and Lumb, G.A.: Metabolic studies of renal
     osteodystrophy I Calcium, phosphorus and nitrogen metabolism
     in rickets, osteomalacia and hyperparathyroidism, complica-
     ting chronic uremia and in the osteomalacia of the adult
     Fanconi syndrome. Medicine, 41:1, 1962.

42. Liu, S.H., and Chu, H.I.: Studies of calcium and phosphorus
     metabolism with special reference to pathogenesis and
     effects of dihydrotachysterol (A.T.10) and iron. Medicine
     (Baltimore) 22:103, 1943.

43. Kaye, M., Chatterjee, G., Cohen, G.F., and Sagar, S.: Arrest
     of hyperparathyroid bone disease with dihydrotachysterol in
     patients undergoing chronic haemodialysis. Annals Int. Med.
     73:225, 1970.

44. Colodro, I.H., Brickman, A.S., Coburn, J.W., Osborn, T.W.,
     and Norman, A.W.: Comparative effects of 25 (OH)-vitamin D_3
     in normal and uremic man. Abstract, Kidney Int. 8:398, 1975.

45. Brickman, A.S., Coburn, J.W., Norman, A.W., and Massry, S.G.:
     Short-term effects of 1,25-dihydroxycholecalciferol on dis-
     ordered calcium metabolism of renal failure. Amer. J. Med.
     57:28, 1974.

46. Brickman, A.S., Sherrard, D.J., Jowsey, J., Singer, F.R.,
     Baylink, D.J., Maloney, N., Massry, S.G., Norman, A.W., and
     Coburn, J.W.: 1,25-Dihydroxycholecalciferol. Effect on
     skeletal lesions and plasma parathyroid hormone levels in
     uremic osteodystrophy. Arch. Intern. Med. 134:883, 1974.

47. Chalmers, T.M., Davie, M.W., Hunter, J.O., Szaz, K.F., Pelc, B., and Kodicek, E.: 1-alpha-hydroxycholecalciferol as a substitute for the kidney hormone   1,25-dihydroxycholecalciferol in chronic renal failure.   Lancet, II:696, 1973.

48. Catto, G.R.D., MacLeod, M., Pelc, B., and Kodicek, E.: 1-hydroxycholecalciferol: A treatment for renal bone disease. B.M.J., 1:12, 1975.

49. Beale, M.G., Chan, J.C.M., Oldham, S.B., and DeLuca, H.F.: Reversal of renal osteodystrophy (RO) by 1-Alpha hydroxy-vitamin D_3 (1α-OH-D_3).   Kidney Int. 8:(6),397, 1975.

50. Rutherford, W.E., Hruska, K., Blondin, J., Holick, M., Deluca, H., Klahr, S., and Slatopolsky, E.: The effect of 5,6-Trans Vitamin D_3 on calcium absorption in chronic renal disease.   J. Clin. Endo., 40:13, 1975.

51. Delano, B.G., Baker, R., Gardner, B., and Wallack, S.: A trial of calcitonin therapy in renal osteodystrophy.   Nephron II:287, 1973.

INTESTINAL PHOSPHATE ABSORPTION IN NORMAL AND UREMIC MAN: EFFECTS OF 1,25(OH)$_2$-VITAMIN D$_3$ AND 1α(OH)-VITAMIN D$_3$

J.W. Coburn, A.S. Brickman, D.L. Hartenbower,
and A.W. Norman
VA Wadsworth Hospital, UCLA School of Medicine,
and University of California Riverside
Los Angeles and Riverside, California

The action of vitamin D on the intestinal absorption of phosphorus has not been studied extensively in man. Limitations in the use of ^{32}P labeled phosphate have restricted observations in large part to those of net absorption derived from metabolic balance techniques. Using such methods, Stanbury and Lumb (1) and Stanbury (2) reported that pharmacologic doses of vitamin D promoted equimolar increments in the net absorption of calcium and phosphorus in patients with advanced renal failure and severe bone disease. Such a relationship between the absorption of calcium and that of phosphorus supports the viewpoint that phosphate transport across the intestine is dependent upon that of calcium. Recent studies in the rat and chick indicate that vitamin D or its active forms stimulates intestinal transport of phosphorus independent of an effect on calcium (3,4). In the present study, we have evaluated the effect of treatment with 1,25-dihydroxy-vitamin D$_3$ (1,25 (OH)$_2$D$_3$) or 1α-hydroxy-vitamin D$_3$ (1α(OH)D$_3$) on net absorption of phosphorus in patients with advanced renal failure and normal volunteers. The results in man indicate that both analogs of vitamin D enhance the intestinal net absorption of phosphorus.

MATERIALS AND METHODS

Sixteen metabolic balance studies were carried out in patients with advanced renal failure and four in normal male volunteers. The mean age was 55 years, with a range from 47 to 69 years. Mean endogenous creatinine clearance averaged 10.6±2.4 (S.E.) ml/min in the uremic patients, one of whom was anephric. Metabolic balance studies were carried out precisely as described previously (5). The subjects underwent dietary equilibration on the metabolic unit and received diets providing calcium and phosphorus in amounts similar to those present in their usual diet. The molar ratios of calcium:phosphorus in the diets ranged from 0.23 to 0.52 in 15 studies without supplemental dietary calcium; the ratio was 1.49 to 2.45 in 5 studies in uremic patients given added calcium. Four patients received the same amounts of aluminum hydroxide gel each day throughout the study. After equilibration periods of 14 to 28 days, stool and urine collections were initiated. The stool collections were made over 4 to 7 day periods; 2 to 5 control periods were collected before treatment with $1,25(OH)_2D_3$ of $1\alpha(OH)D_3$. Brilliant blue was given as an intermittent stool marker, and some subjects received barium sulfate as an internal stool marker (5). Control Values represent mean values over 2 to 5 periods, and Treatment Values are the last 1 or 2 periods during administration of the vitamin D sterol. Net absorption for both calcium and phosphorus is calculated as the difference between dietary intake and fecal excretion; endogenous fecal secretion of calcium and phosphorus was not measured.

The $1,25(OH)_2D_3$ or $1\alpha(OH)D_3$, dissolved in 1:1 ethanol:1,2-propanediol, was given daily by mouth. The quantities given ranged from 0.325 to 13 nmoles/day (equivalent to 5 to 200 I.U. of vitamin D_3), with the duration of treatment, 6-25 days. Eleven studies were carried out with $1,25(OH)_2D_3$ and 9 with $1\alpha(OH)D_3$. Biosynthesized $1,25(OH)_2D_3$, employed in 10 studies, was prepared as previously described (6), and chemically synthesized $1,25(OH)_2D_3$ was provided through the courtesy of Dr. M. Uskokovic, Hoffmann-La-Roche, Nutley, New Jersey. The $1\alpha(OH)D_3$ was synthesized by a modification of the method reported by Mitra et al (7).

Informed consent was obtained from each subject prior to the initiation of the study. The methods for analysis of phosphorus, calcium and creatinine have been previously described. Some of the results in 10 studies were previously reported (8) without attention to phosphorus metabolism.

RESULTS

Both $1,25(OH)_2D_3$ and $1\alpha(OH)D_3$ augmented net phosphorus absorption in normal subjects and in patients with renal failure (Table I). The changes in net absorption of phosphorus varied directly with the dose of sterol given and paralleled the increments in net calcium absorption (Figure 1). In uremic patients, the increase in net phosphorus absorption ranged from 0.6 to 12.0 mmoles/day (mean ± S.E.: 3.9±.82 mmoles/day); in the normal subjects, net absorption increased by 1.8 to 7.4 mmoles/day (mean ± S.E.: 3.9±.27 mmoles/day). The changes in net absorption of calcium ranged from -.9 to +12.4 (4.4±0.95 mmoles/day) and from -1.5 to 6.5 (3.1±1.9 mmoles/day) in uremic and normal subjects, respectively.

Table I. Dose of $1,25(OH)_2D_3$ or $1\alpha(OH)D_3$ and effect on fecal phosphate and net phosphate absorbed.

Study No.	Sterol	Dose nmol/l	Diet P	Fecal P		Fraction Absorbed	
			mmol/day				
				C	E	C	E
NORMAL SUBJECTS							
1	$1,25(OH)_2D_3$	.325	58.8	21.2	19.4	.64	.67
2	"	1.625	58.8	21.2	18.9	.64	.67
3	"	6.5	32.1	7.9	3.7	.78	.89
4	"	6.5	57.4	27.2	19.9	.35	.48
CHRONIC RENAL FAILURE							
5	$1,25(OH)_2D_3$	.325	20.2	6.3	5.8	.69	.71
6	"	.325	32.5	9.7	8.8	.70	.73
7	$1\alpha(OH)D_3$	1.625	21.5	9.2	7.5	.57	.65
8	"	1.625	30.0	11.3	9.3	.62	.69
9	"	1.625	23.2	11.8	9.2	.49	.60
10	$1,25(OH)_2D_3$	1.625	32.5	9.7	7.0	.70	.79
11*	$1\alpha(OH)D_3$	6.5	20.8	9.2	6.8	.56	.67
12	"	6.5	29.0	9.2	6.9	.68	.76
13	"	6.5	28.8	9.5	5.7	.67	.80
14	$1,25(OH)_2D_3$	6.5	29.0	8.6	7.3	.70	.75
15*	"	6.5	24.3	16.5	7.8	.39	.68
16*	"	6.5	18.4	17.4	5.4	.05	.71
17*	"	6.5	36.7	23.8	14.1	.36	.62
18	$1\alpha(OH)D_3$	13.0	20.9	9.2	5.8	.56	.72
19	"	13.0	29.0	8.5	6.3	.71	.78
20	"	13.0	23.7	9.5	5.9	.30	.45

*Receiving aluminum hydroxide throughout balance of study.

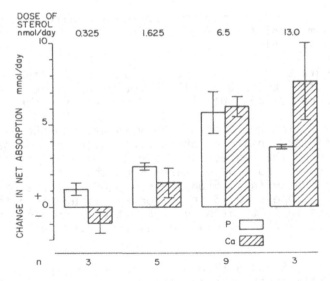

Figure 1. Changes in net absorption of calcium and phosphorus according to daily dose of $1,25(OH)_2D_3$ or $1\alpha(OH)D_3$. Data in normal subjects and patients with renal failure are combined (mean ± SEM).

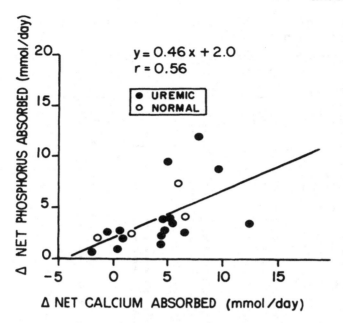

Figure 2. Relation between change in net absorption of phosphorus and that of calcium in all subjects treated with 1,25(OH)$_2$D$_3$ or 1α(OH)D$_3$.

The change in net absorption of phosphorus was directly related to those of calcium with: Δ net P absorption = 0.46 (Δ net Ca absorption) - 2.0 mmoles (Figure 2).

When a regression analysis was applied to the studies with dietary Ca:P ratios below 0.51, the formula was: Δ net P absorption = 0.75 (Δ net Ca absorption) - 1.3 mmoles, r = 0.65.

In figure 3, the relationship between net phosphorus absorption and the dietary intake of phosphorus in the uremic patients is superimposed on the regression slope observed in uremic patients, both personal cases and studies taken from the literature (9). Following treatment with 1,25(OH)$_2$D$_3$ or 1α(OH)D$_3$ the slope was 0.71 compared to the slope of 0.46 in all untreated uremic patients. Also, the values in 4 "treated" uremic patients exceeded the 95% confidence limits for individual values for untreated uremic patients.

In studies 1, 5 and 9 (Table I), the net phosphorus absorption increased slightly in the absence of an increase in net absorption of calcium. These subjects were receiving only 0.325 nmoles/day of 1,25(OH)$_2$D$_3$ or 1.625 nmoles/day of 1α(OH)D$_3$.

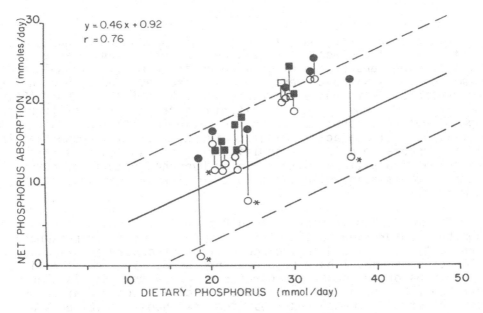

Figure 3. Relationship between net phosphorus absorption and dietary phosphorus intake in patients with advanced renal failure receiving either 1,25(OH)₂D₃ or 1α(OH)D₃. Open symbols represent control measurements, closed symbols indicate measurements during treatment with either 1,25(OH)₂D₃ (circles) or 1α(OH)D₃ (squares). The asterisk indicates those patients receiving constant daily amounts of aluminum hydroxide. The regression line for uremic patients is adapted from personal cases and studies taken from the literature (9).

During treatment of the uremic patients, urinary phosphorus excretion decreased by 2.4-6.3 mmoles/day in 9 studies but changed by 1.4 mmoles/day or less in 6 studies. Urinary phosphorus increased during treatment in each study in normal subjects. The fraction of filtered phosphorus excreted in the urine (C_P/C_{Cr}) decreased in the uremic patients during treatment; this change was not evident in the patients receiving the lower doses of the sterols, 0.325 or 1.625 nmoles/day, or in those exhibiting an increase in serum P by > 0.6 mM. However, the ratio, C_P/C_{Cr}, decreased from 0.72±.067 to 0.54±.087, a significant reduction of 19.7±7.5%, in the patients treated with larger doses of 1,25(OH)₂D₃ or 1α(OH)D₃ (6.5 to 13 nmoles/day) and not exhibiting an increase in serum P.

DISCUSSION

The present data indicate that $1,25(OH)_2D_3$ and $1\alpha(OH)D_3$, in quantities that are near to physiologic amounts, can enhance the net intestinal absorption of phosphorus in normal individuals and uremic patients without overt skeletal disease. These observations are consistent with those of Stanbury and Lumb (1), Stanbury (2), and Stamp (10), who found that vitamin D_2 or dihydrotachysterol can augment net phosphorus absorption in patients with renal failure or nutritional osteomalacia. Also, Caniggia et al (11) found that the plasma appearance of orally administered ^{32}P labeled phosphate increased in 3 patients with X-linked hypophosphatemia or nutritional osteomalacia following 1 month of therapy with vitamin D_2, 15 mg/day.

The mechanism whereby vitamin D sterols may enhance intestinal phosphate absorption is uncertain. A direct effect on phosphate transport, itself, and an indirect action secondary to stimulation of calcium transport have both been proposed. In studies of intestinal transport of phosphate carried out in vitro, Harrison and Harrison (12) found that a decrease in calcium concentration by the addition of EDTA to the media bathing the mucosa inhibited phosphate transport; similar results were obtained by Helbock et al (13). Stanbury and Lumb (1) noted an equimolar relationship between net absorption of calcium and phosphorus following treatment of patients with nutritional osteomalacia or uremia with pharmacologic doses of vitamin D_2 or dihydrotachysterol. Such observations provide support for a dependence of phosphate transport on that of calcium.

More recently, data from several laboratories indicate that vitamin D sterols may exert a direct action on phosphate transport. With studies in vitro, Kowarski and Schachter (14) observed that varying the calcium concentration on the luminal surface had no effect on the intestinal transport of phosphate. Wasserman and Taylor (3) found no suppression of vitamin D_3-stimulated phosphate transport after adding EGTA to a mucosal perfusate in situ. Chen et al found that both $25(OH)D_3$ and $1,25(OH)_2D_3$ augmented phosphate transport independent of their effect on calcium (4). Also Walling and Kimberg found that $1,25(OH)_2D_3$ stimulated active phosphate transport independent of calcium (15). These findings indicate that the phosphorus transport that is vitamin D-stimulated may not require calcium as a co-ion.

Studies in experimental animals indicate that mechanism of phosphate transport in the intestine may differ considerably from those of calcium. Phosphorus absorption occurs more rapidly than calcium in studies which allow comparison of the rate of absorption

of the two ions (3,16). Absorbed phosphorus is rapidly incorporated into the phospholipids of the intestinal mucosa (17).

A phosphate-binding protein, analogous to that for calcium,
has not been identified (3). Other studies have demonstrated that
intestinal phosphate transport occurs against a electrochemical
gradient, that the process is inhibited by metabolic poisons or
anoxia, and that the transport process is saturable (3,12). Such
observations indicate that an active process is responsible, at
least in part, for phosphorus absorption. Finally, observations
by Kowarski and Schachter(14) and Hurwitz and Bar (18) suggest
that vitamin D exerts a greater relative effect on calcium transport in the duodenum and on phosphorus in the jejunum.

Due to its inherent limitations, the metabolic balance technique does not measure true absorption of calcium or phosphorus nor
separate the independent effects of vitamin D sterols on net absorption of calcium and phosphorus. Net phosphorus absorption was enhanced in the absence of an increase in net calcium absorption in
3 of the present studies employing low doses of $1,25(OH)_2D_3$ or
$1\alpha(OH)D_3$. However, the increase in net absorption of phosphorus
was related to that of calcium in the present report, with a ratio
of 0.46 for all studies and 0.75 for studies with dietary Ca/P
ratios of 1:2 to 1.4.

The net absorption of phosphorus has been shown to be slightly
reduced in patients with advanced renal failure (1,9). The present
studies confirm such data and indicate that $1,25(OH)_2D_3$ can raise
the net absorption of phosphorus to values seen in normal. Such
observations are consistent with the postulate that the malabsorption of phosphorus seen in uremia may be due to reduced synthesis
of $1,25(OH)_2D_3$. The increase in net phosphorus absorption in uremia following treatment with small doses of $1,25(OH)_2D_3$ or $1\alpha(OH)D_3$
may have important consequences with the use of these compounds in
the long-term management of azotemic osteodystrophy. Data from our
laboratory suggest that hyperphosphatemia may develop with long-
term administration of $1,25(OH)_2D_3$, 1 μg/day, particularly after
healing and remineralization of severe skeletal disease (unpublished observations).

In normal subjects, urinary phosphate rose in association with
increased net phosphate absorption produced by $1,25(OH)_2D_3$; a
slight increase in filtered phosphate may have accounted for the
urinary losses. A decrease in the fraction of filtered phosphate
excreted in the urine was noted in uremic patients treated with
larger amounts of $1,25(OH)_2D_3$ or $1\alpha(OH)D_3$. Treatment with these
quantities of $1,25(OH)_2D_3$ can lower the plasma iPTH levels in
uremic patients (19), and inhibition of PTH secretion may have
accounted for the enhanced tubular reabsorption of phosphate.

REFERENCES

1. Stanbury, S.W. and Lumb, G.A.:   Metabolic studies of renal
    osteodystrophy. I. Calcium, phosphorus and nitrogen metabol-
    ism in rickets, osteomalacia and hyperparathyroidism compli-
    cating chronic uremia and in osteomalacia of the adult
    Fanconi Syndrome. Medicine 41:1, 1962.
2. Stanbury, S.W.: The phosphate ion in chronic renal failure.
    IN. D.J. Hioco, Ed., Phosphate Inorganique, Biologie et
    Physiopathologie, International Symposium. (Sandoz), Paris,
    p. 187, 1970.
3. Wasserman, R.H. and Taylor, A.N.: Intestinal absorption of
    phosphate in the chick: Effect of vitamin D_3 and other para-
    meters. J. Nutrit. 103:586, 1973.
4. Chen, T.C., Castillo, L., Korycka-Dahl, M., and DeLuca, H.F.:
    Role of vitamin D metabolites in phosphate transport of rat
    intestine. J. Nutrit. 104:1056, 1974.
5. Kopple, J.D. and Coburn, J.W.: Metabolic studies of low
    protein diets in uremia. II. Calcium, phosphorus and
    magnesium. Medicine 52:597, 1973.
6. Norman, A.W., Midgett, R.J., Myrtle, J.F., and Nowicki, H.G.:
    Studies on calciferol metabolism. I. Production of vitamin
    D metabolite 4B from 25-OH-cholecalciferol by kidney homogen-
    ates. Biochem. Biophys. Res. Commun. 42:1082, 1971.
7. Mitra, M.N., Norman, A.W., and Okamura, W.: Studies on vita-
    min D and its analogs. I. Synthesis of 1α-hydroxycholes-5-
    ene. J. Organic Chem. 39:2931, 1974.
8. Brickman, A.S., Coburn, J.W., Massry, S.G., and Norman, A.W.:
    1,25 Dihydroxy-vitamin D_3 in normal man and patients with
    renal failure. Ann. Intern. Med. 80:161, 1974.
9. Coburn, J.W., Hartenbower, D.L., Brickman, A.S., Massry, S.G.,
    and Kopple, J.D.: Intestinal absorption of calcium, magnesi-
    um and phosphorus in chronic renal insufficiency. In D.S.
    David, Ed. Calcium Metabolism in Renal Disease, John Wiley
    & Sons, New York, 1977 (In Press).
10. Stamp, T.C.B.: The intestinal absorption of phosphorus. Its
    relation to calcium absorption and to treatment with vitamin
    D in osteomalacia, parathyroid dysfunction and chronic renal
    failure. Abstracts, Medical Research Society, London, 1972,
    p. 16P.
11. Caniggia, A., Sennari, C., Bencini, M., and Palazzuoli, V.:
    Intestinal absorption of radiophosphate in osteomalacia
    before and after vitamin D treatment. Calcif. Tissue Res.
    2:299, 1968.
12. Harrison, H.E. and Harrison, H.C.: Intestinal transport of
    phosphate: Action of vitamin D, calcium and potassium.
    Amer. J. Physiol. 201:1007, 1961.

13. Helbock, H.J., Forte, J.G., and Saltman, P.: The mechanism of calcium transport by rat intestine. Biochim. Biophys. Acta. 126:81, 1966.

14. Kowarski, S. and Schachter, D.: Effects of vitamin D on phosphate transport and incorporation into mucosal constituents of rat intestinal mucosa. J. Biol. Chem. 244:211, 1969.

15. Walling, M.W. and Kimberg, D.V.: Effects of 1α,25-Dihydroxy-vitamin D_3 and solanum glaucophyllum on intestinal calcium and phosphate transport and on plasma Ca, Mg, and P levels in the rat. Endocrinology. 97:1567, 1975.

16. Cramer, C.F.: In vivo measurement of radiophosphorus and radiostrontium absorption in rats. Proc. Soc. Exptl. Biol. Med. 100:364, 1959.

17. Thompson, V. and DeLuca, H.F.: Vitamin D and phospholipid metabolism. J. Biol. Chem. 239:984, 1963.

18. Hurwitz, S. and Bar, A.: Site of action of vitamin D. Amer. J. Physiol. 222:761, 1972.

19. Brickman, A.S., Sherrard, D.J., Jowsey, J., Singer, F.R., Baylink, D.J., Maloney, N., Massry, S.G., Norman, A.W., Coburn, J.W.: 1,25-Dihydroxycholecalciferol. Effect on skeletal lesions and plasma parathyroid hormone levels in uremic osteodystrophy. Arch. Intern. Med. 134:883, 1974.

THE EFFECT OF PLASMA PHOSPHATE ON THE ACTION OF 1αOHD$_3$ IN HAEMODIALYSIS PATIENTS

M. Peacock,[*] A.M. Davison[**] and G.S. Walker[**]

[*] M.R.C. Mineral Metabolism Unit, The General Infirmary, Great George Street, Leeds LS1 3EX, England.

[**] Department of Renal Medicine, St. James's Hospital, Leeds LS9 7TF, England.

INTRODUCTION

The most potent natural metabolite of vitamin D, 1α,25 di-hydroxy vitamin D (1,25(OH)$_2$D) is produced by the action of renal 1αhydroxylase on 25 hydroxy vitamin D [1]. Patients with renal failure have decreased synthesis and undetectable plasma concentrations of 1,25(OH)$_2$D [2,3]. The failure of 1,25(OH)$_2$D production probably accounts for most, but not all, of the calcium malabsorption of chronic renal failure since it is corrected by small doses of oral 1,25(OH)$_2$D [4]. Synthetic 1αhydroxy vitamin D$_3$ (1αOHD$_3$), which is converted to 1,25(OH)$_2$D$_3$ in the body [3], does not require the renal 1αhydroxylase and is also able in small doses to correct the calcium malabsorption of renal failure [5].

A raised plasma phosphate concentration is a feature of renal failure and has been incriminated as an important factor in metastatic calcification [6] and secondary hyperparathyroidism [7]. It is common practice therefore to attempt to control plasma phosphate in patients with renal failure, even those on haemodialysis, with oral phosphate binders. A raised plasma phosphate concentration is also known to inhibit 1,25(OH)$_2$D production [8]. Furthermore therapeutic doses of 1αOHD$_3$ increase not only calcium but also

phosphorus absorption and raise the plasma calcium and phosphate[5].
The present study was designed to investigate the effect of plasma
phosphate and $1\alpha OHD_3$ on calcium and phosphorus absorption in patients with chronic renal failure on haemodialysis.

Material and Methods

This study was undertaken on 35 unselected patients on maintenance haemodialysis.   Dialysis was performed with a Meltec
Multipoint 1 sq. metre for six hours thrice weekly employing a
dialysate calcium of 1.5 mmol/l.   All patients received a free
diet apart from fluid and potassium restriction.   The average
daily intake of calcium was 15 mmol and of phosphorus 30.6 mmol.

Group 1 consisted of 20 patients who were studied before and
after therapy with $1\alpha OHD_3$.   Group 2 consisted of 15 patients who
were studied in a basal state, following treatment with Aludrox to
reduce the plasma phosphate to 1.6 mmol/l or less and again after
$1\alpha OHD_3$ therapy.   The dose of $1\alpha OHD_3$ was determined for each patient by starting with 2µg daily and then repeating the radiocalcium
absorption 7 - 14 days later.   If the radiocalcium absorption had
not increased to within the normal range the dose was increased by
1µg increments until the absorption was normal or hypercalcaemia
developed.

Plasma for calcium, phosphate and alkaline phosphatase was
obtained after an overnight fast some 36 hours following the previous haemodialysis and was measured by standard Auto-Analyzer
techniques (normal ranges, calcium 2.25 - 2.60 mmol/l, phosphate
0.8 - 1.3 mmol/l, alkaline phosphatase 4 - 13 KA units).

Radiocalcium absorption and phosphorus absorption were estimated in the fasting state following a combined oral dose of ^{45}Ca
and ^{32}P in a carrier of 20mg calcium [9] (as calcium chloride) and
50mg phosphate (as disodium hydrogen phosphate) at pH 5.0 (in press).
Absorption studies were performed 36 hours following the preceding
haemodialysis.

Soft tissue metastatic calcification was assessed radiologic-
ally and corneal calcification by slit lamp examination.

Results

Dose of 1αOHD$_3$

In Group 1 thirteen patients responded to a daily dose of 2µg of 1αOHD$_3$. In five patients the dose had to be increased to 3µg daily and in two patients a dose of 4µg daily was required. In one patient 4µg of 1αOHD$_3$ did not increase the calcium absorption to within the normal range and his dose was not increased further. In Group 2 ten patients responded to a daily dose of 2µg and two patients required 3µg daily. Two patients became hypercalcaemic although their calcium absorption had not increased to within the normal range, one whilst receiving 2µg daily and one whilst receiving 3µg daily. The remaining patient in this group defaulted from therapy and is not included in the analysis.

Plasma calcium   (Fig. 1)

There was no significant difference between the initial plasma calcium concentration of Group 1 and Group 2. In Group 1 the plasma calcium rose from 2.65 $\pm$ 0.04 mmol/l to 2.90 $\pm$ 0.38 mmol/l following oral 1αOHD$_3$ for two weeks (p<0.01). In Group 2 after treatment with Aludrox there was a small but non-significant increase in the plasma calcium from 2.59 $\pm$ 0.04 mmol/l to 2.69 $\pm$ 0.05 mmol/l. However, giving 1αOHD$_3$ to this group resulted in a significant increase to 2.87 $\pm$ 0.10 mmol/l after two weeks therapy (p<0.05). Following two months treatment with 1αOHD$_3$ the plasma calcium in Group 1 was not significantly changed from the two week value but in Group 2 it had increased significantly to 3.12 $\pm$ 0.08 mmol/l (p<0.025), which was significantly higher than the two month value of Group 1 (p<0.025).

Plasma Phosphate   (Fig. 2)

There was no significant difference in the basal plasma phosphate in the two groups (Group 1 1.97 $\pm$ 0.12 mmol/l, Group 2 1.95 $\pm$ 0.11 mmol/l). In Group 1 the plasma phosphate rose significantly to 2.31 $\pm$ 0.10 mmol/l after two weeks therapy with 1αOHD$_3$ (p<0.005). In Group 2 the plasma phosphate fell significantly

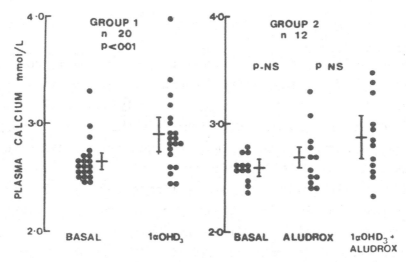

Fig. 1.   The plasma calcium before and on $1\alpha OHD_3$ in Group 1
          patients.   The plasma calcium before, on Aludrox and on $1\alpha OHD_3$
          with Aludrox in Group 2 patients.   The mean $\pm$ 2 S.E. and the
          significance between treatments are shown.

to 1.50 ± 0.14 mmol/l after treatment with Aludrox (p<0.001).
Following the addition of $1\alpha OHD_3$ therapy there was a small but non-
significant increase in the plasma phosphate to 1.59 ± 0.14 mmol/l.

After two months therapy there was no significant difference
in the plasma phosphate of either group compared with the concentration obtained two weeks after commencing $1\alpha OHD_3$ therapy.

Plasma Alkaline Phosphatase

There was no significant difference in the mean plasma alkaline phosphatase between Group 1 and 2 (11.6 and 9.6 respectively)
and there was no significant change following treatment with $1\alpha OHD_3$.

Radiocalcium Absorption

In Group 1 the mean radiocalcium absorption was 0.25 ± 0.03
(normal range 0.3 - 1.2) and only five patients had values within
the normal range.   Following therapy with $1\alpha OHD_3$ the radiocalcium
absorption increased to 0.87 ± 0.09 (p<0.001) with only one patient
remaining below the normal range in spite of receiving 4µg $1\alpha OHD_3$

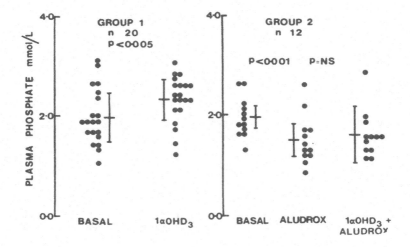

Fig. 2. The plasma phosphate before and on 1αOHD$_3$ in Group 1
patients. The plasma phosphate before, on Aludrox and on
1αOHD$_3$ with Aludrox in Group 2 patients. The mean $\pm$ 2 S.E.
and the significance between treatments are shown.

orally daily. In Group 2 there was no significant change in
radiocalcium absorption after Aludrox therapy. However, following the addition of 1αOHD$_3$ the radiocalcium absorption increased
to 0.61 $\pm$ 0.12 (p<0.005). There was no relationship in either
group between the plasma calcium or plasma phosphate concentration
and the radiocalcium absorption either before or on 1αOHD$_3$ therapy.

Radiophosphorus Absorption

Malabsorption of radiophosphorus was present in both Groups
1 and 2 (normal range 0.4 - 1.3). In Group 1 following 1αOHD$_3$
there was a small but non-significant increase in radiophosphorus
absorption. In Group 2 there was a small but non-significant increase in the radiophosphorus absorption during treatment with
Aludrox. Following the addition of 1αOHD$_3$ there was again a further but non-significant increase. When both Groups were pooled,
however, a significant rise from a basal absorption of 0.31 to
0.47 on 1αOHD$_3$ was seen (p≼0.01). Furthermore, regression

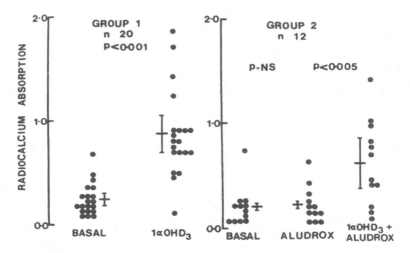

<u>Fig. 3.</u> The radiocalcium before and on $1\alpha OHD_3$ in Group 1
patients. The radiocalcium before, on Aludrox and on
$1\alpha OHD_3$ with Aludrox in Group 2 patients. The mean $\pm$ 2 S.E.
and the significance between treatments are shown.

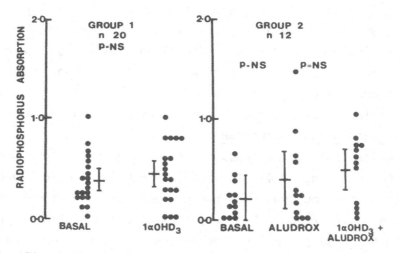

<u>FIG. 4.</u> The radiophosphorus before and on $1\alpha OHD_3$ in Group 1
patients. The radiophosphorus before, on Aludrox and on
$1\alpha OHD_3$ with Aludrox in Group 2 patients. The mean $\pm$ 2 S.E.
and the significance between treatments are shown.

analysis showed that there was a direct relationship between radiophosphorus and radiocalcium absorption both in the basal state
(r = 0.433, p<0.01) and following treatment with $1\alpha OHD_3$ (r = 0.51,
p<0.01).

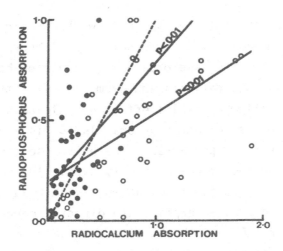

FIG. 5. The relationship between radiophosphorus and radiocalcium
        absorption in patients before (●) and after (o) $1\alpha OHD_3$ therapy.
        The line of equality is indicated by the dotted line.

Complications of Therapy

Pruritus developed or became more severe in 14 patients in
Group 1.   In three this symptom became severe enough for the patients to stop taking $1\alpha OHD_3$ therapy.   In Group 2 seven patients
complained of mild pruritus but in no patient was this severe.
In individual patients the pruritus was not related to the plasma-
calcium or plasma phosphate following therapy with $1\alpha OHD_3$.

Corneal calcification developed or increased in severity in
seven patients in Group 1, whilst this occurred in only one patient
in Group 2.

Metastatic calcification became apparent or more marked in
eight patients in Group 1.   In nine patients in this group the

appearances remained unchanged while in one patient they appeared
to improve.   In Group 2 seven patients have had an adequate radiological examination and in none of these patients has metastatic
calcification appeared or increased in severity.

DISCUSSION

This study confirms that patients with chronic renal failure
on maintenance haemodialysis have calcium malabsorption.   The
malabsorption is of the same order as that of non-haemodialysed
chronic renal failure patients and haemodialysis itself therefore
seems to have little beneficial effect on calcium absorption.
The malabsorption is corrected by oral $1\alpha OHD_3$ in a dose of 2-4µg/
day in the majority of patients.   There is also significant malabsorption of phosphorus which is only partially corrected with
$1\alpha OHD_3$ treatment.   It is clear, as we have already shown[5], that
calcium and phosphorus absorption are directly correlated both
before and after $1\alpha OHD_3$;with the effect on calcium absorption almost twice that on phosphorus absorption.   The rise in plasma
calcium and phosphate following $1\alpha OHD_3$ is likely to be largely due
to the increase in absorption although it was noticeable that some
patients, especially those in Group 2, had increases in plasma calcium and phosphate without a measureable change in absorption.
This may imply that in these cases there was an increase in bone
resorption with little effect on gut absorption.

A high plasma phosphate concentration is known to inhibit
$1,25(OH)_2D_3$ production[8], but in this study lowering the plasma
phosphate from high to high-normal levels did not seem to increase
the production of $1,25(OH)_2D_3$ as reflected by calcium absorption.
Following this same argument it seems unlikely that a high plasma
phosphate concentration plays a role in the malabsorption of renal
failure.   Lowering plasma phosphate appears to decrease the response of the gut to $1\alpha OHD_3$ (Fig. 3).   This however may only be
due firstly to the inclusion of several patients in Group 2 who
had become hypercalcaemic although their calcium absorption had
not increased into the normal range, and secondly that fewer

patients in Group 2 received a dose of $1\alpha OHD_3$ greater than $2\mu g$ as compared to Group 1.

Hypercalcaemia was a greater problem in the group of patients treated with aluminium hydroxide. This was not obvious two weeks after commencing therapy but by two months the mean plasma concentration of this group was significantly greater than those patients not given aluminium hydroxide. It is interesting to note that in Group 1 more patients required a dose greater than $2\mu g$ daily than patients in Group 2.

The complications of therapy were more marked in the patients in Group 1 in spite of the fact that two months after commencing therapy the mean plasma calcium in this Group was lower than Group 2. The main difference between these two groups was the plasma phosphate concentration which was maintained significantly lower in those patients on aluminium hydroxide than in patients of Group 1. It is likely that the lower incidence of complications is attributed to the lower phosphate concentration.

Conclusions

The conclusion of this study are:-

1. In haemodialysis patients there is malabsorption of calcium and phosphorus.

2. The malabsorption of calcium can be corrected and the malabsorption of phosphorus partially corrected by the administration of $1\alpha OHD_3$.

3. There is a direct relationship between the absorption of calcium and phosphorus which is maintained following therapy with $1\alpha OHD_3$. The action of $1\alpha OHD_3$ on calcium absorption is approximately twice that on phosphorus absorption.

4. The increase in calcium and phosphorus absorption is associated with a rise in plasma calcium and phosphate.

5. Reduction of the plasma phosphate by aluminium hydroxide does not increase calcium absorption, but does prevent the rise in plasma phosphate following $1\alpha OHD_3$ therapy.

6. Extra-skeletal calcification as manifest by corneal calcifi-
    cation, pruritis and radiological soft tissue calcification
    are more frequent in patients in whom the plasma phosphate
    is not reduced by aluminum hydroxide therapy.

ACKNOWLEDGEMENTS

Support from the Yorkshire Kidney Research Fund to Dr. G.S.
Walker is gratefully acknowledged.

REFERENCES

1. FRASER, D.R. and KODICEK, E. Unique biosynthesis by kidney
    of a biologically active vitamin D metabolite. Nature 228,
    764 - 766. 1970.

2. MAWER, E.B., BACKHOUSE, J., TAYLOR, C.M., LUMB, G.A. and
    STANBURY, S.W. Failure of formation of 1:25 dihydrocholecal-
    ciferol in chronic renal insufficiency. Lancet 1, 626 -
    628. 1973.

3. HAUSSLER, M.R. Vitamin D_3: Metabolism, mode of action and
    assay of circulating hormonal form. pp25 - 42. in: Vitamin D
    and problems related to uremic bone disease. Ed. Norman,
    A.W., Schaefer, K., Grigoleit, H.G., V. Herrath, D. and
    Ritz, E. Walter de Grayter, Berlin, New York, 1975.

4. BRICKMAN, A.S., COBURN, J.W. and NORMAN, A.W. Action of
    1,25-dihydroxycholecalciferol, a potent metabolite of vitamin
    D_3, in uremic man. New Eng. J. Med. 287, 891 - 895. 1972.

5. PEACOCK, M., NORDIN, B.E.C., GALLAGHER, J.C. and VARNAVIDES,
    C. Action of 1αHydroxy vitamin D_3 in man. pp 611 - 617.
    in: Vitamin D and problems related to uremic bone disease.
    Ed. Norman, A.W., Schaefer, K., Grigoleit, H.G., V. Herrath,
    D. and Ritz, E. Walter de Grayter, Berlin, New York, 1975.

6. MALLICK, N.P. and BERLYNE, G.M. Arterial calcification after
    vitamin D therapy in hyperphosphataemic renal failure.
    Lancet 2, 1316 - 1319. 1968.

7. SLATOPOLSKY, E. and BRICKER, N.S.   The role of phosphorus
    restriction in the prevention of secondary hyperparathyroid-
    ism in chronic renal disease.   Kidney International 4,
    141 - 145. 1973.

8. BOYLE, I.T., GRAY, R.W. and DELUCA, H.F.   Regulation by
    calcium of in vivo synthesis of 1,25 dihydroxycholecalciferol
    and 21,25 dihydroxycholecalciferol. Proc. Nat. Acad. Sci.
    2131 - 2134. 1971.

9. BULLAMORE, J.R., GALLAGHER, J.C., WILKINSON, R., NORDIN,
    B.E.C. and MARSHALL, D.H.   The effect of age on calcium
    absorption. Lancet 11, 535 - 537. 1970.

EVIDENCE FOR A RELATIONSHIP BETWEEN PLASMA IMMUNOREACTIVE

CALCITONIN AND BONE DISEASE IN CHRONIC RENAL FAILURE

J.A. Kanis[1], G. Heynen[2], M. Earnshaw[3], R.G.G.Russell[3],

C.G. Woods[3], P. Franchimont[2], S. Gaspar[2], D. Oliver[1],

and J.G.G. Ledingham[1].

The Renal Unit, Churchill Hospital[1] and the Nuffield
Orthopaedic Centre[2], Oxford and the Radioimmunoassay
Laboratory[3], University of Liege.

In experimental animals a major effect of the administration
of calcitonin (CT) is to inhibit bone resorption and this property
has led to its use in man to suppress excessive bone turnover in
Paget's disease and other disorders (1-4). On the other hand,
the role of endogenous CT in the pathogenesis of bone disease has
remained unresolved. The present studies were designed to
examine the relationships between plasma immunoreactive CT (iCT),
parathyroid hormone (iPTH) and bone disease in chronic renal
failure.

METHODS

Biochemical determinations were done on plasma samples taken
from 28 normal subjects and 80 patients with chronic renal failure
on thrice-weekly intermittent haemodialysis (Kiil Multipoint,
15-24h/wk). Transiliac bone biopsies were also taken from 53 of
the patients for quantitative histology of cancellous bone using
methods described previously (5). Fifty-three of the patients
were treated at the Oxford Renal Unit (dialysate calcium 1.53
mmol/1) and the rest at Liege (dialysate calcium 1.82 - 1.95 mmol/
1), but data from the two centres did not differ. None of the
patients had received barbiturates, anticonvulsants, vitamin D,
its analogues or metabolites for at least 1 year.

With the exception of the hormone assays, biochemical
measurements were done on the Vicker's autoanalyser.   The assay
for iCT measures both small CT (corresponding to the elution
profile of synthetic human CT on Sephadex G-50 column chromatography) and big CT (6-8).   Plasma iPTH was measured using an
antibody (Wellcome Laboratories, London AS 211/32) reported as
having mainly N-terminal specificity (8, 9), though others (10)
have shown it to be equally reactive to the N- and C- terminal
portions of the PTH molecule.

RESULTS

I   Relationship between Plasma iPTH and iCT

The distribution of levels of both hormones taken just before
a dialysis treatment was logarithmic (Fig.1).   Levels of plasma
iPTH and iCT were measured in 10 patients at intervals of 4 to 11
months.   The log-transformed values from each individual patient
showed a high degree of consistency for both iPTH (mean difference
+0.6;   range -3.7 to +4.3% of initial value) and iCT (-1.4;   -16.6
to +11.5%).   There was a negative correlation between plasma iPTH
and iCT in 52 dialysed patients ($r = -0.41$; $P < 0.005$).   In
contrast there was a positive correlation between plasma iPTH and
iCT in 28 normal subjects ($r = +0.72$; $P < 0.001$, Fig.1).

II   Inter-relationships of Plasma iPTH, iCT and
Alkaline Phosphatase (AP)

In the dialysed patients plasma AP correlated positively with
levels of iPTH ($r = +0.72$; $P < 0.001$) and negatively with plasma
iCT ($r = -0.40$; $P < 0.005$).   On the basis of a bimodal distribution of plasma AP, patients were divided into two groups
according to their activity of AP ('high AP group';   'low AP
group').

There was no difference in plasma calcium or phosphate
between the two groups though the relationships of iPTH with iCT
differed markedly (Fig.1).   In the 'low AP group' the correlation
of iPTH with iCT was positive ($r = +0.40$; $P < 0.05$) and the
regression lines seen in this group and normal subjects did not
differ.   A common regression with 95% confidence limits was
calculated (Fig.1).

In the 'high AP group' the relationship of iPTH with iCT
differed in two important respects from the 'low AP group' and
normal subjects.   This ('high AP') group had significantly lower

plasma levels of iCT (2.49 ± SEM 0.10 and 3.11 ± 0.08 $\log_{10}$ ng/l
respectively; t = 4.93, P< 0.001) and higher levels of iPTH
(3.62 ± 0.10 and 2.99 ± 0.007 $\log_{10}$ ng/l respectively; t = 5.17,
P< 0.001), than the 'low AP group'. Secondly, there was a negative correlation between plasma iPTH and iCT (r = 0.46; P< 0.02,
Fig.1) in contrast to the direct relationship seen in the other
groups. The use of a ratio of iPTH over iCT gave a better
discrimination of patients with normal and increased AP than the
use of iPTH or iCT alone (t = 5.58; P< 0.001).

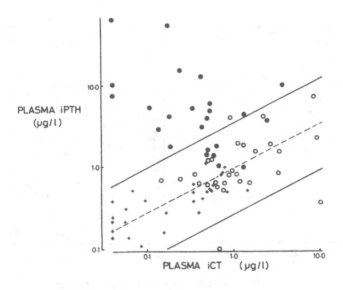

Fig. 1

The relationships between immunoreactive parathyroid hormone
(iPTH) and calcitonin (iCT) in normal subjects (+) and in
dialysed patients with normal (0) and increased (●) activities of
plasma alkaline phosphatase. Hormone concentrations are plotted
on logarithmic scales. The lines show the common regression
(dashed) with 95% confidence limits (continuous) of values from
normal subjects and those patients with chronic renal failure
with normal levels of plasma alkaline phosphatase.

III Relationship of Bone Histology with Plasma iCT and iPTH

Significant positive correlations were found between plasma iPTH (and plasma AP) and osteoblastic activity, resorbing trabecular surface, calcification front, and marrow fibrosis, whereas plasma iCT was negatively correlated with these measurements.   Thus, as was seen with plasma AP, patients with increased osteoblastic activity and fibrosis of bone had higher iPTH and lower iCT levels than patients with lower bone turnover.   The presence or absence of osteomalacia was not associated with any difference in the levels of these hormones.   Partial correlation analysis showed that the correlations of osteoblastic activity with plasma iPTH and iCT were independent of each other (Fig.2) and that the apparent correlation of iPTH with iCT was dependent upon osteoblastic activity.

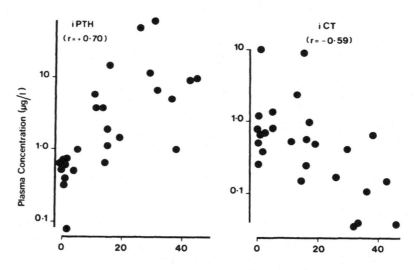

Fig. 2

The correlations between osteoblastic activity (osteoblastic surface X 100/total trabecular surface) with (a) plasma immunoreactive parathyroid hormone (iPTH) (P< 0.001) (b) plasma immunoreactive calcitonin (iCT) (P< 0.005).   Hormone concentrations are plotted on a logarithmic scale.   The correlation coefficients and significance levels are based on log transformed values.   The partial correlations between osteoblastic activity and hormone concentrations were;   iPTH = +0.56 (P< 0.01), iCT = -0.40 (P< 0.05).

IV Effects of Bilateral Nephrectomy

Plasma AP fell rapidly after nephrectomy in 10 patients whose initial plasma AP were above normal (10 patients). In contrast plasma AP in patients whose initial activity was normal showed no change or small increases (Fig.3). Comparable studies were done in a control group of 17 dialysed but non-nephrectomised patients undergoing arterial shunt surgery who showed no post-operative change in plasma AP irrespective of their initial plasma AP.

Histological measurements from paired biopsies were taken before and from 0.5 to 12 months after nephrectomy in 11 patients. The operation was associated with a decrease in resorbing and active osteoblastic surfaces, in the calcification front, and in bone fibrosis when measurements taken within 4 months of nephrectomy were compared with pre-operative values (Fig.4). Thereafter the differences between pre- and post-operative biopsies decreased and where increases in bone turnover were found, as judged by these histological indices, plasma AP also rose.

Measurements of iPTH and iCT in 7 patients before and 5 - 9 days after nephrectomy showed no significant change in iPTH but

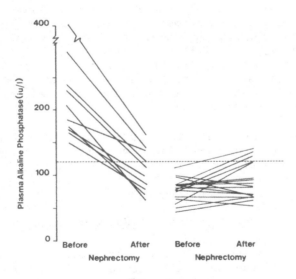

Fig. 3

Plasma alkaline phosphatase before and 2 months after bilateral nephrectomy in patients with increased (left) and normal (right) pre-operative activities of AP. The horizontal line represents the upper limit of normal.

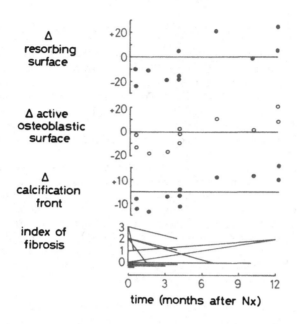

Fig. 4

The difference in histological measurements from iliac bone biopsies taken before and after nephrectomy.   Changes in the resorbing surface (% total trabecular surface), active osteoblastic surface (% osteoid surface), and calcification front (% osteoid surface; toluidine blue) are plotted against the time interval after nephrectomy that the second bone biopsy was taken.   Bone fibrosis (semiquantitative) is shown as lines connecting values observed before and after nephrectomy.

plasma iCT increased markedly (P < 0.02;   Fig.5).   Though sub-sequent levels of iCT (unpaired data) were still increased they did not differ significantly from pre-operative values.

DISCUSSION

Biological Relevance of Hormone Assays

Interpretation of the results of the radioimmunoassays is difficult because of the uncertain nature of the immunoreactive fragments.   However, the assay for iPTH used in this study, though probably N-terminal selective, can distinguish normal from hyper-parathyroid serum (9) and in patients with primary hyperparathyroid-ism plasma levels are in direct proportion to weight of parathyroid

tissue (8).   Similarly plasma levels of iCT, using the present
assay, are related to other biological measurements such as plasma
phosphate (in normal subjects (8) but not in patients with chronic
renal failure), and change appropriately with calcium or EDTA
infusion and pentagastrin injection (8).   In the study described
here striking correlations of both hormones were found with histological and indirect estimates of bone turnover.   These data
suggest that both radioimmunoassays are measuring fragments of
biological relevance, even though the fragments may not themselves
possess biological activity.

Calcitonin and Bone Disease

     In patients with chronic renal failure high plasma levels of
iPTH and iCT could both be found.   In normal subjects and in
dialysed patients without renal bone disease plasma levels of iPTH
and iCT were directly proportional to each other.   The increased
plasma iCT associated with high levels of iPTH might therefore
serve to protect skeletal tissue from excessive resorption.
There are several observations in support of this possibility.

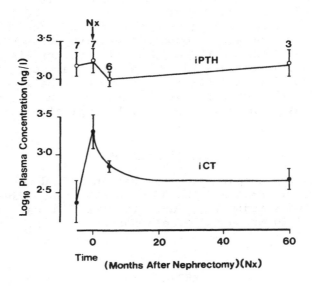

Fig. 5

Mean plasma levels of iPTH and iCT ($\pm$ SEM) before and at intervals
after nephrectomy (N_x).   The numbers refer to the number of
observations at each time.

Patients with renal bone disease, judged by histological methods or by plasma AP, characteristically had higher plasma levels of iPTH and lower levels of iCT than the other patients or normal subjects (Fig.1 and 2).   Secondly the negative correlation between plasma iCT and osteoblastic activity (Fig.2) was not spurious in the sense that partial correlation analysis confirmed that the correlation was independent of iPTH and indeed that plasma iCT contributed to the significance of the relationship of iPTH with osteoblastic activity.   Thirdly, a 70 fold range of plasma iPTH and a 40 fold range of iCT were found in patients with normal bone turnover.   Thus observations that plasma concentrations of iPTH do not accurately reflect histological findings (11) may be due in part to a failure to account for the secretion of CT.   In support of this, the use of an iPTH/iCT ratio allowed a better discrimination of patients with and without bone disease than did the measurement of iPTH or iCT alone.   Finally, the decreased bone turnover seen immediately after nephrectomy (Fig.3) was associated with increases in plasma iCT without significant changes in plasma iPTH.

General Conclusions

These results suggest that endogenous calcitonin may be an important regulator of osteoblastic function and hence bone turnover in chronic renal failure.   Low levels of endogenous CT may be one reason for increased bone turnover in patients with chronic renal failure.   Although there is still considerable debate about the meaning of immunoassays for PTH and CT, particularly with regard to the biological activity of immunologically reactive materials (12), the correlations demonstrated in this study suggest that these assays can provide data of biological relevance.

Acknowledgements

This work was supported by the National Fund for Research into Crippling Diseases and the Belgian FRSM (No. 20305).   J.A.K. is in receipt of a Medical Research Council Clinical Fellowship. We are grateful to Mr. G. MacDonald for his help with the statistics.

REFERENCES

1. Queener, S.F., and Bell, J.H.:   Calcitonin; A general survey. Metabolism. 24:555, 1975.

2. Shai, F., Baker, R.K., and Wallach, S.: The clinical and
    metabolic effects of porcine calcitonin on Paget's disease of
    bone. J. Clin. Invest. 50:1927, 1971.

3. Kanis, J.A., Horn, D.B., Scott, R.D.M., and Strong, J.A.:
    Treatment of Paget's disease of bone with synthetic salmon
    calcitonin. Brit. Med. J. 3:727, 1974.

4. Deftos, L.J., and Neer, R.: Medical management of the
    hypercalcaemia of malignancy. Ann. Rev. Med. 25:322, 1974.

5. Heynen, G., Kanis, J.A., Earnshaw, M., Russell, R.G.G., and
    Woods, C.G.: Plasma immunoreactive calcitonin and bone
    disease in patients on haemodialysis. Proc. Europ. Dial.
    Transpl. Ass. 13:000, 1977.

6. Heynen, G., Franchimont, P.: Human calcitonin radioimmuno-
    assay in normal and pathological conditions. Europ. J. Clin.
    Invest. 4:213, 1974.

7. Heynen, G., Hendrick, J.C., and Franchimont, P.: Hetero-
    geneity of calcitonin in human serum. Vitamin D and problems
    related to uraemic bone disease. Eds. Norman, A.W.,
    Schaefer, K., Grigoleit, H.G., Herrath, D.V., and Ritz, E.
    p. 475. de Gruyter, Berlin, 1975.

8. Franchimont, P., and Heynen, G.: Parathormone and calcitonin
    radioimmunoassay in various medical and osteoarticular dis-
    orders. Masson Inc. New York, 1976.

9. Woo, J., and Singer, F.R.: Radioimmunoassay for human para-
    thyroid hormone. Clin. Chim. Acta, 54:161, 1974.

10. Barling, P.M., Hendy, G.N., Evans, M.C., and O'Riordan,
    J.L.H.: Region - specific immunoassays for parathyroid
    hormone. Endocrinol. 66:307, 1975.

11. Ritz, E., Mehls, O., Malluche, H., Krempien, B., Schmidt-
    Gayk, H., Heimberg, H.: Unanswered problems in uraemic bone
    disease. Vitamin D and problems related to uraemic bone
    disease. Eds. Norman, A.W., Schaefer, K., Grigoleit, H.G.,
    Herrath, D.V., Ritz, E., p 497. de Gruyter, Berlin. 1975.

12. Tashjian, A.H., Wolfe, H.J., Voekel, E.F.: Human calcitonin.
    Amer. J. Med., 56:840, 1974.

HYPOPHOSPHATAEMIA AND OSTEOMALACIA IN HAEMODIALYSIS PATIENTS NOT TAKING PHOSPHATE BINDERS

K. Y. Ahmed, Z. Varghese, E. A. Meinhard, R. A. Baillod
R. K. Skinner, M. R. Wills and J. F. Moorhead.

Departments of Nephrology and Chemical Pathology,
Royal Free Hospital, London, N.W.3.

The association of hypophosphataemia with osteomalacia in dialysis patients has been previously described in association with the administration of oral phosphate binders[1]. Hypophosphataemia unassociated with the use of oral phosphate binders is a rare finding in patients on regular haemodialysis. Bishop et al[2] reported that the dialysis process itself was associated with a negative phosphate balance, although Verberckmoes et al[3] reported a positive balance in 6 patients on haemodialysis. In the present study we report the development of persistent hypophosphataemia and osteomalacia in four long-term haemodialyis patients, despite the withdrawal of Aludrox for periods of two years or more. Biochemical, radiological and histological studies were undertaken to reveal the factors responsible for the persistence of the hypophosphataemia. The effect of treatment with Dihydrotachysterol (DHT), is evaluated and the possible contribution of the hypophosphataemia to the development of osteomalacia in haemodialysis patients is discussed.

PATIENTS AND METHODS

The 4 patients studied were 3 males and 1 female. Their ages ranged from 27 to 42 years. They had been on maintenance haemodialysis treatment for periods of $3\frac{1}{2}$ to 7 years, using a Kiil dialyser for 24 to 30 hours per week. The dialysate calcium concentration was 7 to 7.5mg/100ml. Initially, moderate doses of aluminium hydroxide had been required (2 to 3g/day) to reduce the raised plasma inorganic phosphate concentration, but it was withdrawn when their plasma phosphate levels fell below 3mg/100ml. Their diet contained an average of 2,000 calories, 46g protein, 400mg of calcium and 650mg of phosphate without added vitamin D. Biochemical investigations included regular estimations of plasma calcium, phosphate, proteins, alkaline phosphatase activity, hydroxyproline[4] and serum 25-hydroxycholecalciferol[5]. Serum i-PTH was measured using Wellcome antibodies raised in Guinea Pigs against bovine PTH (AS 211/32) and human PTH reference standard provided by the MRC. Blood samples were collected 36 to 48 hours after dialysis without haemostasis and after overnight fasting.

Intestinal phosphate absorption was measured using the method of Condon et al[6]. Fasting patients were given 17.4g of Disodium hydrogen phosphate B.P.(1.5g of elemental phosphorus) dissolved in 200ml of water by mouth in 2 minutes. Blood samples were collected before and 30, 60, 90, 150, 210 and 270 minutes after giving the oral phosphate. The patients were not allowed to eat or drink until the end of the test. Results from 12 control subjects provided data for a normal range of phosphate absorption profiles in which the rise above baseline phosphate value in each sample was plotted against time (Fig 1.) The phosphate absorption profile for each patient was then compared with the composite control profile. The area under the curve represents an index of intestinal phosphate absorption.

Intestinal calcium absorption was measured using oral ^{47}Ca[7]. Radiological skeletal surveys were done at six monthly intervals for evidence of fractures, Looser's zones, sub-periosteal erosions and ectopic calcification. An iliac crest bone biopsy was taken from all patients before starting DHT therapy. The specimens were processed according to the method of Tripp and MacKay[8] and counterstained with Ehrlich's haematoxylin. Quantitative histological data was obtained for the tissue volume proportion (Vv%) of trabecular osteoid, mineralised bone, total bone and the percentage of trabecular surface (Sv%), covered by osteoblasts and osteoclasts using a computerised morphometric technique[9].

After completing the baseline investigations the patients began a course of DHT in an oral dose of 0.25mg daily. Regular biochemical monitoring continued and absorption studies were repeated after 2 months on all patients. The 2 patients who did not show significant improvement were then given 0.5mg and 0.75mg DHT for a further 2 months before again repeating the absorption studies.

RESULTS

Before starting DHT therapy all patients had bone pains,

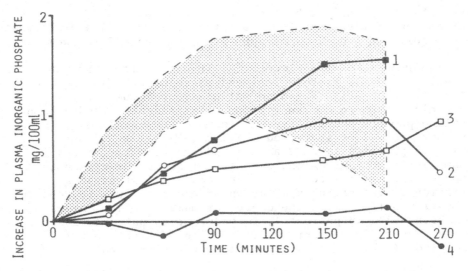

Figure 1.   Phosphate absorption profile before treatment with D.H.T.

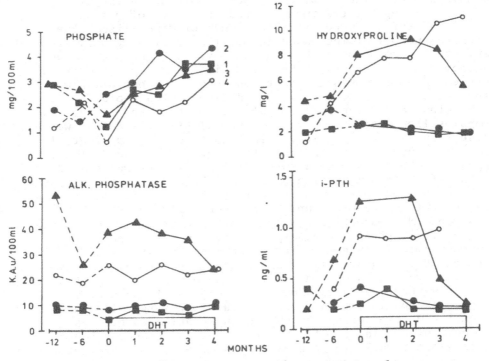

Figure 2.   Pre-treatment and treatment values.

particularly in their ribs and feet. Two complained of muscle
weakness and fatigue and the one with the lowest plasma phosphate
values suffered from loss of appetite and generalised weakness.

The results of the biochemical investigations are shown
in Table I and the histological and radiological findings in
Table II. All patients had normal plasma calcium and low
inorganic phosphate concentrations. In patients 3 and 4 both
alkaline phosphate activity and plasma hydroxyproline
concentrations were increased. Serum i-PTH (Fig 2.) was
normal in patients 1 and 2 and raised in patients 3 and 4.
Serum 25-HCC concentrations were either normal or raised when
compared with normal control values adjusted for seasonal
variations. Intestinal absorption of phosphate was reduced in
all patients (Fig 1.). The degree of malabsorption varied
from being mild in patient 1, to moderate in patients 2 and 3
and was severe in patient 4. The degree of impairment in ^{47}Ca
absorption (Table I) paralleled that of the phosphate.

During the 2 years of hypophosphataemia multiple rib
fractures and Looser's zones were noticed in patients 1, 2 and
3, while patient 4 had very early subperiosteal erosions in
the phalanges (Table II). No ectopic calcification was noted
in any patient. The iliac crest bone biopsies taken just
before starting DHT treatment showed an excess of osteoid
in all patients, but not at the expense of mineralized bone
which was normal or increased in all (Table II, Fig 3.). In
patient 3 osteoid volume had doubled over a 2 year period when
another previous biopsy, taken from him 2 years previously, was
reassessed. Increasingly severe phosphate malabsorption was
associated with increasingly marked excess of osteoid.
Trabecular coarsening and irregularity were marked in the
biopsies from patients 3 and 4. Osteoclastic resorption was
present in all the biopsies, slight in those from patients 1
and 2, but more marked in those from patients 3 and 4 (Table II,
Fig 3.). When phosphate absorption studies were repeated 2
months after treatment with 0.25mg DHT (Fig 4.), patients 1 and
2 showed marked improvement. Patients 3 and 4 did not show any
significant improvement and we're given daily doses of 0.5 and
0.75mg of DHT respectively. Two months later a marked improvement in their phosphate absorption studies was found (Fig 4.).
The biochemical changes during 4 months of treatment are
summarised in Fig 2. Plasma phosphate levels rose steadily
to normal values in all patients by the end of the fourth month.
Similarly there was a marked improvement in all parameters
studied except in patient 4 whose plasma hydroxyproline and
serum i-PTH rose during the DHT administration. There was
evidence of healing of all the fractures and Looser's zones.
There was a remarkable clinical improvement in all patients,
bone pain decreased and general weakness and appetite improved.

TABLE I

Results of Biochemical and ^{47}Ca Absorption Studies on Hypophosphataemic Dialysis
Patients Before Treatment with DHT

Patient No.	PLASMA				SERUM	^{47}Ca ABSORPTION STUDIES % OF ORAL DOSE PER LITRE OF PLASMA AT 3 HRS
	Calcium (mg/100ml)	Inorganic Phosphate (mg/100ml)	Alkaline Phosphatase KAu/100ml	Hydroxyproline (mg/l)	25-Hydroxychole-calciferol ng/ml	
1	10.2	1.2	4	2.5	58.7	0.83
2	10.4	2.5	8	2.5	50.6	0.44
3	9.6	1.7	39	8.1	82.3	0.34
4	10.4	0.6	26	6.7	30.8	0.25
NORMAL RANGE	9.7 ± 0.7	3.6 ± 0.9	3 - 13	1.6 ± 1.2	26.8 ± 18.4	0.6 - 1.8

TABLE II

| Pt. No. | Radiology | | | | Quantitative Histology on Iliac Crest Bone Biopsy | | | | |
| | Fractures Looser's zones | Sub-periosteal Erosions | Ectopic Calcif | | Vv% | | | Sv% | |
					Osteoid	Mineralised	Total Bone	Blasts	Clasts
1	Ribs & L Foot	None	None		2.3	24.8	27.1	2	2
2	Ribs	None	None		5.1	23.8	24.9	4	2
3	Ribs	None	None		17.8	36.8	54.6	12	6
4	None	Early in Both Hands	None		20.7	27.4	48.1	10	3
Normal Values					Up to 0.5	$20 \overset{+}{-} 4$	$20.5 \overset{+}{-} 4$	0.5	0.5

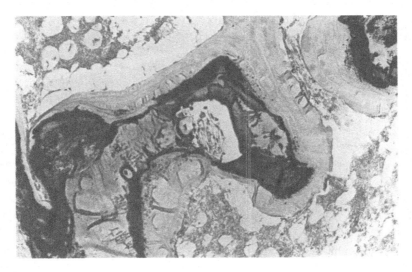

Fig 3. Bone Biopsy - Trabecular bone, in patient 4, shows
marked osteoid excess, with some osteoclastic
resorption (T & M, x 100)

DISCUSSION

Although in patients with renal osteodystrophy there is
malabsorption of both calcium and phosphate[10], a decrease in
the amount of phosphate available for bone mineral formation
has not generally been considered to be a crucial factor in
the development of osteomalacia in haemodialysis patients.
Hypophosphataemic osteomalacia in these patients has been
described when excessive oral phosphate binders were ingested.
In the patients described here the plasma inorganic phosphate
continued to fall for 2 years despite the withdrawal of
Aludrox. All these patients had normal pre-dialysis plasma
calcium and normal or raised levels of 25-HCC. It seems
likely, therefore, that the osteomalacia resulted from phosphate
depletion and hypophosphataemia. Persistence of hypophosphataemia in these patients was due to combination of low dietary
phosphate, phosphate malabsorption and phosphate loss on
dialysis. A normal diet contains an average 1,000 to 1,200/mg
of phosphate per day. The protein restricted diet of patients
with chronic renal failure contains an average of only 600mg
per day. Phosphate loss during dialysis can be substantial
and leads to a negative phosphate balance as shown by Bishop

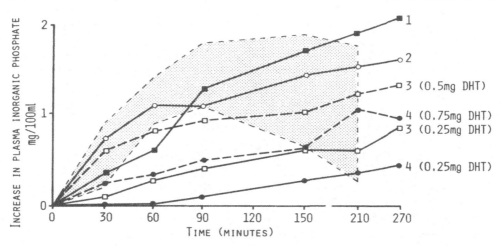

Figure 4.   Phosphate absorption profile after treatment with D.H.T.

et al[2].   However, their patients had normal or high pre-
dialysis plasma phosphate values during the period of the
study.   Our patients' dialysis regime was similar to theirs
and it is very likely that the continuous use of phosphate
free dialysate was associated with a similar loss of phosphate.
Negative phosphate balance and phosphate malabsorption has
been previously demonstrated in undialized chronic renal
failure patients before receiving vitamin D supplements[10].
Phosphate malabsorption has been shown in the patients studied
here, using a simple oral sodium phosphate loading technique.
This test appears to be valuable in the follow-up of these
patients.

The malabsorption of the phosphate and calcium in these
patients with normal levels of 25-hydroxycholecalciferol
suggests that a more active metabolite of vitamin D is required
for adequate absorption.   The vitamin D analogue, dihydrotachysterol (DHT) has been shown to cause direct stimulation of
phosphate transport in the jejunum[11] and an increase in bone
mineralization when given to patients with chronic renal
failure[10].   It has also been suggested that the rotation of its
A ring 180° places the 3β-hydroxyl function in a position
comparable to the 1-hydroxylation by the kidney[12].   The DHT dosage
used in this study (up to 0.75mg) appeared to be effective
in correcting both the calcium and phosphate malabsorption.   It
has to be stressed however that doses used for each patient
should be adjusted in order to avoid inadequate or excessive
dosages.

This study suggests the possible importance of hypophosphataemia in development of osteomalacia in haemodialysis patients. It also shows that hypophosphataemia and phosphate depletion can result not only from the use of oral phosphate binders but also from the combination of intestinal phosphate malabsorption and loss during dialysis. It is the long term effect of these two factors that probably maintains patients in negative phosphate balance. Phosphate depletion can be a serious problem in the long term haemodialysis patient, therefore the use of dihydrotachysterol and the addition of phosphate containing salts to dialysate should be considered for the future management of similar patients.

REFERENCES

1. Baker, L.R.I., Ackrill, P. et al: Iatrogenic osteomalacia and myopathy due to phosphate depletion. Br. Med. J. 3: 150-152, 1974.

2. Bishop, M.C., Ledingham, J.G.G., and Oliver, D.O.: Phosphate deficiency in haemodialysed patients, Proc. Europ. Dial. Transpl. Assoc. 8:106-114, 1971, Pitman Medical, London.

3. Verberckmoes, R., Hombroek, A.M. et al: Calcium, magnesium and phosphate balance studies in patients under maintenance haemodialysis. Proc. Europ. Dial. Transpl. Assoc. 6:269, 1969, Pitman Medical, London.

4. Varghese, Z., Moorhead, J.F. et al., "Plasma hydroxyproline in renal osteodystrophy" Proc. Europ. Dial. Transpl. Assoc. 10:187, 1973, Pitman Medical, London.

5. Haddad, J.G., Chyu, K.J.: Competitive protein binding radio assay for 25-hydroxycholecalciferol. J. Clin. Endocrinol. Metab. 33:992, 1971.

6. Condon, J.R., Nassim, J.R., and Rutter, A.: Defective intest. phosphate absorption in familial and non-familial hypophosphataemia. Br. Med. J. 3:138-141, 1970.

7. Agnew, J.E., Kehayoglou, A.K., and Holdsworth, C.D.: Comparison of three isotopic methods for the study of calcium absorption. Gut 10:590-597, 1969.

8. Tripp, E.J., and MacKay, E.H.: Silver staining of bone prior to decalcification for quantitative determination of osteoid in sections. Stain Technol. 47:129-136, 1972.

9. Meinhard, E.A., Wadbrook, D.S. et al: Computer card morphometry in uraemic bone disease. In "Vitamin D and Problems Related to Uraemic Bone Disease". Proc. of 2nd Workshop on Vit. D, Wiesbaden, 547-552, Walter de Gruyter, Berlin, 1974.

10. Stanbury, S.W., and Lumb, G.A.: Metabolic studies of renal osteodystrophy. Medicine 41:1-31, 1962.

11. Harrison, H.E., Harrison, H.C., and Lifshitz, F.: Inter-relation of vitamin D and parathyroid hormone. The response of vitamin D depleted and thyroparathyroid ectomised rats to ergocalciferol and dihydrotachysterol. In "Parathyroid hormone and thyrocalcitonin (Calcitonin) R. V. Talmage and L. F. Belanger, Eds. Amsterdam, Excerpta Medica, Page 455-463, 1968.

12. Hollick, R.B., and Deluca, H.F.: Metabolites of dihydrotachy-sterol in target tissues. J. Biol. Chem. 247:91-97, 1972.

EFFECTS OF 25-HYDROXYCHOLECALCIFEROL ON CALCIUM METABOLISM IN CHRONIC RENAL FAILURE[*]

J.M. Letteri, L.M. Kleinman, K.N. Ellis, R. Caselnova,
M. Akhtar, and S.H. Cohn.
Department of Medicine, Nassau County Medical Center,
East Meadow, NY, USA, and Brookhaven National Laboratories,
Upton, NY, USA

Abnormalities of vitamin D metabolism, secondary hyperparathyroidism, acidosis and other less well defined factors are postulated to be important factors in the genesis of altered calcium (Ca) metabolism of chronic renal failure (CRF) and renal osteodystrophy. This study quantitatively characterizes a number of parameters of Ca metabolism in patients with CRF before and after oral administration of pharmacologic quantities of 25-hydroxycholecalciferol (25-OHD$_3$). A previously formulated compartmental model is used to quantitate certain parameters of Ca metabolism. The model consists of a number of compartments of variable size and intercompartmental transfer rates (1). The experimental data required for this analysis were obtained from a ^{47}Ca tracer kinetic study, a Ca balance study, and the retention of ^{47}Ca in the body as measured by whole body counting techniques. Total body (TB) Ca and phosphorus (P) stores were measured by neutron activation analysis (NAA) and compared to values obtained in normal subjects by methods previously described by this laboratory (2).

The effects of 25-OHD$_3$ on Ca metabolism in patients with CRF were assessed from the changes in ^{47}Ca kinetics, Ca balance, and the whole body stores of Ca and P. In addition, plasma concentrations of 25-OHD$_3$ and immunoreactive parathyroid hormone (PTH) were assayed serially to determine the relationship between the compartmental ^{47}Ca kinetic analysis and some of the endocrine factors which contribute to the altered Ca metabolism in CRF.

[*]Supported by the United States Energy Research and Development Agency and the Kidney Foundation of New York, Inc.

METHODS

Patients

Eight patients, ranging in age from 17 to 54 years, with modest to severe CRF, plasma creatinine ranging from 1.6 mg/100 ml to 13.7 mg/100 ml, not requiring peritoneal or hemodialysis were studied. All patients were prescribed aluminum hydroxide gels and $CaCO_3$ prior to the study but the degree of adherence to this therapy was variable. Skeletal radiographic examination revealed renal osteodystrophy in all patients. Biochemical composition of the plasma of the patients is shown in Table I.

Experimental Design

Two groups of patients were studied. Group I comprised six patients who received 160 µg/day of 25-OHD_3 for six weeks. Group II comprised two patients who received 100 µg daily for two weeks (3) and then a mean daily intake of 40 µg of 25-OHD_3 for a total of six months. During the period of administration of 25-OHD_3 all patients received aluminum hydroxide gels to control plasma P concentration. Dietary Ca and P intake averaged 500 mg/day and 800 mg/day respectively for Group I, and 700 mg/day and 800 mg/day respectively for Group II.

^{47}Ca Kinetic and Compartmental Analysis

After 7 - 10 days of equilibration to a constant diet on a metabolic ward, ^{47}Ca (20 µCi , specific activity 140 mCi/gm) was administered I.V. to each patient. The plasma activity was measured at 1 hour, 6 hours, and thereafter every 24 hours for a period of 10 days. The whole body level of ^{47}Ca was measured daily with the Brookhaven whole body counter. Stool and urine were collected over 24 hours and analyzed for stable and ^{47}Ca.

Calcium Balance

In 6 of the 8 patients Ca balance was measured on the metabolic research ward of the Brookhaven National Laboratory Hospital. The methods were essentially those outlined by Refeinstein, Albright and Wells (4). Diet and feces were ashed in a muffle furnace before Ca analysis. Daily lots of stool were analyzed and average daily fecal Ca excretion calculated. Urine and serum were analyzed directly. Fecal and dietary Ca was determined by atomic absorption spectrometry; urine and plasma Ca, P, urea nitrogen (BUN), creatinine (Cr) and bicarbonate (HCO_3) were measured with an auto analyzer. Plasma 25 OHD_3 was measured by a competitive protein binding assay (5,6,7). Plasma immunoreactive parathyroid

hormone (PTH) was measured by radioimmunoassay (8,9). Total body
levels of Ca and P were measured by NAA.

   After the conclusion of the initial control study the patients
were maintained on the above described Ca and P diet and aluminum
hydroxide gels. 25-OHD$_3$ was then administered for 6 weeks to
patients in Group I, and for 6 months to patients in Group II at a
dose of 160 μg/day and 40 μg/day respectively. Ca balance, ^{47}Ca
kinetics, and whole body stores of Ca and P were then remeasured.

   The details of the compartmental analysis of the tracer
kinetics data have been previously presented (1). The compartmental model has been shown to fit ^{47}Ca tracer kinetic data studies
in man. The Berman simulation analysis and modelling (SAAM) program was used to adjust the parameters of the above mathematical
model to the data (10). The program by an iterative system obtained the best coefficient for a given set of differential equations
describing the model. The set of coefficients is then used to
determine the desired parameters of the system, the size of the
compartments and the transfer rates between them. The flow rates
(ρs) are then calculated from the product of the transfer rate
and the compartment size.

RESULTS

Effects of 25-OHD$_3$ on the

Biochemical Composition of Plasma in Renal Failure

   Prior to 25-OHD$_3$ administration plasma Ca, P and total
alkaline phosphatase (total A.P.) averaged 9.1 $\pm$ 0.4 mg/100 ml,
4.9 $\pm$ 0.6 mg/100 ml and 14 $\pm$ 4 I.U./liter respectively for Group I,
and 9.5 mg/100 ml, 3.8 mg/100 ml and 23 I.U./liter respectively for
Group II (Table I). Although no significant difference in mean
plasma Ca and P concentrations were noted, plasma Ca increased in
4 patients more than 0.5 mg/100 ml following 25-OHD$_3$ administration.
No change in total A.P. was noted after 25-OHD$_3$ therapy in either
group. Mean plasma 25-OHD$_3$ increased (P < 0.0025) following 25-OHD$_3$
administration, from 35 $\pm$ 9 ng/ml to 128 $\pm$ 9 ng/ml. A lower
than normal 25-OHD$_3$ plasma level was noted in only one patient prior
to 25-OHD$_3$ administration (11,12). Immunoreactive PTH was elevated
(13) in all but one patient in Group I (normal value 305 $\pm$ 119
picograms/ml) and was elevated in all patients in Group II (normal
value < 40 μleq/ml) (Table I). In Group I, after 25-OHD$_3$ administration, PTH decreased in three patients and increased in one
patient with a mean decrease of 150 picograms/ml. In Group II, PTH
increased in one patient and decreased in the other patient following 25-OHD$_3$ (Table I).

TABLE I

Biochemical Characteristics of Patients Before and After 25-Hydroxycholecalciferol Administration

	Ca**	Phos	Total A.P.	$25\ OHD_3^*$	PTH*
			PLASMA		
	------ mg/100 ml ------		IU/liter	nanograms/ml	picograms/ml
Group I					
Mean C	9.1 (0.4)	4.9 (0.6)	14.3 (3.6)	37.1 (11.5)	2500
Mean X	9.8 (0.2)	4.7 (0.5)	14.1 (5.6)	96.5 (4.6)	2350 (819)
N = 6				$P < 0.0005$	
Group II					μleq/ml
Mean C	9.5	3.8	23	29	747
Mean X	9.9	4.2	22	209	1152
N = 2					

* = determinations kindly done by Dr. S. Arnaud at the Mayo Clinic and Dr. M. Roginsky at the Nassau County Medical Center.   C = before administration of 25 OHD$_3$.   X = following administration of 25 OHD$_3$. **See text for description of terms.

Effect of 25-OHD$_3$ on Ca^{47} Kinetics

The mean values of the compartment size and transfer rates relative to 1000 g of TB Ca before and after 25-OHD$_3$ administration for both groups are shown in Table II. Prior to 25-OHD$_3$ administration the size of compartment 2, and the accretion and exchange rates were increased (P $<$ 0.05) when compared to predicted normal values. The size of compartment 2 and the accretion rates were variable but were related to TB Ca. In patients with normal or slightly decreased TB Ca values, accretion rate and compartment 2 were essentially normal. In patients with low TB Ca stores, compartment 2 and accretion were markedly elevated. In Group I patients following 25-OHD$_3$ administration, accretion and resorption increased with a marked increase in the accretion/resorption ratio from 1.05 to 2.18. In Group II however, accretion remained unchanged or decreased despite an increasing or unchanged resorption rate. Short term administration of 25-OHD$_3$ effects an increase in the accretion/resorption ratio; in patients treated with a longer course of 25-OHD$_3$ a decreased accretion/resorption ratio was noted.

Endogenous fecal Ca decreased in all patients from 0.135 $\pm$ 0.020 g/day/Kg TB Ca to 0.081 $\pm$ 0.017 g/day/Kg TB Ca after 25-OHD$_3$ administration (P $<$ 0.05). No consistent change in compartment 1 and 2 was observed.

Effects of 25-OHD$_3$ on Ca Balance

Prior to 25-OHD$_3$, calcium balance was positive in two patients (+ 114 mg/day and + 222 mg/day), essentially zero in 2 others (+ 25 mg/day and + 29 mg/day) and markedly negative in two patients (- 189, and - 143 mg/day) (Table III). During 6 weeks of 25-OHD$_3$ administration (Group I), Ca balance became positive in all patients. In patients receiving the drug for 6 months however (Group II), Ca balance remained negative or decreased from + 222 to + 102 mg/day. Absorption of Ca across the G.I. tract increased significantly in Group I. In Group II no significant change occured in Ca absorption following ingestion of 25-OHD$_3$. Urinary Ca excretion increased in Group I from 44 $\pm$ 14 mg/day to 81 $\pm$ 23 mg/day.

Effect of 25-OHD$_3$ on TB Ca and TB P

Table IV depicts the TB Ca and TB P measurements obtained by NAA and whole body counting. Prior to administration of 25-OHD$_3$ the TB P/Ca was increased (P $<$ 0.025). In Group I, TB Ca was approximately 10% lower than predicted normal values (Table IV). TB P decreased in all but two patients in Group I after ingestion of 25-OHD$_3$ but TB Ca remained essentially unchanged. The TB P/Ca ratio in Group II, decreased from 0.8 to 0.5 following 25-OHD$_3$ ingestion.

TABLE II

Comparison of Radiocalcium Kinetics Before and
Following 25 Hydroxycholecalciferol Administration

	Compartment[a], g/kg of TBCa			Transfer Rates[b] g/day/kg of TBCa			
	1	2	1 & 2	Urine $\rho41$	Stool $\rho51$	Accretion $\rho31$	Exchange $\rho12, 21$
Group I N = 6							
Mean C	2.84	4.17	7.01	0.147	0.135	1.168	6.12
SEM	0.69	0.99	1.55	0.085	0.028	0.399	2.14
Mean X	3.27	4.64	7.92	0.099	0.085	1.323	7.66
SEM	0.52	1.22	1.69	0.020	0.024	0.482	2.63
Group II N = 2							
Mean C	1.93	2.70	4.64	0.023	0.133	0.478	2.95
Mean X	1.90	1.79	3.68	0.049	0.067	0.374	4.71
Group III N = 23							
Normal mean	2.86	2.14	5.00	0.150	0.134	0.405	1.72
SEM	0.13	0.17	0.22	0.001	0.002	0.024	0.36

[a]Compartments are designated as follows: Compartment 1 represents the pool of Ca in isotopic equilibrium one hour after injection. Compartment 2 represents the physiologic pool of Ca in isotopic equilibrium within three days. [b]The transfer constants are designated as follows: Urine = urinary Ca excretion ; Stool = the endogenous fecal Ca excretion rate; Accretion = $\rho31$ the rate of accretion into bone and extra osseous calcification. Exchange = $\rho21$, $\rho21$, the rate of transfer of Ca from compartment 2. [c]Normal values to TB_{Ca} of 1000g based on height and weights (14, 15).

TABLE **III**
CALCIUM BALANCE IN CHRONIC RENAL FAILURE (mg/day)[a]

GROUP	INTAKE	TOTAL FECAL	ENDO FECAL	NET FECAL	ABSORPTION
I N=4					
Mean C	511	458	91	380	137(27%)[b]
SEM	22	60	16	42	46
X	549	234	56	198	351*(62%)**
II N=2					
Mean C	733	671	97	574	159(17%)
X	651	614	53	561	89(11%)

GROUP	URINE	ACCRETION RATE	RESORPTION RATE	Ca BALANCE	ACCRETION RESORPTION
I					
Mean C	51	807	806	-5	1.05
SEM	17	211	340	65	0.06
X	89	1439	988	208	2.18
SEM	30	339	460	108	1.00
II					
Mean C	22	340	300	39	1.24
X	52	288	304	-16	1.07

[a]Intake=Intake of Ca in diet; Total fecal= Total fecal Ca excretion; Endo fecal=Endogenous fecal Ca excretion into the gastrointestinal (GI) tract; Net Fecal=Total fecal - endogenous fecal Ca excretion; Absorption=Net absorption of Ca across the GI tract; Urine=Urinary Ca excretion; Accretion Rate=bone formation rate or transfer of Ca from compartment 1 to compartment 3; Resorption Rate=Bone resorption rate; Ca Balance=Ca Intake - total fecal excretion and urinary Ca excretion. [b]Net absorption of Ca across the GI tract as percentage of Ca intake in diet. C=prior to administration of 25OHD3. X=following administration of 25OHD3. *P < 0.05 **P < 0.025

TABLE IV

Body Composition in Chronic Renal Insufficiency Before
and Following 25-Hydroxycholecalciferol Administration

	TB_P	TB_{Ca}	P/Ca	$\dfrac{TB_{Ca}}{TB_{Ca_E}}$
	g	g		
Group I				
Mean C (SEM)	591 (54)	771 (90)	0.83** (.14)	0.89* (.06)
Mean X	559 (43)	770 (95)	0.79 (.12)	0.89 (.06)
N = 6				
Group II				
Mean C	630	777	0.80	1.028
Mean X	393	780	0.50	1.031
N = 2				
Group III				
Normal mean[a]	472	1015	0.47	1.000
SEM	29	53	0.02	0.010
N = 14				

Group I = 6 weeks 25-OHD$_3$; Group II = 6 months 25-OHD$_3$; TB$_P$ = total body phosphorus; TB Ca = total body calcium; P/Ca = ratio of TB$_P$/TB$_{Ca}$; TB$_{Ca}$/TB$_{Ca_E}$ = ratio of measured TB$_{Ca}$ to estimated TB$_{Ca}$. C = before administration of 25-OHD$_3$. X = after administration of 25-OHD$_3$. a = normal value from Letteri et al (16). *P < 0.05, **P < 0.025 compared to Group III.

DISCUSSION

Although resistence to vitamin D effects on Ca absorption and healing of the osteomalacic components of uremic bone disease have been noted (17), short term administration of 25-OHD$_3$ (160 μg/day for 6 weeks) to patients with decreased TB Ca stores and increased exchangeable Ca pools and transfer rates (Group I) was associated with an increase in Ca absorption, a more positive Ca balance, and an increased accretion/resorption ratio (18,19). The increase in Ca absorption was attended by a significant decrease in endogenous fecal Ca excretion suggesting that net Ca transfer from blood to intestinal lumen was decreased with 25-OHD$_3$ administration. Longer term administration of 25-OHD$_3$ to 2 patients with higher total body Ca stores than patients in Group I was associated with continued negative Ca balance or less positive Ca balance despite increasing plasma levels of 25-OHD$_3$ induced by administration of 40 μg/day of 25-OHD$_3$ for 6 months to these 2 patients. Thus, Ca absorption may not be stimulated by pharmacologic doses of 25-OHD$_3$ in some patients with renal osteodystrophy. Despite the resistance to increasing Ca absorption, endogenous fecal Ca excretion decreased in these 2 patients to the same extent observed in patients in Group I in whom 25-OHD$_3$ increased net Ca absorption. 25-OHD$_3$ increased the mean accretion/resorption ratio in Group I but not Group II patients. Short term administration may be associated with increased bone and other calcified tissue formation out of proportion to the increased release of Ca from bone and other calcified tissues (resorption). This could be related to the suppression of PTH since decreasing levels of PTH were noted in some patients. A direct effect of 25-OHD$_3$ on bone and calcified tissue formation rates cannot be excluded.

In Group II patients, with near normal pre-treatment exchangeable Ca kinetics and transfer rates and near normal TB Ca stores, 25-OHD$_3$ administration was not associated with increasing Ca absorption, or increased accretion/resorption ratios. The mechanism responsible for this relative resistance is unclear. We have previously described a relationship between TB Ca and exchangeable Ca pools (Compt. 2) and accretion rate in renal failure (16). As TB Ca decreases below predicted normal values, accretion and the size of Compt. 2 increases. The present studies extend these observations. In 4 patients with low TB Ca stores, 25-OHD$_3$ stimulated Ca absorption, increased accretion, and the size of exchangeable Ca pools. In 3 of 4 patients with normal TB Ca stores, no significant change in Ca absorption, or accretion or the size of compartment 2 was noted. It appears that TB Ca stores may be an important modulating influence in determing the response of the parameters of Ca metabolism measured in this study to the administration of 25-OHD$_3$.

REFERENCES

1. Cohn, S.H., Bozzo, S.R., Jesseph, J.E., Constantinides, C., Heune, D.R., and Gusmano, E.A.: Formation and testing of a compartmental model for calcium metabolism in man. Radiat. Res. 26:319, 1965.

2. Cohn, S.H., Dombrowski, C.S., and Fairchild, R.G.: In vivo neutron activation analysis of calcium in man. Int. J. Appl. Rad. Isotopes 22:127, 1970.

3. Slatopolsky, E.: Studies with 25-hydroxycholecalciferol in patients with chronic renal disease. IND number 8900 report to the F.D.A., March 5, 1974.

4. Reifenstein, E.C., Jr., Albright, F. and Wells, S.L.: The accumulation, interpretation and presentation of data pertaining to metabolic balances notably those of calcium, phosphorus and nitrogen. J. Clin. Endocrin. 5:367, 1945.

5. Haddad, J.G. and Chyu Kyung, J.A.: Competitive protein binding radioassay for 25-hydroxycholecalciferol. J. Clin. Endocrin. 33:992, 1971.

6. Bligh, E.G., Dyer, W.J.: A rapid method of total lipid extraction and purification. Canad. J. Biochem. 37:911, 1959.

7. Holick, M.F., DeLuca, H.F.: A new chromatographic system for vitamin D_3 and its metabolites. Resolution of a new vitamin D_3 metabolite. J. Lipid Res. 12:460, 1971.

8. Kleerekoper, M., Ingham, J.P., Mc Carthy, S.W. and Posen, S.: Parathyroid hormone assay in primary hyperparathyroidism. Experience with a radioimmunoassay based on commercially available reagents. Clin. Chem. 20:369, 1974.

9. Arnaud, C.D., Tsao, H.S., and Littledike, T.: Radioimmunoassay of human parathyroid hormone in serum. J. Clin. Invest. 50:21, 1971.

10. Berman, M. and Weiss, M.F.: Users manual for SAAM (simulation, analysis and modelling). Natl. Institute Arthritis Metabolic Disease, Bethesda, Md., 1967.

11. Bec, P., Louvet, J., Boayard, F.: Plasma 25-hydroxycholecal-
    ciferol in normal subjects and patients on chronic hemodialysis
    (abstract). Clin. Res. 19:732, 1972.

12. Shen, H., Baylini, C.D., Sherrard, D.: Serum 25-hydroxychole-
    calciferol in patients with uremic bone disease. Clin. Res.
    21:204, 1973.

13. Reiss, E., Canterbury, J.M., and Kanter, A.: Circulating para-
    thyroid hormone concentration in chronic renal insufficiency.
    Arch. Intern. Med. 124:417, 1969.

14. Heaney, R.P., Mauer, G.C.H., Bronner, F., Dymlying, J.F.,
    Lafferty, F.W., Nordin, B.E.C., Rich, C.: A normal reference
    standard for radiocalcium turnover and excretion in humans.
    J. Lab. Clin. Med. 64:21, 1964.

15. Cohn, S.H., Bozzo, S.R., Jesseph, J.E., Constantinides, C.,
    Huene, R., Gusmand, E.A.: Formulation and testing of a
    compartmental model for calcium metabolism in man. Radiat.
    Res. 26:319, 1965.

16. Letteri, J.M., Ellis, K.J., Orofino, D.P., Ruggieri, S.,
    Asad, S.N. and Cohn, S.H.: Altered calcium metabolism in
    chronic renal failure. Kid. Int. 6, 45, 1974.

17. Brickman, A.S., and Norman, A.W.: Treatment of renal osteo-
    dystrophy with calciferol (vitamin D) and related steroids.
    Kid. Int. 4, 161, 1973.

18. DeLuca, H.F., Avioli, A.V.: Treatment of renal osteodystrophy
    with 25-hydroxycholecalciferol. Arch. Intern. Med. 126:896,
    1970.

19. Henning, H.V., Hesch, R.D., Husken, W.S., Quellhorst, E.,
    Scheler, F.: Treatment of renal osteodystrophy with vitamin
    D and 25-hydroxycholecalciferol: Effects on plasma calcium
    and phosphate and the intestinal calcium absorption. Proc.
    Europ. Dial. Transpl. Assoc. 9:150, 1972.

BONE DISEASE, HYPOPHOSPHATEMIA AND HYPERPARATHYROIDISM AFTER RENAL TRANSPLANTATION

Nielsen, H.E., Christensen, M.S., Melsen, F., and
Tørring, S.
First Medical University Clinic, Kommunehospitalet,
Institute of Pharmacology, University of Aarhus, and
University Institute of Pathology, Amtssygehuset,
8000 Aarhus C, Denmark

Aseptic necrosis of bone and spontaneous fractures are frequent and sometimes disabling complications to renal transplantation (1, 2, 3,). The pathogenesis of these bone affections is not
known, but several factors have been proposed as pathogenic, for
example steroid-induced osteoporosis (4), secondary hyperparathyroidism (5), ischemia of bone (1) and hypophosphatemic osteomalacia (6).

We have analysed the serum concentrations of parathyroid hormone (PTH), calcium and phosphorus and the bone morphology in 78
long-term survivors after renal transplantation, in order to
elucidate the significance of hypophosphatemia and hyperparathyroidism for the development of bone lesions after renal transplantation.

PATIENTS

Seventy-eight long-term survivors after renal transplantation
(RT) with a creatinine clearance at or above 50 ml per min were
studied. The mean survival after RT was 4.1 years, range ½-11 years.
The mean age of the patients was 40 years, range 17-65 years, and
the mean daily dose of prednisone 5.1 mg. The usual daily dose of
azathioprine was 2 mg per kg body weight. Twenty of the recipients
developed radiological bone lesions after RT: aseptic necrosis of
bone in 14 and spontaneous fractures in 6.

In 16 patients with mild renal insufficiency caused by various
kidney diseases biochemical measurements were performed.

METHODS AND INVESTIGATIONS

Fasting serum concentrations of calcium (corrected for individual variation in protein binding), phosphorus and creatinine were measured by autoanalyser methods. Serum parathyroid hormone (s-PTH) was measured in a sensitive radioimmunoassay on extracts of serum (7). Radiological examination of the skeleton was performed. In 20 long-term survivors an iliac crest bone biopsy was performed and a quantitative histological analysis was made using a point-counting technique (8). In order to evaluate the degree of mineralization in bone we measured (9): osteoid surfaces (OS) in per cent of total trabecular bone surfaces, relative osteoid volumen (OV) in per cent of total trabecular bone volume. The rate of mineralization was measured after double tetracycline labelling as the calcification rate in trabecular bone (CR). Bone resorption was expressed as the trabecular osteoclastic resorption surfaces (RS) in per cent of total trabecular bone surfaces.

For comparison of mean values the Student´s t-test or the Mann-Whitney rank sum test were used.

RESULTS

Table I shows biochemical values in 78 long-term survivors compared to normal control subjects. The transplanted patients showed a decrease in mean serum phosphorus ($p < 0.001$), an increase in mean serum PTH ($p < 0.001$) and an increase in mean serum creatinine ($p < 0.001$). No difference was found in serum calcium.

Table I. Biochemical values in renal transplanted (RT) patients with a serum creatinine concentration at or below 2 mg/100 ml compared to normal controls.

	s-Calcium corr.prot. mg/100 ml	s-Phosphorus mg/100 ml	s-PTH pg/ml	s-Creatinine mg/100 ml
RT patients n=78	9.95	2.93	109	1.24
Normal controls n=64	9.86	3.57	67	0.90
t-test	n.s.	$p < 0.001$	$p < 0.001$	$p < 0.001$

Table II compares the biochemical values in 16 renal transplanted patients with those found in 16 patients with a comparable
mild renal insufficiency caused by a number of kidney diseases. Both
groups of patients had a similar decrease in mean serum phosphorus
and an equal elevation of s-PTH. Serum calcium was decreased in
the non-transplanted patients (p<0.01) compared to both transplanted patients and control subjects.

Table II. Biochemical values in renal transplanted (RT) patients
compared to patients with mild renal insufficiency caused by various
kidney diseases.

	s-Calcium corr.prot. mg/100 ml	s-Phosphorus mg/100 ml	s-PTH pg/ml	s-Creatinine mg/100 ml
RT patients n=16	9.95	2.97	117	1.69
Mild renal failure n=16	9.64	3.06	119	1.75
Mann-Whitney rank sum test	p<0.01	n.s.	n.s.	n.s.

Table III compares the biochemical values found in the transplanted patients with subnormal serum phosphorus and a normal
serum phosphorus. The two groups had identical serum concentrations of calcium, creatinine and PTH.

Table IV compares the biochemical values in transplanted
patients with and without radiological bone lesions. No difference
were found in the serum concentrations of calcium, phosphorus or
creatinine. In the group with bone lesions s-PTH was lower
(p<0.01) than in the group without bone lesions.

Quantitative measurements of bone histology showed that the
amount of osteoid (OS and OV) was increased (p< 0.01) in the transplanted patients compared to normal subjects and the calcification
rate decreased (p<0.01).

Table V shows that the amount of uncalcified tissue (OS and
OV) is correlated to low serum phosphorus. Bone resorption (RS)
was slightly increased.

Table III. Biochemical values in renal transplanted (RT) patients
with hypophosphatemia compared to RT patients with normal serum
phosphorus.

	s-Calcium corr.prot. mg/100 ml	s-Phosphorus mg/100 ml	s-PTH pg/ml	s-Creatinine mg/100 ml
s-Phosphorus >2.7 mg/100 ml n=58	9.92	3.19	108	1.24
s-Phosphorus <2.7 mg/100 ml n=20	10.06	2.20	110	1.23
t-test	n.s.		n.s.	n.s.

Table IV. Biochemical values in renal transplanted (RT) patients
with and without bone lesions following renal transplantation.

	s-Calcium corr.prot. mg/100 ml	s-phosphorus mg/100 ml	s-PTH pg/ml	s-Creatinine mg/100 ml
20 RT patients with bone lesions	9.95	2.97	87	1.18
58 RT patients without bone lesions	9.96	2.96	115	1.25
t-test	n.s.	n.s.	p<0.01	n.s.

Table V. Amount of uncalcified bone (Osteoid surface and Osteoid volume) in iliac crest bone biopsies in renal transplanted patients with high and low serum phosphorus.

	Osteoid surface (%)	Osteoid volume (%)
s-Phosphorus <3.0 mg/100 ml n=10	27.5	3.65
s-Phosphorus >3.0 mg/100 ml n=10	20.1	2.00

Osteoid surface = per cent of trabecular bone covered with osteoid.
Osteoid volume = amount of osteoid in per cent of total amount of trabecular bone.

DISCUSSION

Secondary hyperparathyroidism has been reported to persist for several years after renal transplantation (5,10,11,12,13) and has been claimed to be a causal factor in the development of bone abnormalities after renal transplantation (5). However, in this study serum parathyroid hormone was singificantly lower in long-term survivors with radiological bone lesions than in those without. Histological signs of hyperparathyroidism, i.e. increased bone resorption, were minimal. The frequency of radiological bone lesions in patients with posttransplant hypercalcemia was not different from that found in normocalcemic long-term survivors (14). The small elevation of s-PTH in long-term survivors may be due to the mild reduction in kidney function in these patients.

In accordance with other studies (6) we found a high frequency of hypophosphatemia in the long-term survivors. The mean serum phosphorus was equally decreased in a group of non-transplanted patients with a similar degree of renal insufficiency and in the long-term survivors. No correlation was found between serum phosphorus and serum parathyroid hormone. The hypophosphatemia cannot be explained by the mild hyperparathyroidism also found in these patients. The phypophosphatemia is probably caused by a primary renal phosphate loss as suggested by Moorhead et al. (6). In accordance with this, Massry et al. (15) found an increased fractional phosphate excretion in long-term survivors after RT. Our preliminary investigations of phosphate excretion also indicate an increased phosphate elimination after transplantation.

The bone morphometry in the long-term survivors showed an increase in the amount of uncalcified bone matrix (osteoid) which was inversely correlated to the level of serum phosphorus. However, the significance of osteomalacia for the development of bone lesions after RT is not clear. In an investigation of aseptic necrosis after RT (2) we found that the amount of osteoid was not significantly increased in patients with aseptic necrosis of bone compared to patients without. However, a highly significant (p<0.01) reduction in the amount of trabecular bone was present in the patients with aseptic necrosis compared to the long-term survivors without this bone lesion. The calcification rate was decreased in the long-term survivors. Aseptic necrosis of bone after RT is probably due to bone compression in osteopenic bone. The osteopenia may be the result of both pretransplant osteodystrophy and post-transplant steroid-induced decreased bone formation, perhaps aggravated by hypophosphatemic osteomalacia.

SUMMARY

Long-term survivors after renal transplantation (RT) show:
1) decreased s-phosphorus
2) increased s-PTH
3) no correlation between s-PTH and s-phosphorus
4) increased amount of non-mineralized bone (osteomalacia), inversely correlated to s-phosphorus
5) decreased amount of trabecular bone (osteopenia)
   in RT patients with aseptic necrosis of bone.

Conclusion: aseptic necrosis of bone after RT is mainly due to osteoid-induced osteopenia, perhaps aggravated by hypophosphatemic osteomalacia.

REFERENCES

1. Harrington, K.D., Murray, W.R., Kountz, S.L., and Belzer, F.O.: Avascular necrosis of bone after renal transplantation. J. Bone Jt.Surg. 53:203, 1971.

2. Nielsen, H.E., Melsen, F., and Christensen, M.S.: Aseptic necrosis of bone following renal transplantation. Clinical and biochemical aspects and bone morphometry. To be published.

3. Pierides, A.M., Simpson, W., Strainsby, D., Alvarez-Ude, F., and Uldall, P.R.: Avascular necrosis of bone following renal transplantation. Quart.J.Med. 19:459, 1975.

4. Solomon, L.: Drug-induced arthropathy and necrosis of the femoral head. J.Bone Jt.Surg. 55B: 246, 1973.

5. Chatterjee, S.N., Friedler, R.M., Berne, T.V., Oldham, S.B., Singer, F.R., and Massry, S.G.: Persistent hypercalcemia after successful renal transplantation. Nephron 17:1, 1976.

6. Moorhead, J.F., Wills, M.R., Ahmed, K.Y., Baillod, R.A., Varghese, Z., and Tatler, G.L.V.: Hypophosphatemic osteomalacia after cadaveric renal transplantation. Lancet 1:694, 1974.

7. Christensen, M.S.: A sensitive radioimmunoassay of parathyroid hormone in human serum using a specific extraction procedure. Scand.J.clin.Lab.Invest. vol. 36, in press, 1976.

8. Bordier, P., Matrajt, H., Moravet, L., and Hioco, D.: Mesure histologique de la masse et de la resorption des travées osseuse. Path.Biol. 12:1238, 1964.

9. Courpront, P.: Données histologique quantitative sur le vieillessement osseux humans. Thése, Lyon, 1972.

10. Bernheim, J., Touraine, J.L., Labeeuw, M., Pozet, N., and Traeger, J.: Blood parathormone levels and sensitivity of parathyroid glands to hypercalcemia after successful renal transplantation. Proc. XIIth Congress of EDTA, 477, 1976.

11. David, D.S., Sakai, S., Brennan, B.L., Riggio, R.A., Cheigh, J., Stenzel, K.H., Rubin, A.L., and Sherwood, L.M.: Hypercalcemia after renal transplantation. Long-term follow-up data. New Engl. J.Med. 289:398, 1973.

12. Geis, W.P., Popovtzer, M.M., Corman, J.L., Halgrimson, C.G., Groth, C.G., and Starzl, T.E.: The diagnosis and treatment of hyperparathyroidism after renal homotransplantation. Surg. Gynecol.Obstet. 137:997, 1973.

13. Kleerekoper, M., Ibels, L.S., Ingham, J.P., McCarthy, S.W., Mahony, J.F., Stewart, J.H., and Posen, S.: Hyperparathyroidism after renal transplantation. Brit.Med.J. 3:680, 1975.

14. Christensen, M.S., Nielsen, H.E., and Tørring, S.: Hypercalcemia and parathyroid function after renal transplantation. Acta med. Scand., in press.

15. Massry, S.G., Coburn, J.W., Lee, D.B.N., Jowsey, J., and Kleeman, C.R.: Skeletal resistance to parathyroid hormone in renal failure. Studies in 105 human subjects. Ann.Intern.Med. 78:357, 1973.

SCINTIGRAPHIC SKELETAL CHANGES IN DIALYSIS AND KIDNEY TRANSPLANTED PATIENTS

Madsen, S., Ølgaard, K., Heerfordt, J.,
Brix, E. & Vistisen, L.
Nephrological, Orthopaedic and Radiological
Dept.
Rigshospitalet and The Niels Bohr Institute
Copenhagen, Denmark

Metabolic bone disorders exhibit great problems in dialysis as well as in kidney transplanted patients. Bone scintigraphy using technetium-polyphosphate^{99m} (Tc-PP) has recently been shown superior to X-ray in early detection of metabolic skeletal changes [1]. This investigation presents the results obtained by this method, used in a material of consecutive dialysis and kidney transplanted patients.

MATERIAL
The clinical data of 3o uremic patients on regular hemodialysis are given in Table I. In 14 of these patients an unsuccessful kidney transplantation had previously been performed. In 12 patients the kidney graft was removed after less than 1 month and in the last 2 patients after 2 and 36 months, respectively. During transplantation, the patients had been treated with an average total of 8583 mg prednisone (range 4o-24345 mg). The average dose per day was 2o5 mg prednisone (range 2o-454 mg). The clinical data of 1o5 kidney transplanted patients are given in Table II. As a reference a control material consisting of the Tc-PP scintigrams in 3o normal persons were investigated (Table I).

METHODS
Tc-PP whole body scintigraphy was carried out with a dual probe 5-inch Elscint whole body rectilinear scanner with photorecorder and video-display processor. The collimators used have a nearly depth-independent respon-

Table I. Clinical data of 3o uremic patients on regular
hemodialysis and of 3o normal persons.

	NO	AGE (YEARS)	TIME ON HEMODIA-LYSIS (MONTHS)	PREVIOUS KIDNEY TRANSPLAN-TATION	ANEPHRIC PATIENTS	UREMIC POLY-NEUROPATHY
PATIENTS ON HEMODIALYSIS	30	44 (24 - 60)	25 (3 - 63)	14	8	10
NORMAL PERSONS	30	41 (22 - 61)	-	-	-	-

Table II. Clinical data of lo5 kidney transplanted
patients.

AGE YEARS	CREATININE CLEARANCE ML/MIN	HYPERTENSION NO	HYPERCALCEMIA NO	HYPOPHOSPHATEMIA NO
41.3 (20 - 62)	53.8 (4 - 102)	28	8	13

TIME ON DIALYSIS MONTHS	TIME AFTER TRANSPLANTATION MONTHS	TRANSPLANTATIONS PER PATIENT NO	TOTAL DOSE OF PREDNISONE G	REJECTIONS PER PATIENT NO
12.2 (0 - 62)	39.5 (2 - 75)	1.2 (1 - 3)	19.589 (0 - 36.617)	1.0 (0 - 4)

se over a range of 3-5 inches; this prevents the errors
in interpretation which may be caused by the "tomogra-
phic" effect of a fine focus collimator, if the position of the patient is not strictly symmetrical.
      The ^{99m}Tc generator was delivered from Amersham,
and the stannous polyphosphate kits from Diagnostic Isotopes Inc. In preparation and use of Tc-PP the direc-
tions of the manufacturer were followed; almost all doses were administered less than 1 h after preparation,
and in no case later than 2 h after preparation. The
whole body scintigraphy was performed 2-3 h after intravenous administration of 12 mCi Tc-PP. Four h postinjec-
tion, 5o-6o% of the ^{99m}Tc-PP is accumulated in the skeleton and 3o% of the remaining is bound to plasma proteins and 3o% bound to the erythrocytes. Presuming a
normal kidney function the renal excretion is approximately 25% after 4 h. The physical half-life of ^{99m}Tc
is 6 h. The total radiation dose to an adult with normal kidney function is less than 2oo mrad and the dose
to the critical organs (i.e., urinary tract, gonads,
skeleton) is 2oo-5oo mrad. In patients with chronic renal failure and no renal elimination of Tc-PP, the ra-

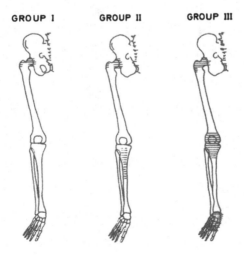

GROUP I   GROUP II   GROUP III

Fig. 1.   Schematic generalized scintigraphic classifi-
          cation.
          Increasing severity of the scintigraphic chan-
          ges from group I to group III.

diation dose is only slightly higher than in normal subjects, as the short physical half-life of ^{99m}Tc is major
determinant in calculation of radiation dose (2).

CLASSIFICATION OF SCINTIGRAMS
The scintigraphic changes were classified as A) <u>focal</u>
(number of foci with increased uptake of the tracer in
the skeleton) and B) <u>generalized</u> (increased symmetrical
uptake of the tracer in the legs). According to the number of foci, the <u>focal</u> changes were subdivided into
group 0, 1, 2 and 3.

The <u>generalized</u> changes were classified into 4
groups according to the degree of generalized symmetrical increased uptake of the radiopharmaceutical in the
cancellous bone of the legs, i.e. in the metaphyses of
the femur and tibia, the trochanteric region, the proximal part of the tibial diaphysis, the tarsus and the
proximal part of the metatarsus (Fig. 1).

<u>Group 0.</u> No generalized scintigraphic changes
(Fig. 2). All 3o normal persons were included in this
group.

<u>Group I.</u> Abnormal symmetrical accentuation of the
uptake throughout the femoral head, with a fading extension to the femoral neck and the trochanteric region.

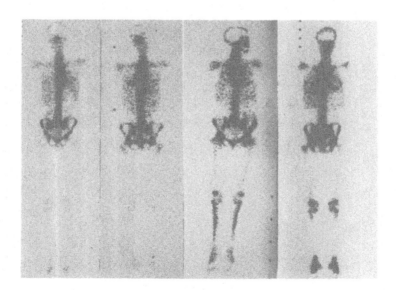

<u>Fig. 2.</u>   Scintigrams from 4 patients on regular hemo-
           dialysis, showing the <u>generalized</u> scintigra-
           phic classification from group 0 (left) to
           group III (right).

Table III. Results from scintigraphy of 3o uremic
patients on regular hemodialysis.

GENERALIZED SCINTIGRAPHIC CHANGES	NO	AGE	TIME ON HEMODIALYSIS	PREVIOUS KIDNEY TRANSPLANTATION	ANEPHRIC PATIENTS	UREMIC POLYNEUROPATHY
		YEARS	MONTHS	%	%	%
GROUP 0	3	34	15	33.3	0	33.3
GROUP I	9	41	25	22.2	33.3	11.1
GROUP II	5	52	33	20.0	20.0	20.0
GROUP III	13	45	23	76.9	30.8	53.9
TOTAL	30	44	25	46.7	26.7	33.3

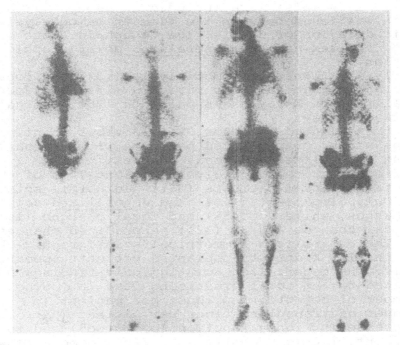

Fig. 3.   Scintigrams from kidney transplanted patients showing generalized and focal changes
with increasing severity from left to right.

Group II. In addition, a diffusely increased uptake in the proximal half of the tibial shaft, without
extension to the tibial condyles, but with a clear maximum uptake in the region of the tibial tuberosity.
Group III. Severe scintigraphic changes. The uptake
in the femoral head is considerably more intensive than
in group I, and further a severe symmetrical uptake is
present in the femoral and tibial condyles, the tarsus
and the proximal part of the metatarsus (Fig. 2).

RESULTS
Hemodialysis patients. Twentyseven of the 3o patients
on regular hemodialysis (9o%) had generalized scintigraphic changes. In 13 patients (47%) the scintigraphic
changes could be classified as severe (group III) (Table
III). The frequency of previously unsuccessfully kidney
transplanted patients (treated with on average total of
8.5 g prednisone, (mean 2o5 mg/day) were significantly
higher (p < o.ol) in group III, than in the other dialysis patients. Seven of the lo patients with uremic po-
lyneuropathy and the 3 patients with surgically verified
hyperparathyreoidism were included in group III. No correlation was found between the time on hemodialysis, pre-
dialytic duration of uremia, age, anephric state of the
patient, the sex and the generalized scintigraphic classification.
      Only 4 patients on hemodialysis (13%) had focal
scintigraphic changes. Four patients (13%) had focal
abnormalities on X-ray and 8 patients (26%) had halisteresis on X-ray.
Kidney transplanted patients. Fig. 3 shows scintigrams
from the kidney transplanted patients with gradually increasing generalized and focal changes.
      In contrast to the dialysis patients, 4o of the
kidney transplanted patients (38%) had normal scintigrams. Only 5l patients (49%) had generalized scintigraphic changes, while 47 (45%) had focal changes (14 (13%)
only focal changes and 33 (32%) generalized changes as
well). The generalized symmetrical scintigraphic changes in the lo5 kidney transplanted patients appear from
Table IV. The generalized scintigraphic findings were
correlated to the total prednisone dose (p < o.oo5),
the number of rejection episodes per patient (p < o.oo5),
the number of transplantations per patient (p < o.o5),
the decrease in kidney function (p < o.oo5) and to the
focal scintigraphic classification (p < o.ool). The radiographic halisteresis was parallel to the generalized
scintigraphic changes although with a lower frequency.
      The focal scintigraphic changes in the lo5 kidney

Table IV. <u>Generalized</u> scintigraphic changes. Results from scintigraphy of lo5 kidney transplanted patients.

GENERA-LIZED SCINTIGRA-PHIC CHAN-GES	NO	AGE Years	TIME ON DIALY-SIS Months	TIME AFTER TRANS-PLAN-TATION Months	TRANS-PLAN-TATIONS PER PATIENT No	REJEC-TIONS PER PATI-ENT No	TOTAL PREDNI-SONE DOSE g	CREATI-NINE CLEAR-ANCE ml/min	HALI-STERE-SIS ON X-RAY %	FOCAL CHAN-GES ON X-RAY %	FOCAL CHANGES ON SCINTI-GRAPHY %
Group 0	54	38.6	lo.1	38.2	1.1	o.8	17.9	58.7	27.8	16.7	25.9
Group I	11	4o.o	13.o	37.2	1.2	o.8	16.9	52.8	36.4	9.1	36.4
Group II	24	49.o	12.3	43.2	1.2	1.2	22.2	52.1	54.2	58.3	62.5
Group III	16	39.8	18.o	4o.o	1.4	1.8	23.4	4o.2	68.8	62.5	87.5
Total no.	lo5	41.3	12.2	39.5	1.2	1.o	19.6	53.8	4o.9	32.4	44.8

Table V. <u>Focal</u> scintigraphic changes. Results from scintigraphy of lo5 kidney transplanted patients.

FOCAL SCINTI-GRAPHIC CHANGES	NO	AGE Years	TIME ON DIALY-SIS Months	TIME AFTER TRANS-PLAN-TATION Months	TRANS-PLAN-TATIONS PER PATIENT No	REJEC-TIONS PER PATI-ENT No	TOTAL PREDNI-SONE DOSE g	CREATI-NINE CLEAR-ANCE ml/min	HALI-STERE-SIS ON X-RAY %	FOCAL CHAN-GES ON X-RAY %	GENERA-LIZED SCINTI-GRAPHIC CHANGES %
0	58	41.2	lo.4	39.3	1.1	o.8	17.8	56.5	32.8	0	31.0
1	27	38.8	16.7	37.5	1.2	1.3	2o.6	51.8	4o.7	55.6	51.9
2	15	45.7	11.9	41.9	1.3	1.3	23.2	5o.8	66.7	93.3	93.3
≥ 3	5	4o.4	9.4	41.8	1.2	2.o	24.o	41.8	6o.o	loo	loo
Total no.	lo5	41.3	12.2	39.5	1.2	1.o	19.6	53.8	4o.9	32,4	48.6

transplanted patients appear from Table V. The _focal_
changes correlated to the number of rejection episodes
per patient (p < o.oo5) and to the total dose of prednisone (p < o.ol). The focal changes on X-ray paralel-
led the _focal_ scintigraphic changes. Fourteen of the
patients had femoral head necrosis on X-ray, in 9 cases
ipsilateral to the graft, in 2 cases contralateral to
the graft, while 3 patients were bilaterally transplanted.

None of the other investigated parameters could be
correlated either to the _generalized_ or to the _focal_
changes.

DISCUSSION
Bone scintigraphy is a highly sensitive indicator of
focal and generalized skeletal disorders (3) and reflects the osseous metabolic turnover (4). The mechanism of the accumulation of Tc-PP in the bones is still
controversial (4, 5). The method is superior to X-ray
in early detection of metabolic skeletal changes (1).

The present investigation shows that the frequency
of the _generalized_ skeletal disorder seen in patients
on regular hemodialysis, decreases from 9o to 5o% after
a successful kidney transplantation. This suggests an improvement of the renal osteodystrophy after regain in
kidney function. The improvement is a long lasting slow
process as signs of renal osteodystrophy still may be
present several years after transplantation (6) and may
be influenced and changed by many factors, primarily
the prednisone treatment and a decrease in kidney function due to rejection episodes. Thus in both dialysis
and kidney transplanted patients a highly significant
correlation was found between the severity of the _gene-
ralized_ scintigraphic changes and the total prednisone
dose given to the patients.

After a kidney transplantation the pattern of the
scintigraphic skeletal disorders is modified from predominantly _generalized_ changes to _focal_ changes as well.
Both kinds of changes showed highly significant correlation to the total dose of prednisone, suggesting that
glucocorticoids is an important etiological factor in
the developement of _focal_ and maintenance of _generalized_
skeletal lesions after a kidney transplantation.

SUMMARY
[99m]Technetium-polyphosphate bone scintigraphy was performed in 3o uremic patients on regular hemodialysis
and in lo5 kidney transplanted patients. The pathological scintigraphic changes were classified as either

1) <u>generalized</u>, symmetrical or 2) <u>focal</u> accumulation of the tracer in the bones.

In the 3o hemodialysis patients 27 (9o%) showed <u>generalized</u>, symmetrical accumulation and 4 of these (13%) had <u>focal</u> changes too. A preponderance of previous unsuccessfully kidney transplanted patients was found in the group of dialysis patients exhibiting the most severe <u>generalized</u> changes.

In the lo5 kidney transplanted patients 4o (38%) had normal scintigrams, while 51 (49%) had <u>generalized</u>, symmetrical uptake. In these 51 patients 33 (32%) had <u>focal</u> uptake too, while in the entire group 14 (13%) had <u>focal</u> uptake alone. The patients with <u>focal</u> uptake had evidence of femoral head necrosis in 14 cases, in 9 ipsilateral to the kidney graft, in 2 contralateral to the graft, while 3 patients were bilaterally transplanted. Significant correlations were found between the total dose of prednisone and both kinds of scintigraphic changes.

It is concluded that the high frequency of <u>generalized</u> skeletal changes in uremic patients decreases after a successful transplantation, and it is suggested that intensive steroid treatment during a short-lasting unsuccessful kidney transplantation may aggravate uremic osteodystrophy. The frequent appearance of <u>focal</u> changes after a kidney transplantation suggests that a bone disease of a different etiology now is superimposed, but still connected to the prednisone treatment.

REFERENCES

1. Rosenthall, L. & H., Kaye, M.: J. nucl. Med. 16: 33, 1975.

2. Ølgaard, K., Heerfordt, J. & Madsen, S.: Nephron, in press (1976).

3. Charkes, N.D., Valentine, G. & Cravitz, B.: Radiology lo7: 563, 1973.

4. Sy, W.M. & Mittal, A.K.: J. nucl. Med. 15: 536, 1974.

5. Castronovo, F.P. & Callahan, R.J.: J. nucl. Med. 13: 823, 1972.

6. Pierides, A.M., Ellis, H.A., Peart, K.M., Simpson, W., Uldall, P.R. & Kerr, D.N.S.: Proc. Eur. Dial. Transpl. Ass. 11: 481, 1974.

INDEX